Chagas Disease: Diagnosis and Treatment

Chagas Disease: Diagnosis and Treatment

Editor: Malcolm Clark

MURPHY & MOORE
www.murphy-moorepublishing.com

www.murphy-moorepublishing.com

MURPHY & MOORE

Cataloging-in-Publication Data

Chagas disease : diagnosis and treatment / edited by Malcolm Clark.
p. cm.
Includes bibliographical references and index.
ISBN 978-1-63987-100-1
1. Chagas disease. 2. Chagas disease--Diagnosis. 3. Chagas disease--Treatment. 4. Trypanosomiasis. I. Clark, Malcolm.
RC124.4 .C43 2022
616.936 3--dc23

Murphy & Moore Publishing,
1 Rockefeller Plaza,
New York City, NY 10020, USA

ISBN 978-1-63987-100-1 (Hardback)

Contents

Preface VII

Chapter 1 **Silent Information Regulator 2 from *Trypanosoma cruzi* is a Potential Target to Infection Control** 1
Luís Gaspar, Terry K. Smith, Nilmar Silvio Moretti, Sergio Schenkman and Anabela Cordeiro-da-Silva

Chapter 2 **Eco-Epidemiology of Chagas Disease in Chile** 37
Mauricio Canals Lambarri, Andrea Canals Cifuentes, Salvador Ayala, Valentina Tapia-Garay and Dante Cáceres Lillo

Chapter 3 **The Mouse Model as a Tool for Histological, Immunological and Parasitological Studies of *Trypanosoma cruzi* Infection** 59
María Elena Villagran-Herrera, José Alejandro Martínez-Ibarra, Manuel Sánchez-Moreno, Hebert Luis Hernández-Montiel, Ricardo Francisco Mercado-Curiel, Nicolás Camacho-Calderón and José Antonio de Diego-Cabrera

Chapter 4 **Chagas Cardiomyopathy: Role of Sustained Host-Parasite Interaction in Systemic Inflammatory Burden** 77
Rodolfo A Kölliker-Frers, Matilde Otero-Losada, Gabriela Razzitte, Mariela Calvo, Justo Carbajales and Francisco Capani

Chapter 5 **Efficacy and Safety of Chagas Disease Drug Therapy and Treatment Perspectives** 101
Wilton H. Kawaguchi, Leticia Bonancio Cerqueira, Mariana Millan Fachi, Michel L. Campos, Iara J. Messias Reason and Roberto Pontarolo

Chapter 6 **Biochemical, Cellular, and Immunologic Aspects during Early Interaction between *Trypanosoma cruzi* and Host Cell** 132
Rosa Lidia Solís-Oviedo, Víctor Monteon, Ruth López and Ángel de la Cruz Pech-Canul

Chapter 7 **Slowed Development of Natural Products for Chagas Disease: How to Move Forward?** 144
Javier Varela, Hugo Cerecetto and Mercedes González

Chapter 8 **Transmitter Insect of Chagas Disease in Northwest Mexico: A Comparative Study of the Cuticular Hydrocarbons Profile of Three Populations of *Triatoma rubida*: Peridomestic, Domestic and Sylvatic** 161
Edgar Alfonso Paredes González, Gerardo Álvarez Hernandez and Jesús Ortega-García

Chapter 9 **Antiparasitic Mechanisms of the Human Placenta** 182
Castillo Christian, Ana Liempi, Lisvaneth Medina, Ileana Carrillo and Ulrike Kemmerling

Chapter 10 **New Approaches for Chagas Disease Chemotherapy** ... 191
Guadalupe García Liñares

Chapter 11 **Physiology and Pathology of Infectious Diseases: The Autoimmune Hypothesis of Chagas Disease** ... 211
Armanda Moreira Mattoso-Barbosa, Renato Sathler-Avelar, Jordana Grazziela Alves Coelho-dos-Reis, Olindo Assis Martins-Filho, Andrea Teixeira-Carvalho and Danielle Marchetti Vitelli-Avelar

Permissions

List of Contributors

Index

Preface

The purpose of the book is to provide a glimpse into the dynamics and to present opinions and studies of some of the scientists engaged in the development of new ideas in the field from very different standpoints. This book will prove useful to students and researchers owing to its high content quality.

Chagas disease is a tropical disease which is caused by a parasite known as Trypanosoma cruzi. The symptoms do not manifest themselves in the early stages of the disease. Severe cases of this disease can result in heart diseases and digestive complications. Infection can be caused by a kissing bug's bite. It can spread from one person to another through organ transplantation, blood transfusion, vertical transmission and consumption of contaminated food. The diagnosis of Chagas disease is conducted by examining fresh anticoagulated blood under a microscope. The parasites can also be viewed directly by staining thin and thick blood smears with Giemsa. The treatment of this disease involves antiparasitic drugs and symptomatic treatment. This book is a compilation of chapters that discuss the most vital concepts and emerging trends related to the diagnosis and treatment of Chagas disease. It aims to shed light on some of the unexplored aspects of this disease and the recent researches in this field. This book will serve as a reference to a broad spectrum of readers.

At the end, I would like to appreciate all the efforts made by the authors in completing their chapters professionally. I express my deepest gratitude to all of them for contributing to this book by sharing their valuable works. A special thanks to my family and friends for their constant support in this journey.

Editor

1

Silent Information Regulator 2 from *Trypanosoma cruzi* is a Potential Target to Infection Control

Luís Gaspar, Terry K. Smith, Nilmar Silvio Moretti, Sergio Schenkman and Anabela Cordeiro-da-Silva

Abstract

Human trypanosomiasis is a neglected tropical disease caused by protozoan parasites of the genus *Trypanosoma*. *Trypanosoma brucei* is responsible for sleeping sickness, also called African trypanosomiasis, while *Trypanosoma cruzi* causes Chagas disease, or American trypanosomiasis. Together, these diseases are responsible for significant mortality, morbidity and lost productivity in the endemic regions. There are no vaccines and treatments rely on drugs with limited efficacy, high cost, serious side effects and long administration periods. Since these diseases affect mostly the poor, there is no economic interest in the development of new drugs by pharmaceutical companies, and hopes for new treatments rely on public initiatives, public-private partnerships or philanthropic programs. The first step in the discovery of new drugs involves the identification of active molecules as starting points for further development, by either employing whole cells or by specific molecular target screenings. Research efforts undertaken by the authors' groups have focused on exploiting both strategies in the search for new molecules for trypanosomiasis drug discovery. In this chapter, we focus on Chagas disease and the recently uncovered potential of using sirtuins as targets for infection control.

Keywords: *Trypanosoma cruzi*, Chagas disease, sirtuins, drug discovery, chemotherapy

1. Introduction

Despite the efforts of many individuals and organizations over the years, human trypanosomiasis remains one of the most neglected diseases in the world. Chagas disease in particular, is a leading cause of disease and disability in Latin America, with thousands of deaths every year [1]. The negligence is particularly patented by the lack of new drugs. Indeed, the available treatment options, benznidazole and nifurtimox (**Figure 1**), were discovered more than 40 years ago. Different strategies have been employed to control the disease, but the most impactful so far has been the control of the transmitting vector led by the World Health Organization (WHO) and Pan American Health Organization (PAHO). Vector control has caused the reduction of cases from a staggering 24 million in the 1980s to about 6 million nowadays [1, 2], with some countries considered to be free of domestic vectorial transmission. Continued and rigorous implementation of the disinfestation programs in the remaining zones should decrease even further the global numbers of *Trypanosoma cruzi* vectorial transmission. Also, the screening of donor blood and transplant organs in endemic regions and other parts of the world has greatly reduced the

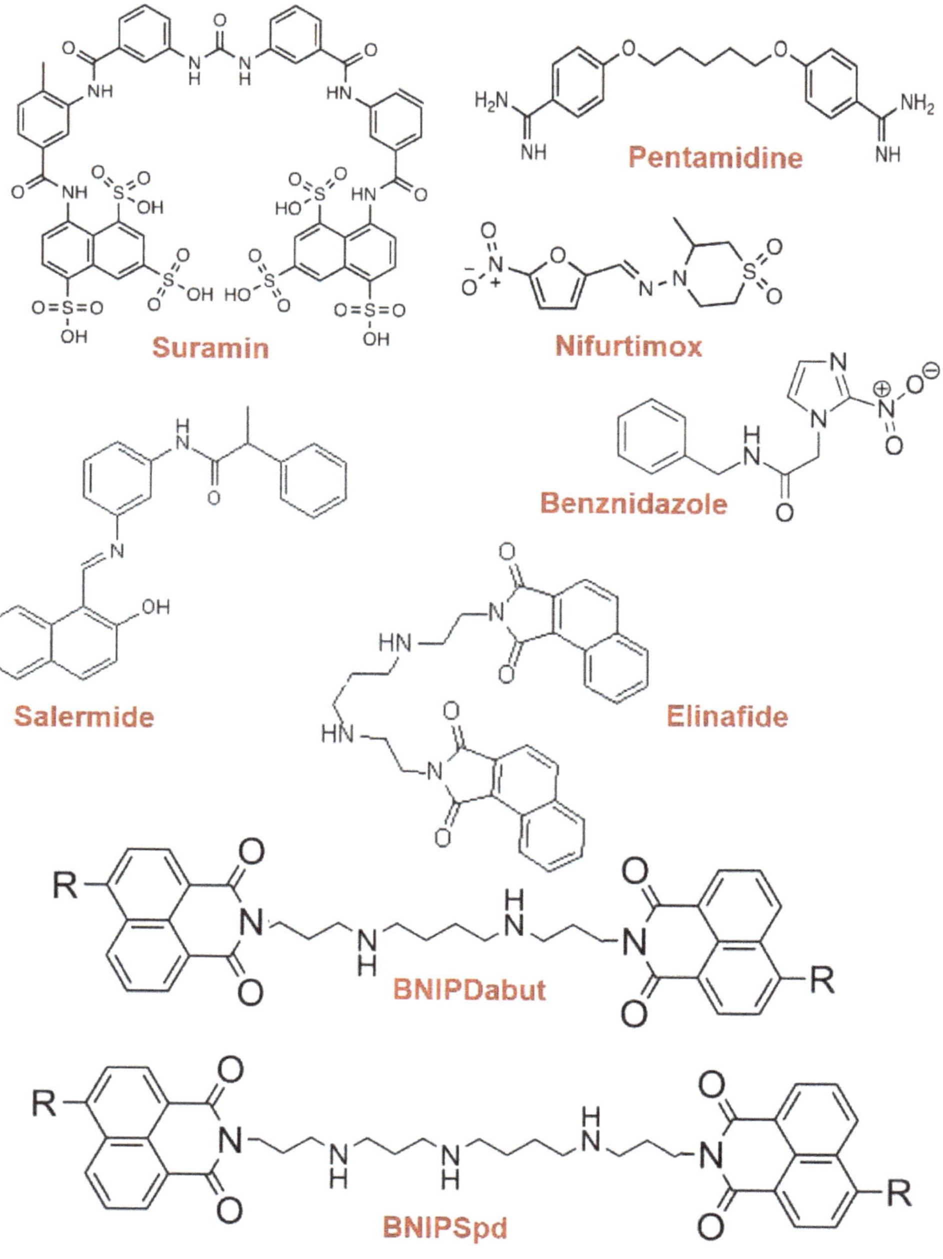

Figure 1. Various trypanocidal agents.

number of cases transmitted by this route. Whereas the global interruption of the domestic cycle will be a major breakthrough and reduce to a minimum the number of new cases of Chagas disease, complete eradication of the parasite, however, is unlikely to be achieved due to the huge natural reservoir of *T. cruzi* and the many species of triatomines capable of its transmission in the sylvatic environment [3–5].

What then, stands in the way of disease control for Chagas? First, no major technological advances are required to interrupt vectorial transmission responsible for the majority of new cases; second, decades of research in the molecular understanding of *T. cruzi* biology, the particularities of pathogenesis of the disease or the dynamics of immune response against the parasite have failed to translate into therapeutic alternatives; and finally, vaccination, either preventive or therapeutic, has remained an elusive achievement. The answer lies in new therapeutics. New, safer, cheap, easy to administer and efficacious drugs that are able to treat not only new cases, but also the millions of people already affected by the chronic stage and indeterminate form of the disease. There is growing evidence that chronic manifestations are ultimately related with inflammation resulting from parasite persistence [6, 7] and effective treatment of these cases would be highly beneficial to stop the development of symptomatology.

Active drug discovery efforts for Chagas disease have been restricted, until some years ago, to just a very limited number of groups, mostly based in academia. As a consequence, results have been sporadic, slow, ineffective and highly dependent upon intermittent funding, failing to deliver an alternative treatment. Chagas disease is as much neglected by the pharmaceutical industry as it is by research funding organizations, whose majority of funds are directed to developed world diseases.

Only recently has drug discovery for Chagas been met with concerted, focused efforts. While still not privately embraced by pharmaceutical companies, public-private partnerships have been set up with the objective of bringing together the biology expertise from academia and the technical expertise, facilities and resources from pharmaceutical industries. One organization that is leading the efforts to find new therapies for neglected diseases, including human trypanosomiasis, is the Drugs for Neglected Diseases Initiative (DND*i*), that has been involved in coordinating activities from early drug discovery to the launch and conclusion of clinical trials for some candidates like inhibitors of ergosterol biosynthesis of *T. cruzi*. The Bill and Melinda Gates Foundation, a non-governmental organization devoted to human development in underdeveloped countries, has committed to help control neglected diseases by signing The London Declaration on Neglected Diseases together with the WHO, the World Bank and 13 leading pharmaceutical industries. The Declaration states that by 2020 the signers will achieve, among other ambitious milestones, the eradication of Human African trypanosomiasis (HAT) and the control of American trypanosomiasis. Since then, other initiatives have been launched with the objective of boosting the research in new drugs for *Trypanosomal* diseases, like the European Commission Seventh Framework Program (FP7) consortia NMTrypI and KINDReD. The recent award of the Nobel Prize in Physiology or Medicine 2015 to William C. Campbell, Satoshi Omura and Youyou Tu is a recognition of the importance of drug discovery for parasitology and should further increase the awareness of neglected diseases by the international community.

Pharmaceutical research and drug discovery for infectious disease have historically began with what would be classified today as phenotypic assays, and can be traced to the pioneering work of Paul Ehrlich in the nineteenth century, while testing the effect of different dyes in trypanosomes [8]. Cultures of the microorganism of interest, bacteria or parasites, were incubated with a compound of interest, and the selective staining of the dyes was monitored by microscopy. Products of such "dye therapy" approaches were in the origin of well-known chemicals like the crystal violet dye that was proposed to be used in blood banks of endemic areas to kill *T. cruzi* parasites present in transfusion blood as a way to reduce transmission by this route [9]. Another example is trypan blue, that is still widely used as a cell biology reagent and that was the starting point for the design of the colorless analogue Suramin, a drug still in use today for the treatment of HAT and infected animals as well [10]. Such early whole cells drug screening principles were also central to the development of nifurtimox and benznidazole (**Figure 1**) in the 1960s and 1970s, by the pharmaceutical companies Bayer and Roche, respectively [11].

With the genomic era there was a dramatic shift in the way new drugs are discovered. The past 20 years have witnessed incredible advancements in genomics, proteomics, structural biology, computational chemistry and structure based drug-design, that coupled with high-throughput screening and combinatorial chemistry have helped to shape the reductionist mentality "one gene—one protein—one drug" [12]. However, the complexity of many diseases and the capacity of adaptation to adverse conditions, like the presence of a xenobiotic, evidenced by many living cells, have brought the more naïve phenotypic whole-cell screening strategies back to the spotlight. With modern phenotypic approaches, the effect of a pure molecule in a fully intact whole living organism, bacteria, parasites or human-derived cell lines, results in the identification of hit compounds that are potentially useful as scaffolds for further medicinal chemistry optimization.

While early phenotypic screenings for *T. cruzi* sometimes used the insect-specific epimastigote stage due of its extracellular nature and ease to culture, the use of reporter genes expressed during the clinically relevant stage of the disease, the intracellular amastigotes, has met a widespread application. The first of such assays was based upon the β-galactosidase-expressing parasites that made possible the detection of anti-*T. cruzi* activity by a colorimetric reaction [13]. Later, tdt-tomato and luciferase genes were also constitutively expressed in parasites, allowing more sensitive measurement of a fluorescent or luminescent signals, respectively [14].

However, the use of genetically unmodified parasites has always been an attractive pursuit, made available only recently due to technologic advancements. Such cell-based assays were developed by researchers at Institut Pasteur Korea and have met widespread use [15–18]. This assay employed the use of wild type parasites of *T. cruzi* infecting a non-modified cell line and the imaging of the resulting infection (in the amastigote stage) by high-content analysis (HCA) microscopy. Furthermore, the assay was developed in the 384-well format, allowing a high throughput testing of compounds. Preliminary cell toxicity is concomitantly determined by quantifying the ratio of host cell nuclei, a clear advantage since it reduces the need of an independent assay to assess this parameter. Using this screening assay, the authors of this chapter have also screened a library of 4000 kinase/phosphatase-like inhibitors that allowed the identification of 11 compounds with strong anti-parasitic activity and selectivity, suitable for follow up hit-to-lead optimization (unpublished results). In addition, a complementary assay developed for phenotypic profiling also allowed the identification of several compounds that interfered with the development and intracellular differentiation of *T. cruzi*. Compounds that hindered the differentiation from trypomastigotes to amastigote and the replication of amastigotes inside host cells are among the examples of "phenotypic" hits discovered (unpublished results). Due to the complex genetics and still many unknown aspects of *T. cruzi* biology, these types of compounds have the potential to constitute important chemical genomic tools that may help answering fundamental questions like: what triggers stage differentiation and what are the pathways involved? What factors are responsible for parasite persistence? How are amastigotes kept dormant for years to decades in host cells, hidden from the immune system? Due to the nature of the chemical library, it is likely that the compounds target kinases, of which the *T. cruzi* genome has 190 annotated potential members [19]. *T. cruzi* and other Trypanosomatids have a relatively big kinome when compared with other parasites that undergo several stage differentiations and contact with distinct environments, like *Plasmodium* spp. [20, 21]. One hypothesis is that while in metazoa and yeast the ultimate targets of many signaling cascades are transcription factors, which then trigger the expression of new sets of genes, Trypanosomatids have constitutive transcription of a majority of genes in large polycistronic units, hinting at a greater role of post-translational modifications (PTMs) like phosphorylation and acetylation.

2. Sirtuins: family and functions

Post-Translational Modifications (PTMs) represent one of the major mechanisms in regulating protein function in all life forms. Through phosphorylation, acetylation, methylation, glycosylation and ubiquitination, cells greatly extend the possibilities beyond the coding genome [22]. PTMs can change the enzymatic activity of a protein, change its subcellular localization, interfere with protein complexes assembly, increase or decrease its stability and induce interactions with DNA and RNA [22, 23].

Discovered half a century ago and largely ignored for the following years, lysine acetylation has re-emerged in the last two decades as a highly important PTM [24, 25]. Initial studies had focused in the role of lysine acetylation in the regulation of chromatin structure and gene expression, but with the advances in proteomic approaches, it was possible to begin to explore the function of lysine acetylation in non-histone proteins [24, 25].

Studies based on proteomic analysis to describe the lysine-acetylated proteins repertoire of an organism, called acetylome, have shown the presence of lysine acetylation in proteins from different cellular compartments and involved in different biological processes in several organisms [26]. Because of that, lysine acetylation has been placed by some authors in the same level of biological relevance as phosphorylation [24, 25]. In fact, studies of the acetylome of mammalian cells revealed acetylation sites in 1750 different proteins [27], a number close to the about 2000 proteins found to be phosphorylated [28].

The "acetyl code" is maintained by three different protein types: the "writers", lysine acetyltransferases (KATs) that add acetyl groups to proteins, the "erasers", lysine deacetylase (KDACs) that remove acetyl groups, and "readers", proteins that specifically recognize and bind acetyl-lysine groups [26].

KDACs in particular have been the focus of great interest by the scientific community due to their many roles in cell function and disease. KDACs are interchangeably called histone deacetylases (HDACs), because the first discovered reactions catalyzed by these proteins were the removal of acetyl groups in histone tails [24, 29].

HDACs are separated into four different classes based upon sequence homology (class I, II, III and IV) and two different families: the histone deacetylase family and the sirtuin family, the latter being all class III HDACs. While the first family has a limited set of molecular targets, mainly composed of histones, sirtuins have a variety of substrates ranging from metabolic enzymes to structural proteins, as well as histones [30–32]. The sirtuin family seems to be ubiquitous throughout all kingdoms of life. The number of genes coding for sirtuins within an organism ranges from as little as one in bacteria, to seven in vertebrates [33]. The sirtuin family is further classified in 5 subclasses (I, II, III, IV and V) [34].

The most common reaction catalyzed by sirtuins is deacetylation. This reaction is of upmost biological importance as there is a clear relation between the acetylation status of several proteins and their cellular functions [35–38]. The deacetylase reaction requires (nicotinamide adenine dinucleotide) NAD^+, an acetylated lysine residue and produces deacetylated lysine, nicotinamide and 2′-O-acetyl-ADP-ribose (OAADPR) [39]. Studies on the kinetics and biochemical properties of the enzymes revealed binding to the acetyl-lysine substrate prior to NAD^+. This is followed by nicotinamide cleavage from NAD^+, that is the first product released, followed by deacetylated lysine and OAADPR [40] (**Figure 2A**). All sirtuins are strictly NAD^+ dependent, a distinct characteristic that distinguishes them from other deacetylases. In fact, SIRT6 is a sirtuin capable of tightly binding to NAD^+ without the requirement of an acetylated substrate, indicating that it may function as a NAD^+ sensor [41].

Besides being an endogenous product of the deacetylation reaction, nicotinamide is also a well-known inhibitor of sirtuins. Nicotinamide is an amide of nicotinic acid (vitamin B3) and is part of common enzyme co-factors like NAD^+ and NADP (nicotinamide adenine dinucleotide phosphate) [42]. Intracellular physiological levels of nicotinamide in some mammalian cells seem to be in the range similar to the IC_{50}'s of some sirtuins reinforcing the hypothesis that some sirtuins may act as NAD^+ and nicotinamide sensors [43, 44].

OAADPR is another product of the deacetylation reaction [45] (**Figure 2A**). Early studies characterizing this molecule found that quantitative microinjection into starfish oocytes led to a blockage of oocyte maturation, indicating for the first time that OAADPR can evoke a biological activity [46]. There is now mounting evidence that OAADPR can elicit downstream responses that might synergize or antagonize the biological functions of sirtuin genes. So far, OAADPR has demonstrated to be related with functions in gene silencing, ion channel modulation and cell redox state maintenance [45].

Another reaction catalyzed by sirtuins is ADP-ribosylation. Although sirtuins were firstly described as ADP-ribosyltransferases (**Figure 2B**), their deacetylase activity has quickly

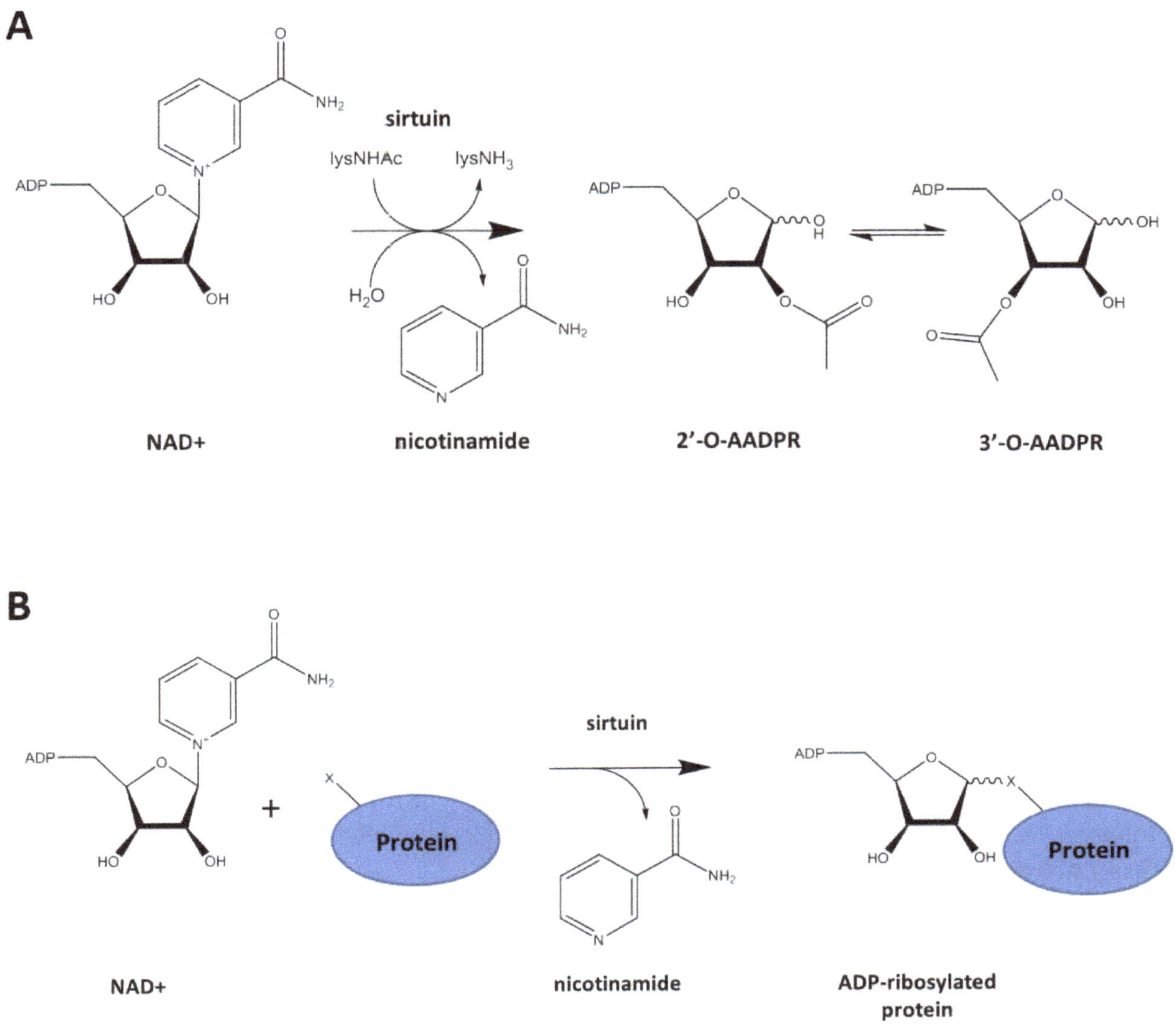

Figure 2. Sirtuin deacetylation and ADP-ribosylation mechanisms. (A) Sirtuins carry out protein deacetylation by removing acyl chains from protein lysine residues. This activity requires the cofactor nicotinamide adenine dinucleotide (NAD^+), such that nicotinamide is released with concomitant production of O-acetyl-ADP-ribose (O-AADPR). There is a sirtuin-independent equilibrium between 2′ and 3′-O-AADPR isomers. The unspecified stereochemistry at the Cl′ position of O-AADPR reflects the fast epimerization observed in solution between α and β-anomers. (B) A number of sirtuins also exhibit ADP-ribosylating functionality. This reaction is also NAD^+-dependent, as the cofactor acts as the source of ADP-ribose. 'X' represents the nucleophilic side-chain of a protein residue.

overshadowed this activity, and as a consequence the biological processes associated to this reaction remains poorly understood [47]. In truth, sirtuins may have just deacetylase activity, both, or be mostly ADP-ribosyltransferases. An example is SIRT4 that is an efficient *in vitro* ADP-ribosyltransferase of histones that only recently was discovered to possess deacetylase activity [48, 49]. There is an active debate on whether ADP-ribosylation is in fact a biologically relevant function of sirtuins, or just an irrelevant side reaction/non-enzymatic artifact [50]. Nevertheless, some of the players in the dynamics of intracellular ADP-ribosylation have only been recently identified and it is becoming apparent that this PTM might be relevant for the modulation of important cell processes and signaling pathways like signal transduction mechanisms, transcription and DNA repair [51]. The ADP-ribose hydrolysis in Trypanosomatids has recently been studied in both *Trypanosoma brucei* and *Trypanosoma cruzi* and found to be mediated by a macrodomain with a conserved catalytic site [52].

Although (de)acetylation is the most common PTM, (de)acylation of other groups can be targeted, like succinyl and malonyl groups. SIRT5 and SIRT6 are some examples of proteins that perform deacylations of lysines other than acetyl groups, and their activities are important regulators of cell functions [53–55].

There is a wealth of information regarding the structural features of sirtuins. To date, some 83 structures of sirtuins are available in the protein databank, many of them co-crystalized with natural ligands or inhibitors. Though the available structures range from bacterial to mammalian sirtuins, the majority of the structures originate from the human genome.

Although the sequence homology can vary significantly between sirtuins, especially between prokaryotic and eukaryotic proteins, there is a conserved catalytic core of about 250 amino acids common to all members in the family [56]. The structure similarity of the *Plasmodium falciparum* PfSir2A with the mammalian SIRT5, despite a sequence homology of just 33% is a clear illustration [56]. This core contains a Rossman fold domain that is a NAD^+ binding site, and a Zn^{2+} binding domain containing four highly conserved cysteine residues arranged in the motif ($CX_2CX_{20}CX_2$). The catalytic site is located inside a hydrophobic channel formed at the interface of these two domains [56].

Whereas in HDACs from class I, II and IV, Zn^{2+} is an active participant in catalysis by producing free acetate and deacetylated lysine, in sirtuins it does not participate in reaction. However, the metal is essential for structural integrity, as was elucidated by the reversible loss of activity in a *P. falciparum* sirtuin where the zinc ion was removed [57]. Interestingly, an exception to the conservation of the $CX_2CX_{20}CX_2$ motif is found on some sirtuins of Trypanosomatids, where one of the cysteines is not present [58]. However, deacetylase activity does not seem to be affected [59]. The molecular mechanism of deacetylation is still not completely elucidated, but it is generally accepted that the first step in the reaction involves the nucleophilic addition of the acetyl oxygen to nicotinamide ribose by a mechanism of S_N2 substitution to produce O-alkylamine intermediate and nicotinamide. Then the acetyl group is transferred to ADP-ribose to form O-acetyl-ADP-ribose and deacetylated lysine [60].

The founding member of the sirtuin family is Sir2 from the budding yeast and was initially identified as part of a protein complex necessary to silence the expression of the mating-type-loci [61, 62]. Subsequently, it was also implicated in transcriptional silencing at telomere proximal sites [63] and ribosomal repeats at the ribosomal DNA (rDNA) locus [64–66]. Sir2 can be associated in distinct protein complexes that vary according to target site. For instance, at telomeres and the mating-type-loci, Sir2 forms a complex with two other homologs, Sir3 and Sir4 [63], while at rDNA locus Sir2 associates with Net1 and Cdc14 to form the regulator of nucleolar silencing and telophase exit—RENT complex [67, 68]. Yeast cells lacking Sir2 present a reduced lifespan that has been correlated with the accumulation of extrachromosomal ribosomal DNA circles originating from illegitimate recombination that are toxic to the cell and have been associated with aging [66, 69, 70].

In mammals, the nuclear SIRT1 is the most extensively studied member among the sirtuin family. The TATA box binding protein-associated factor RNA polymerase I subunit B (TAF_I68) was the first substrate to be identified for SIRT1 in mouse cells. It is a transcription factor necessary for regulating the RNA polymerase I transcriptional complex, where it was shown that deacetylation inhibits transcriptional initiation *in vitro* [71]. Studies on p53, a non-histone substrate, demonstrated that acetylation activates the DNA-binding activity and target gene expression, also increasing its stability [72]. Consistent with this proposed SIRT1 inhibition of p53 function, SIRT1 knockout mice exhibit p53 hyper-acetylation and increased radiation-induced apoptosis, suggesting that SIRT1 can facilitate tumor growth by antagonism of p53 [73]. Still, the fact that SIRT1 can be found either overexpressed or underexpressed in different tumor types, and the finding that it can also function as a tumor suppressor [74] has hindered the clarification of its role in tumorigenesis. SIRT1 also plays an important role in metabolism, and its relation with caloric restriction and life-span extension has received much attention (reviewed in [75–77]). The beneficial effects of caloric restriction have been focused on the insulin-like growth factor-1 (IGF-1) and the target of rapamycin (TOR) pathways [78, 79], but increasing evidence suggest a role of SIRT1 in caloric restriction in mammals as well. For instance, SIRT1 expression was found to be elevated in models of caloric restriction, like fasting mice, low calorie diet in rat, or humans on a 25% caloric restriction diet [80–82]. On the other hand, mice lacking SIRT1 lost the life-span extension benefits of a 40% reduced calorie diet [83]. Despite many studies, the exact molecular mechanisms of SIRT1 in caloric restriction are still to be unraveled.

In vitro studies attribute a role to human SIRT2 in cell cycle regulation through the deacetylation of both tubulin and histone H4 [32, 84, 85]. In particular, it has been found that SIRT2 overexpressing cells were significantly delayed in cell cycle progression through mitosis [86]. Some links with age-related diseases have been described for SIRT2, such has neurodegenerative diseases [87–89], and different kinds of cancer. Mice lacking SIRT2 are prone to the appearance of tumors, an effect believed to be mediated by SIRT2 negative regulation of the anaphase-promoting complex [90]. It was demonstrated that SIRT2 expression is reduced in human gliomas, some of the most frequent malignant tumors in the brain [32, 91].

SIRT3 is the major mitochondrial deacetylase and studies with double knockout mice have revealed high levels of acetylation in protein targets [92, 93]. In addition, it was observed that these mice have impaired production of ATP [92]. When fasting or fed with a high-fat diet, the mice display atypical phenotypes that include cold intolerance and decreased ketone body formation [94, 95]. This strengthened the link with thermogenesis that had been previously demonstrated [96, 97]. In fact, SIRT3 expression is induced in mice in both white and brown adipose tissue upon caloric restriction and exposure of brown adipose tissue to cold temperatures [98]. In addition, SIRT3 also has a role in the deacetylation and activation of fatty acid β-oxidation, amino acid metabolism, electron transport chain and antioxidant defenses [99, 100].

SIRT4 was originally thought to be an unusual sirtuin due to the lack of deacetylase activity [101]. However, it was shown to ADP-ribosylate and down-regulate glutamate dehydrogenase production of ATP and has been implicated in insulin regulation of β-cells [48, 101]. Moreover, SIRT4 has recently been attributed a tumor suppressive function due to its involvement in

DNA damage protection mediated by inhibition of mitochondrial glutamine metabolism, suggesting it might have therapeutic potential for treating glutamine-dependent cancers [102]. This mechanism is inhibited by mammalian target of rapamycin complex 1 (mTORC1) pathway [103]. SIRT4 also coordinates the balance between lipid synthesis and their catabolism by repressing malonyl-CoA decarboxylase, proving that it has, in fact, deacetylase activity [49].

SIRT5 is a NAD^+-dependent protein lysine demalonylase and desuccinylase [104] and also has a deglutarylase activity [105]. It has a deacetylase activity [30], but has preference for acyl-carboxyl negatively charged groups [104, 105]. Some of its functions are related to glycolysis modulation [55]. The succinylome of mammalian cells has revealed many points of succinylation that are possible targets of SIRT5, mostly concentrated on mitochondrial metabolism [54]. SIRT5 also promotes urea cycle function via the regulation of carbamoyl-phosphate synthase [30, 35], and purine metabolism via urate oxidase [106]. Although a global protein hypersuccinylation and elevated serum ammonia during fasting were observed in SIRT5 knockout mouse model, the enzyme deficiency did not lead to any major metabolic abnormalities under either low or high fat diet conditions. These observations suggest that SIRT5 is likely dispensable for metabolic homeostasis under the basal conditions. It remains to be evaluated the role of SIRT5 in extreme conditions [107].

While most mammalian sirtuins have been implicated with metabolism, SIRT6 seems to be the only one with a direct link supporting a defined role in mammalian aging [108]. In fact, mice lacking SIRT6 gene develop a progeroid-like symptom with loss of subcutaneous fat, curved spine and lymphopenia. They develop normally for 2 weeks after birth, but then suffer from acute degeneration processes, ending up dying at 1 month of age [109]. At first considered to not possess deacetylase activity, but solely an ADP-ribosyltransferase activity [110], it was later found that SIRT6 removes both acetyl and long chain acyl groups from target molecules [53, 111]. It is localized in the nucleus, associated with chromatin, where it promotes the specific NAD^+-dependent deacetylation of H3K9 and H3K56 [111–113]. SIRT6 is involved in genome protection by assuring correct telomere maintenance [111, 112], as well as DNA repair by double-strand break repair machinery [114, 115]. Like other sirtuins it also has a role in metabolism by influencing both glycolysis and gluconeogenesis [116–118] and lipid metabolism, by regulating triglyceride synthesis [108, 119]. Conditions like inflammation, heart disease and cancer all seem to be linked with SIRT6 function [120].

SIRT7 is the least studied sirtuin of all the mammalian sirtuins, but recent findings have established new functions and roles for this protein. It is a nucleolar sirtuin [121] and its localization is associated with the main process happening at this sub-nuclear structure, namely rDNA transcription [122]. SIRT7 does not possess a very strong deacetylate activity toward common synthetic and natural peptides [121], which is in agreement with the fact that SIRT7 depletion in mice did not change the global acetylation levels of either nucleus or nucleolus proteome [123], indicating that SIRT7 deacetylase activity is specific to a limited set of proteins. One example is specific deacetylation of H3K18 [31, 124] that underlies its role in chromatin remodeling. Also, SIRT7 has been found to be closely associated with B-WICH complex, a chromatin-remodeling complex [125]. It also has a role in protein synthesis [123, 126] and contributes to cell survival, namely by protecting against genomic insult [127, 128], hypoxia [129] and low glucose induced stress [130]. All the functions described characterize SIRT7 as a pro-survival protein. Indeed, it is currently considered to be an oncogene in all the cancer types studied so far [126, 131, 132].

3. Parasitic sirtuins

Various genome-sequencing projects demonstrated the presence of genes coding for sirtuins in most protozoan parasites of medical importance. An interesting finding was that depending on the protozoan parasite species the number of sirtuins varied (**Table 1**).

Organism	Number of sirtuins	GeneID	Subcellular Localization	Data Source
Trypanosomatids				
Trypanosoma cruzi	2	TcCLB.508207.150 (TcSir2rp1); TcCLB.447255.20 (TcSir2rp3)	cytoplasm (TcSir2rp1); mitochondria (TcSir2rp3)	TriTrypDB (v.34)
Trypanosoma brucei	3	Tb927.7.1690 (TbSir2rp1); Tb927.8.3140 (TbSir2rp2); Tb927.4.2520 (TbSir2rp3)	nucleus (TbSir2rp1); mitochondria (TbSir2rp2, TbSir2rp3)	TriTrypDB (v.34)
Leishmania spp.	3	LinJ.26.0200 (LiSir2rp1); LinJ.23.1450 (LiSir2rp2); LinJ.34.1900 (LiSir2rp3)	cytoplasm (LiSir2rp1); mitochondria (LiSir2rp2, LiSir2rp3)	TriTrypDB (v.34)
Apicomplexa				
Plasmodium spp.	2	PF13_0152 (PfSir2A); PF14_0489 (Sir2B)	nucleus; cytoplasm	PlasmoDB (v34)
Toxoplasma gondii	2	TGVEG_068040; TGVEG_108780	n.d	ToxoDB (v34)
Babesia bovis	1	BBOV_I003070	n.d	PiroplasmaDB (v34)
Others				
Giardia lamblia	5	GL50803_10708; GL50803_10707; GL50803_16569; GL50803_11676; GL50803_6942	n.d	GiardiaDB (v34)
Trichomonas vaginalis	10	TVAG_549940; TVAG_409810; TVAG_026260; TVAG_319320; TVAG_480900; TVAG_190210; TVAG 362260; TVAG_413390; TVAG_146810; TVAG_016210; TVAG_146820; TVAG 256040	n.d	TrichDB (v34)

n.d=not determined

Table 1. Sirtuin genes identified in genome-sequencing programs for parasitic protozoa.

Plasmodium spp. have been shown to contain two sirtuin orthologues, called Sir2A and Sir2B. Sir2A is the most extensively studied homolog, mainly located at the nucleus [133] although it can also shuttle to cytoplasm after posttranslational SUMOylation [134]. Sir2A has been characterized as a mediator of transcriptional silencing at the telomeric regions of chromosomes [133, 135]. The telomeres of *P. falciparum* are rich in gene families involved in antigenic variation such as the *var.* family of genes. These genes are responsible for the expression of parasite-derived *P. falciparum* erythrocyte membrane protein, PfEMP1, responsible for immune evasion in humans [136]. The family of *var.* genes is tightly regulated by sirtuins, with the expression of its members being mutually exclusive [137, 138]. The switch of active *var.* is controlled exclusively at the epigenetic level [137, 139].

PfSir2B is a larger homolog with a molecular weight more than four times the size of Sir2A and is involved in the transcriptional silencing of a complementary subset of *var.* genes with distinct promoter types [140].

Sirtuins from *Leishmania* spp. parasites were among the first to be identified in Trypanosomatids, when a complementary DNA (cDNA) isolated and sequenced from *Leishmania major* showed a high homology with yeast Sir2 [141]. Antibodies raised against this LmSir2 later showed to be reactive against different life cycle stages of *L. major*, but also to *Leishmania amazonensis* and even to the serum of a patient infected with *Leishmania infantum* [142]. Furthermore, the protein was found to be among the secreted material of *L. major* [142].

Overexpression of the Sir2 protein in *L. infantum*, sharing 93% homology to the *L. major* protein, led to an increased survival of amastigotes under axenic conditions [143]. Also, when the overexpression was performed in mammalian fibroblasts, host cells became more permissive to infection by *Leishmania* infection in comparison with wild type cells, hinting at a modulation of host cell by the parasite [144]. Genetic knockouts in *L. infantum* of the Sir2 related protein 1 (Sir2rp1) gene also highlighted the importance of this protein in the parasite. While single knockouts were readily obtainable, double deletion of the alleles was only possible after the rescue by an ectopical copy of the gene, suggesting an essential role for parasite survival [145]. When single-knockouts of *L. infantum* Sir2rp1 were used to infect a macrophage cell line, *in vitro*, it was noted that although they had the same invasive capacity than wild-type parasites, they showed a hindered replication rate leading to diminished infections over-time. Furthermore, the mutant parasite also failed to establish an infection in an *in vivo* mouse model of Leishmaniasis [145]. Cellular and biochemical studies later established LiSir2rp1 has NAD^+-dependent deacetylase with ADP-ribosylation activity that co-localized to the cytoskeleton and potentially interacted with tubulin as well as with HSP83, an orthologue of mammalian HSP90 [146, 147]. The association with cytoskeleton is a characteristic feature of both SIRT2 and HDAC6 in mammalian cells [32, 148]. In addition, an orthologous from *L. amazonensis*, LaSir2rp1 was found to be a glycosylated protein, but whether this is the case for other species remains to be seen [149]. Although the Sir2 related protein 1 has received much attention, no studies have been made for the other two proteins codified by the *Leishmania* species; Sir2 related protein 2 and Sir2 related protein 3.

Sir2rp1 from *L. donovani* has also been implicated in the resistance of amphotericin B, a reference drug in the treatment of visceral Leishmaniasis. When clinical isolates were targeted for gene knockout of the protein, parasites showed a lower level of multi-drug resistant transporter MDR1, lower drug efflux, increased ROS production and increased sensitivity to amphotericin B [150]. On the contrary, overexpression led to a resistant phenotype, thereby suggesting Sir2 as a new resistant marker for visceral Leishmaniasis [150]. Comparative transcriptomic analysis also implicates Sir2 in resistance to miltefosine, another drug used to treat the disease [151]. In addition to its potential as a novel drug target, Sir2rp1 from *Leishmania* spp. has also been suggested as a vaccine [152, 153].

Recently, LiSir2rp2 and LiSir2rp3, the others *Leishmania* sirtuins, were characterized as mitochondrial proteins, and while LiSir2rp3 was demonstrated to not be essential (**Table 1**), attempts to generate LiSir2rp2 knockout cells failed. LiSir2rp2 was implicated in parasite proliferation depending on NAD^+ availability [154].

Trypanosoma brucei, like *Leishmania* spp., has 3 sirtuins annotated in its genome (**Table 1**). The first enzyme to be characterized in the parasite was TbSir2rp1 [155]. The enzyme is localized mainly in the nucleus in association with chromosomes. The protein was shown to possess both deacetylase activity toward endogenous histones while being also able to ADP-ribosylate calf thymus histones and, to a lesser extent, bovine serum albumin (BSA). Up to that time, no ADP-ribosylation had been detected in common members of the sirtuin family like yeast Sir2 or HST2, hence TbSir2rp1 was one of the first enzymes to exhibit this dual activity [156–159]. Furthermore, mutation of a catalytic histidine essential for deacetylase activity also affected ADP-ribosylation activity, suggesting that the two activities were occurring simultaneously. Because of the increased or decreased resistance to DNA damage caused by the alkylating drug methyl methanesulfonate (MMS) in overexpressing or RNAi-induced knockdown *T. brucei* cell lines, respectively, TbSir2rp1 was also considered to have a role in DNA repair in this organism [155].

A later study performed with bloodstream forms (as opposed to insect stage forms in the previous works) characterized TbSir2rp1 and also the other two sirtuins, TbSir2rp2 and TbSir2rp3 that both with mitochondrial localization [160]. TbSir2rp1 was found in the nucleus, but when overexpressed to high levels in *T. brucei* cells, it localizes to the cytoplasm, with toxic effects to the parasite [160]. Besides, gene knockouts for the three proteins caused no growth in parasites maintained in standard conditions [160]. TbSir2rp1 mutants, however, did show an increased sensitivity to MMS damage, confirming the previous results performed with RNA interference (RNAi). The particular localization of TbSir2rp1 led to the investigation of Sir2 mediated telomere gene silencing like the one that occurs in yeast and *Plasmodium* spp., as discussed earlier [161, 162]. Although TbSir2rp1 was found to have a role in telomere DNA repair and telomere silence, it was not required for antigenic variation [160] as described for *Plasmodium* Sir2 [133, 135].

TbSir2rp1 has also been studied as a model sirtuin, with both deacetylase and ADP-ribosylation activity. Biochemical experiments revealed that ADP-ribosylation is 5-fold less active than the deacetylation reaction, and occurs only in the presence of an acetylated substrate by two distinct biochemical mechanisms [163]. Another research group demonstrated that ADP-ribosylation can also occur in arginine, independent of the presence of an acetylated substrate, as supported by mass spectrometry and molecular dynamics simulations [164].

Additional information about parasitic sirtuins can be found in a recent review by Hailu et al. [165].

4. *Trypanosoma cruzi sirtuins*

Although the draft of the *T. cruzi* genome has been published a decade ago [19], it was not until recently that the first experimental studies involving the sirtuins of this parasite have been published. Unlike *Leishmania* spp. and *T. brucei* that possess three Sir2-like proteins, *T. cruzi* only has two coding sequences annotated in its genome, TcSir2rp1 and TcSir2rp3 (**Table 1**).

One study employing parasites overexpressing TcSir2rp1 and TcSir2rp3 by a tetracycline inducible vector characterized some of the features of both proteins [58]. Localization studies employing both wild type parasites and polyclonal sera raised against both proteins, as well as localization of tagged copies in the overexpression mutants with monoclonal antibodies, attributed a cytoplasmic localization to TcSir2rp1 and a mitochondrial to TcSir2rp3 [58]. Both of the proteins' levels are regulated throughout the life cycle of the parasite, with a significant decrease in both at the trypomastigote stage [58]. Overexpression of TcSir2rp1 was responsible for higher metacyclogenesis and higher infectivity of Vero cells. Since metacyclogenesis occurs under nutrient deprivation, it is hypothesized that TcSir2rp1 may function like sirtuins from other organisms that respond to starvation [101, 166, 167]. On the other hand, overexpression of TcSir2rp3 led to a decrease in epimastigote replication time, lower infectivity in Vero cells, increased amastigote replication and normal metacyclogenesis [58]. Due to the oxidizing environment in which amastigotes replicate, it has been suggested that TcSir2rp3 performs protecting functions against oxidative stress like SIRT3 [36]. Both of the overexpressing cell lines reduced the levels of acetylation for particular proteins, as well as protected against the effect of specific sirtuin inhibitors [58].

Moretti and colleagues also independently characterized both of the sirtuins in a simultaneous study [59]. In their study, they show that salermide, a sirtuin inhibitor analogue of sirtinol found to be a strong anticancer molecule, is active against both *in vitro* cultures of epimastigotes, and against an *in vivo* model of infection by *T. cruzi*, albeit at moderate levels [59, 168]. Salermide was also found to be a strong inhibitor of TcSir2rp3 recombinant protein [59]. The authors report the same localization for both proteins, as well as the interference in epimastigote growth, metacyclogenesis, infectivity of host cells and amastigote replication in lines overexpressing the sirtuins. Differently from Ritagliati work [58], in their studies, the overexpression of the cytosolic TcSir2rp1 caused a decreased in the epimastigotes proliferation while TcSir2pr3 increased the growth rate. These differences might be due to the amount of overexpression achieved and parasite strains used [59].

5. Potential of *Trypanosoma cruzi* sirtuins as targets for infection control

A strategy that has been traditionally employed in Chagas disease drug discovery is the target-based approach. One such molecular target that has gained increasing interest as a potential drug targets against parasitic diseases is that of sirtuins [169, 170]. The hypothesis arose by the time that it was demonstrated that sirtuins are life-span regulators in organisms like yeast, flies and worms [70, 171, 172]. Therefore, many groups promptly investigated whether sirtuin orthologues present in parasites could have important functions that could be exploited for novel therapeutic applications.

One important aspect for the viability of targeting sirtuins in parasites is the homology between the protein of interest and other proteins present in the host organisms. Although sirtuins are conserved through evolution [33], significant difference at the sequence level can be found between Trypanosomatid and human homologs. For instance, *T. cruzi* Sir2rp1 shares only 33% identity with mammalian SIRT2, its closest homolog (Multi-way protein alignment, BLOSUM 62) [173].

Another argument that has led to the consideration of *T. cruzi* sirtuins as a drug target is that this family of proteins is considered to possess structural properties adequate to inhibition by small-molecule compounds. In particular, the catalytic site is located inside a hydrophobic channel formed at the interface between the two constituting domains, the Rossman fold containing the NAD^+ binding domain and the Zn^{2+} ion binding domain [56]. Catalytic pockets buried inside the protein are considered an essential feature for target druggability [174].

One last fact that prompted the evaluation of TcSir2rp1 as a drug target was the previous evidence that a class of experimental compounds preferentially inhibited LiSir2rp1 over the human homolog SIRT1 [175]. The possibility to synthetize selective sirtuin inhibitors has been successfully achieved for human homologs, based upon structural knowledge of the catalytic site as has been demonstrated for human SIRT2 [176, 177].

Enzymatic inhibition by small molecule compounds is an essential step in the druggability assessment of novel therapeutic targets [174]. Biochemical studies performed by our research groups evaluated the effect of nicotinamide, a classic non-competitive inhibitor of sirtuins in TcSir2rp1 and TcSir2rp3 (to be published). TcSir2rp1 was shown to be inhibited by nicotinamide, albeit at a relatively high IC_{50} when compared with other sirtuins (4-fold higher for hSIRT1 and 11-fold higher for LiSir2rp1) [175]. Different nicotinamide sensitivities are found among distinct sirtuins, and may explain the differences described [177]. Nicotinamide inhibits deacetylation by binding to a conserved C pocket present in sirtuins that participates in NAD^+ binding and catalysis, where it promotes a base-exchange reaction at the expense of deacetylation [178]. A hypothesis for the high IC_{50} for nicotinamide in TcSir2rp1 could be related with structural characteristics of this conserved C pocket. Structural determination of TcSir2rp1 by X-ray crystallography currently ongoing in our group will certainly highlight these differences. Contrary to previous studies [179], we could not observe any antiparasitic activity of nicotinamide against *T. cruzi* amastigotes for up to a concentration of 2 mM. Several studies report the activity of nicotinamide against parasitic protozoa [180–182], but to our knowledge, none clearly establishes a relation between antiparasitic activity and sirtuin inhibition.

Other biochemical functions and protein interactions have been attributed to Sir2rp1 in related Trypanosomatids, and future experiments should shed light whether it applies to TcSir2rp1. One of the biochemical functions that has been characterized for both TbSir2rp1 and LiSir2rp1 is ADP-ribosylation. Both orthologous showed to ADP-ribosylate calf thymus histones and BSA [155, 183]. Later studies involving TbSir2rp1 demonstrated that this biochemical function is dependent upon acetylated histones, is coupled to the deacetylase activity of the sirtuin, but occurs at a much lower rate than the latter [163]. In fact, even though ADP-ribosylation has clear functions in both physiological and pathogenic situations when catalyzed by other

ADP-ribosyltransferases [183, 184], the reaction catalyzed by sirtuins is currently challenged to be an unspecific side-reaction [159].

Like the human SIRT2, *L. infantum* Sir2rp1 was also found to be associated with tubulin [146], the major component of Trypanosomatids cytoskeleton formed by an array of subpellicular microtubules that span the whole cell of the parasite [185]. SIRT2 is a tubulin deacetylase that displays a higher affinity for tubulin than for histones [32], and has been found to be linked to regulation of mitotic progression [86], chromatin condensation [186] and cell migration [187]. TcSir2rp1 overexpression in *T. cruzi* was found to increase the deacetylation level of endogenous tubulin [58]. It is interesting to note that Sir2rp1 from *T. cruzi* is a cytoplasmic protein like LiSir2rp1 and not nuclear like TbSir2rp1. Since *T. cruzi* shares some characteristics with *L. infantum* like the amastigote intracellular stage, it should not be ruled out that Sir2rp1 may have functions in the cytoskeleton remodeling necessary for stage differentiation. Several proteins, sirtuins included, have demonstrated the ability to shuttle from the nucleus to the cytoplasm and vice-versa [188, 189]. SIRT2, the closest sirtuin homolog of mammalian cells, is actively exported to the cytoplasm during interphase, but is accumulated in the nucleus from prophase until cytokinesis where it co-localizes with important mitotic structures like centrosomes and the mitotic spindle [190]. Curiously, analysis of TcSir2rp1 by Wregex and cNLS Mapper, bio-computational tools that identify nuclear export signals (NES) and nuclear localization signals (NLS), respectively, indicate the presence of non-canonical NES/NLS in the sequence of this sirtuin [191, 192]. Whether TcSir2rp1 does shuttle to the nucleus during specific phases of *T. cruzi* life cycle, for instance to repair DNA damage like the *T. brucei* orthologue, remains to be reported.

The mitochondrial TcSir2rp3 was found less expressed in *T. cruzi* forms proliferating in mammalian cells. Its expression increased when the parasite transformed in trypomastigotes [59]. The fact that cells overexpressing only the active form, but not the inactive form of TcSir2rp3 showed an increased intracellular growth and failed to transform in to extracellular trypomastigotes [59], suggested that it could also be a drug target to control the infection, although further experiments to generate knockout cell lines need to be performed. We recently identified several compounds that prevented intracellular growth of *T. cruzi* some of them inhibiting specifically TcSir2rp1 or TcSir2rp3 which might indicate the requirement of both enzymes for the parasite (to be published).

6. Naphtalimide derivatives as potential drugs for Chagas disease control

Naphthalimides are a class of compounds that have generated intense interest as active molecules with potential to treat a range of conditions [193]. A naphthalene ring linked to an imide group that forms a third heterocycle composes the basic chemical scaffold of the naphthalimide derivatives. This moiety has a planar nature and is considered to be responsible for the pharmacological activities attributed to compounds derived from this structure, that can be as distinct as anticancer, antibacterial, antiprotozoal, antiviral, analgesic, and anesthetic [193]. Their potential as anticancer compounds has received particular attention, mostly because of their DNA intercalating properties and also to their reported activity as topoisomerase inhibitors [194–196]. Compounds like amonafide and bisnafide have been proposed as anticancer agents and have inclusively reached clinical trials in the past [197, 198]. Elinafide is another derivative with two naphthalimide moieties that has been evaluated in preclinical studies and demonstrated potential against various mouse xenograft models [199]. This last compound was in the origin of the synthesis of the first BNIPs that differed in the alkyl chain linking the naphthalimide and amine group, i.e. a propyl instead of an ethyl chain [200]. These derivatives showed potential activity against breast cancer MCF-7 cell line and actively bound DNA as demonstrated by thermal denaturation measurements, ethidium bromide displacement and DNA gel mobility [200]. Later derivatives that varied in the length of the chain linking the two amines of bisnaphthalimidopropyl groups were also evaluated against cancer cell lines and promastigotes of the parasite *L. infantum* [201]. While screening for enzymatic inhibitors of the recently characterized LiSir2rp1, BNIPs were identified as inhibitors of its deacetylase activity [175]. Furthermore, they were active against intracellular amastigotes, the clinically relevant stage of the parasite present in humans, at concentrations in the single micromolar range [175].

Our groups' previous results demonstrating activity toward *L. infantum* led to the testing of BNIPs as inhibitors of the related Trypanosomatid *T. brucei* and its Sir2rp1 orthologue, TbSir2rp1 [202]. BNIPs revealed to be very potent inhibitors of *in vitro* parasite growth, with one of the compounds, BNIPDabut (**Figure 1**) with an EC_{50} in the range of the reference drug pentamidine. However, when tested against the TbSir2rp1 recombinant enzyme, BNIPDabut had an IC_{50} more than 10^4 times superior to the EC_{50} against the whole cell parasite, indicating that Sir2rp1 inhibition is probably not a major mechanism of action for the compound. Whether BNIPDabut inhibits other *T. brucei* sirtuin enzymes remains to be elucidated. It should be noted that RNAi and gene knockout experiments of the three sirtuins did not led to a deleterious effect, and unlike LiSir2rp1, there is no indication of that these proteins may be essential [155, 160]. The optimal *in vitro* properties of BNIPDabut led to the testing with an *in vivo* model of trypanosomiasis by bioluminescence imaging. Although BNIPDabut maintained a strong trypanocidal activity *in vivo*, as assessed by the decrease in bioluminescent signals to levels similar to those of the reference drug control pentamidine, it was not sufficient for infection clearance, as animals' parasitaemia relapsed shortly after treatment interruption. Nevertheless, BNIPDabut should constitute a scaffold for further consideration in HAT drug discovery [202].

In a different study, BNIP derivatives were also tested against TcSir2rp1 and *in vitro* cultures of *T. cruzi* amastigotes (unpublished results). BNIPs demonstrated to inhibit the deacetylase activity of this enzyme, with BNIPSpd (**Figure 1**) as the most potent compound, showing a dose-dependent effect on inhibition. BNIPSpd also proved to be active and selective against amastigotes of *T. cruzi* in a high content screening (HCS) assay – an assay that takes advantage of computer-assisted image processing of hundreds of microscopic images originating in automated microscopes able to simultaneously capture multiple conditions or drug compounds. In this work, a new set of derivatives was also synthetized in order to improve both solubility and binding to cellular targets, mostly by including cyclic structures and heteroatoms in the carbon chain linking the two naphthalimide groups. The most active compounds were BCNIPP, also a TcSir2rp1 inhibitor, and trans BNIP-1,4-Dacyhex, a derivative of BNIPDabut that weakly inhibited the enzyme. In turn, BNIPDabut had some inhibitory activity on *T. cruzi* amastigotes, with low selectivity, but also did not inhibit TcSir2rp1 at 10 μM. The activity of BNIPSpd in a mice model of Chagas disease using bioluminescent parasites was also determined and found to be absent at the doses tested. An explanation might be the poor pharmacokinetic profile of the compounds, which fails to ever achieve at least the *in vitro* IC_{50} against *T. cruzi* amastigotes.

Altogether, our data indicate that BNIP derivatives may not be acting only by a mechanism of Sir2rp1 inhibition, with other targets contributing to the activity detected. BNIPs were originally designed and developed as anti-cancer agents [203, 204] through DNA intercalation. This property might explain some of the cytotoxic effects verified against host cells, but may also be an important mechanism of activity toward the parasite, especially since trypanosomes are highly susceptible to intercalating agents [205].

Confirmation of the mechanism of action can be undertaken by appropriate target deconvolution experiments [206]. The most common type of such experiments are biochemical methods that employ some variation of biochemical affinity purification, where the compounds are immobilized in a column, and allowed to interact with protein extracts, preferably previously fractionated. After stringent washing steps, the bound proteins are eluted and identified. Such strategy has been employed in the identification of small molecule activators of cryptochrome of mammalian cells [207]. A disadvantage is that there is a bias toward high affinity ligands, and when the target is relatively less abundant or has less affinity, important targets may not be detected. Furthermore, the washing steps may eliminate protein complexes that may be important for appropriate drug activity.

Genetic methods can also be valuable for target deconvolution. Gene knockouts and RNAi screens can be used to try to phenotype a compound's effect [208]. Furthermore, if the mutant is hypersensitive to the compound in question, the evidence that the protein could be the target for the compounds would be strengthened. The validation of trypanothione synthetase and N-myristoyltransferase as drug targets against trypanosomes are examples where the differential sensitivity of an inhibitor in wild type, overexpression, and knockout mutants is clearly illustrated [209, 210]. An additional genetic strategy is based on the generation of resistant cell lines by culturing the parasites in increasing sub-lethal drug concentrations that are posteriorly sequenced to find mutated genes related to the mechanism of action for the compound [208]. Genetic methods have recently been employed in the search of the mechanism of action of oxaboroles [211], a class of compounds in development for HAT, but also active against *T. cruzi* [212, 213].

Chemical genomics can also be applied to the discovery of novel drug targets, as exemplified by the recent characterization of cytochrome b from *T. cruzi*. This enzyme was demonstrated to be selectively targeted in relation to the human homolog by a hit compound coming from a phenotypic screening [214].

7. Perspective

Here we highlighted the potential of sirtuins, particularly in the *T. cruzi* as possible targets of drug development for Chagas disease for the following reasons:

1. The parasite contains only two sirtuins, instead of three present in *Leishmania* spp. and *T. brucei* species, and seven in the human host, which facilitates a more precise design and avoid redundant effects.

2. Several experiments demonstrate the requirement of these enzymes for growth and survival, particularly in intracellular forms of the parasite, which are clinically relevant.
3. There are several compounds already designed to be selective sirtuin inhibitors that could be modified to provide increased specificity and selectivity to the parasite enzyme. Some of these compounds have already defined druggability and specific derivatives can be repurposed more easily.
4. Both sirtuins were produced to perform enzymatic screenings and crystals of TcSir2rp1 have been obtained to be the basis of further medicinal chemistry.

Finally, several lead compounds were identified for *T. cruzi* sirtuin, which can provide the basis for future development. It is also important to note that these possible inhibitors could act synergistically with drugs already in use for treatment, as a novel combinational therapy, opening new avenues to eliminate Chagas disease.

Acknowledgements

This article is a result of the project NORTE-01-0145-FEDER-000012, supported by Norte Portugal Regional Operational Programme (NORTE 2020), under the PORTUGAL 2020 Partnership Agreement, through the European Regional Development Fund (ERDF)".

Author details

Luís Gaspar [1,2], Terry K. Smith [3], Nilmar Silvio Moretti [4], Sergio Schenkman [4] and Anabela Cordeiro-da-Silva [1,2,5*]

*Address all correspondence to: cordeiro@ibmc.up.pt

1 Instituto de Investigação e Inovação em Saúde, University of Porto, Portugal

2 Institute for Molecular and Cell Biology, University of Porto, Porto, Portugal

3 Biomedical Sciences Research Complex, The University, St. Andrews, Fife, Scotland, UK

4 Departament of Microbiology, Imunology and Parasitology, Escola Paulista de Medicina, Federal University of São Paulo, São Paulo, Brazil,

5 Departament of Biological Sciences, Faculty of Pharmacy of University of Porto, Porto, Portugal

References

[1] WHO. Chagas disease in latin america: An epidemiological update based on 2010 estimates. Weekly Epidemiological Record. 2015;**90**(6):33-43

[2] Walsh JA. Estimating the burden of illness in the tropics. In: Warren KS, Mahmoud AAF, editors. Tropical and Geographical Medicine. McGraw Hill Education; 1984. pp. 1073-1085

[3] Knowles LL, Carstens BC. Delimiting species without monophyletic gene trees. Systematic Biology. 2007;**56**(6):887-895

[4] Deane LM. Animal reservoirs of *Trypanosoma cruzi* in Brazil. Revista Brasileira de Malariologia e Doenças Tropicais. 1964;**16**:27-48

[5] Barreto M. Reservatórios do *Trypanosoma cruzi* nas américas. Revista Brasileira de Malariologia e Doenças Tropicais. 1964;**16**:527-552

[6] Tarleton RL. Parasite persistence in the aetiology of Chagas disease. International Journal for Parasitology. 2001;**31**(5–6):550-554. DOI: 10.1016/S0020-7519(01)00158-8

[7] Tarleton RL. Chagas disease: A role for autoimmunity? Trends in Parasitology. 2003; **19**(10):447-451

[8] Wainwright M. Dyes, trypanosomiasis and DNA: A historical and critical review. Biotechnic & Histochemistry. 2010;**85**(6):341-354. DOI: 10.3109/10520290903297528

[9] Docampo R, Moreno SN, Gadelha FR, de Souza W, Cruz FS. Prevention of Chagas' disease resulting from blood transfusion by treatment of blood: Toxicity and mode of action of gentian violet. Biomedical and Environmental Sciences. 1988;**1**(4):406-413

[10] Kennedy PG. The continuing problem of human african trypanosomiasis (sleeping sickness). Annals of Neurology. 2008;**64**(2):116-126. DOI: 10.1002/ana.21429

[11] Gaspar L, Moraes C, Freitas-Junior L, Ferrari S, Costantino L, Costi M, et al. Current and future chemotherapy for Chagas disease. Current Medicinal Chemistry. 2015;**22**(37): 4293-4312. DOI: 10.2174/0929867322666151015120804

[12] Butera JA. Phenotypic screening as a strategic component of drug discovery programs targeting novel antiparasitic and antimycobacterial agents: An editorial. Journal of Medicinal Chemistry. 2013;**56**(20):7715-7718. DOI: 10.1021/jm400443k

[13] Buckner FS, Verlinde CL, La Flamme AC, Van Voorhis WC. Efficient technique for screening drugs for activity against *Trypanosoma cruzi* using parasites expressing beta-galactosidase. Antimicrobial Agents and Chemotherapy. 1996;**40**(11):2592-2597

[14] Canavaci AM, Bustamante JM, Padilla AM, Perez Brandan CM, Simpson LJ, Xu D, et al. *In vitro* and *in vivo* high-throughput assays for the testing of anti-*Trypanosoma cruzi* compounds. PLoS Neglected Tropical Diseases. 2010;**4**(7):e740. DOI: 10.1371/journal.pntd.0000740

[15] Moon S, Siqueira-Neto JL, Moraes CB, Yang G, Kang M, Freitas-Junior LH, et al. An image-based algorithm for precise and accurate high throughput assessment of drug activity against the human parasite *Trypanosoma cruzi*. PLoS One. 2014;**9**(2):e87188. DOI: 10.1371/journal.pone.0087188

[16] Moraes CB, White KL, Braillard S, Perez C, Goo J, Gaspar L, et al. Enantiomers of nifurtimox do not exhibit stereoselective anti-*Trypanosoma cruzi* activity, toxicity, or pharmacokinetic properties. Antimicrobial Agents and Chemotherapy. 2015;**59**(6):3645-3647. DOI: 10.1128/aac.05139-14

[17] Balfour MN, Franco CH, Moraes CB, Freitas-Junior LH, Stefani HA. Synthesis and trypanocidal activity of a library of 4-substituted 2-(1h-pyrrolo[3,2-c]pyridin-2-yl)propan-2-ols. European Journal of Medicinal Chemistry. 2017;**128**:202-212. DOI: 10.1016/j.ejmech.2017.01.040

[18] Moraes CB, Giardini MA, Kim H, Franco CH, Araujo-Junior AM, Schenkman S, et al. Nitroheterocyclic compounds are more efficacious than cyp51 inhibitors against *Trypanosoma cruzi*: Implications for Chagas disease drug discovery and development. Scientific Reports. 2014;**4**:4703-4714. DOI: 10.1038/srep04703

[19] El-Sayed NM, Myler PJ, Bartholomeu DC, Nilsson D, Aggarwal G, Tran AN, et al. The genome sequence of *Trypanosoma cruzi*, etiologic agent of Chagas disease. Science. 2005; **309**(5733):409-415. DOI: 10.1126/science.1112631

[20] Naula C, Parsons M, Mottram JC. Protein kinases as drug targets in trypanosomes and *Leishmania*. Biochimica et Biophysica Acta. 2005;**1754**(1–2):151-159. DOI: 10.1016/j.bbapap.2005.08.018

[21] Ward P, Equinet L, Packer J, Doerig C. Protein kinases of the human malaria parasite *Plasmodium falciparum*: The kinome of a divergent eukaryote. BMC Genomics. 2004;**5**:79-98. DOI: 10.1186/1471-2164-5-79

[22] Walsh CT, Garneau-Tsodikova S, Gatto GJ Jr. Protein posttranslational modifications: The chemistry of proteome diversifications. Angewandte Chemie (International Ed. in English). 2005;**44**(45):7342-7372. DOI: 10.1002/anie.200501023

[23] Lothrop AP, Torres MP, Fuchs SM. Deciphering post-translational modification codes. FEBS Letters. 2013;**587**(8):1247-1257. DOI: 10.1016/j.febslet.2013.01.047

[24] Verdin E, Ott M. 50 years of protein acetylation: From gene regulation to epigenetics, metabolism and beyond. Nature Reviews. Molecular Cell Biology. 2015;**16**(4):258-264. DOI: 10.1038/nrm3931

[25] Kouzarides T. Acetylation: A regulatory modification to rival phosphorylation? The EMBO Journal. 2000;**19**(6):1176-1179. DOI: 10.1093/emboj/19.6.1176

[26] Choudhary C, Weinert BT, Nishida Y, Verdin E, Mann M. The growing landscape of lysine acetylation links metabolism and cell signalling. Nature Reviews. Molecular Cell Biology. 2014;**15**(8):536-550. DOI: 10.1038/nrm3841

[27] Choudhary C, Kumar C, Gnad F, Nielsen ML, Rehman M, Walther TC, et al. Lysine acetylation targets protein complexes and co-regulates major cellular functions. Science. 2009;**325**(5942):834-840. DOI: 10.1126/science.1175371

[28] Olsen JV, Blagoev B, Gnad F, Macek B, Kumar C, Mortensen P, et al. Global, *in vivo*, and site-specific phosphorylation dynamics in signaling networks. Cell. 2006;**127**(3):635-648. DOI: 10.1016/j.cell.2006.09.026

[29] Inoue A, Fujimoto D. Enzymatic deacetylation of histone. Biochemical and Biophysical Research Communications. 1969;**36**(1):146-150

[30] Nakagawa T, Lomb DJ, Haigis MC, Guarente L. SIRT5 deacetylates carbamoyl phosphate synthetase 1 and regulates the urea cycle. Cell. 2009;**137**(3):560-570. DOI: 10.1016/j.cell.2009.02.026

[31] Barber MF, Michishita-Kioi E, Xi Y, Tasselli L, Kioi M, Moqtaderi Z, et al. SIRT7 links h3k18 deacetylation to maintenance of oncogenic transformation. Nature. 2012;**487**(7405):114-118. DOI: 10.1038/nature11043

[32] North BJ, Marshall BL, Borra MT, Denu JM, Verdin E. The human Sir2 ortholog, SIRT2, is an NAD^+-dependent tubulin deacetylase. Molecular Cell. 2003;**11**(2):437-444. DOI: 10.1016/s1097-2765(03)00038-8

[33] Frye R. Evolution of sirtuins from archaea to vertebrates. In: Verdin E, editor. Histone Deacetylases. Humana Press; 2006. pp. 183-202. DOI: 10.1385/1-59745-024-3:183

[34] Frye RA. Phylogenetic classification of prokaryotic and eukaryotic Sir2-like proteins. Biochemical and Biophysical Research Communications. 2000;**273**(2):793-798. DOI: 10.1006/bbrc.2000.3000

[35] Ogura M, Nakamura Y, Tanaka D, Zhuang X, Fujita Y, Obara A, et al. Overexpression of SIRT5 confirms its involvement in deacetylation and activation of carbamoyl phosphate synthetase 1. Biochemical and Biophysical Research Communications. 2010;**393**(1):73-78. DOI: 10.1016/j.bbrc.2010.01.081

[36] Bause AS, Haigis MC. SIRT3 regulation of mitochondrial oxidative stress. Experimental Gerontology. 2013;**48**(7):634-639. DOI: 10.1016/j.exger.2012.08.007

[37] Bharathi SS, Zhang Y, Mohsen AW, Uppala R, Balasubramani M, Schreiber E, et al. Sirtuin 3 (SIRT3) protein regulates long-chain acyl-coa dehydrogenase by deacetylating conserved lysines near the active site. The Journal of Biological Chemistry. 2013;**288**(47):33837-33847. DOI: 10.1074/jbc.M113.510354

[38] Sauve AA. Sirtuin chemical mechanisms. Biochimica et Biophysica Acta. 2010;**1804**(8):1591-1603. DOI: 10.1016/j.bbapap.2010.01.021

[39] Jackson MD, Denu JM. Structural identification of 2′- and 3′-o-acetyl-ADP-ribose as novel metabolites derived from the sir2 family of beta-NAD^+-dependent histone/protein deacetylases. The Journal of Biological Chemistry. 2002;**277**(21):18535-18544. DOI: 10.1074/jbc.M200671200

[40] Borra MT, Langer MR, Slama JT, Denu JM. Substrate specificity and kinetic mechanism of the Sir2 family of NAD^+-dependent histone/protein deacetylases. Biochemistry. 2004;**43**(30):9877-9887. DOI: 10.1021/bi049592e

[41] Pan PW, Feldman JL, Devries MK, Dong A, Edwards AM, Denu JM. Structure and biochemical functions of SIRT6. The Journal of Biological Chemistry. 2011;**286**(16):14575-14587. DOI: 10.1074/jbc.M111.218990

[42] Berger F, Ramirez-Hernandez MH, Ziegler M. The new life of a centenarian: Signalling functions of NAD(P). Trends in Biochemical Sciences. 2004;**29**(3):111-118. DOI: 10.1016/j.tibs.2004.01.007

[43] Smythe GA, Braga O, Brew BJ, Grant RS, Guillemin GJ, Kerr SJ, et al. Concurrent quantification of quinolinic, picolinic, and nicotinic acids using electron-capture negative-ion gas chromatography-mass spectrometry. Analytical Biochemistry. 2002;**301**(1):21-26. DOI: 10.1006/abio.2001.5490

[44] Hagino Y, Lan SJ, Ng CY, Henderson LM. Metabolism of pyridinium precursors of pyridine nucleotides in perfused rat liver. The Journal of Biological Chemistry. 1968;**243**(19):4980-4986

[45] Tong L, Denu JM. Function and metabolism of sirtuin metabolite o-acetyl-ADP-ribose. Biochimica et Biophysica Acta. 2010;**1804**(8):1617-1625. DOI: 10.1016/j.bbapap.2010.02.007

[46] Borra MT, O'Neill FJ, Jackson MD, Marshall B, Verdin E, Foltz KR, et al. Conserved enzymatic production and biological effect of o-acetyl-ADP-ribose by silent information regulator 2-like NAD+-dependent deacetylases. The Journal of Biological Chemistry. 2002;**277**(15):12632-12641. DOI: 10.1074/jbc.M111830200

[47] Frye RA. Characterization of five human cdnas with homology to the yeast Sir2 gene: Sir2-like proteins (sirtuins) metabolize NAD and may have protein ADP-ribosyltransferase activity. Biochemical and Biophysical Research Communications. 1999;**260**(1):273-279. DOI: 10.1006/bbrc.1999.0897

[48] Ahuja N, Schwer B, Carobbio S, Waltregny D, North BJ, Castronovo V, et al. Regulation of insulin secretion by SIRT4, a mitochondrial ADP-ribosyltransferase. The Journal of Biological Chemistry. 2007;**282**(46):33583-33592. DOI: 10.1074/jbc.M705488200

[49] Laurent G, German NJ, Saha AK, de Boer VC, Davies M, Koves TR, et al. SIRT4 coordinates the balance between lipid synthesis and catabolism by repressing malonyl COA decarboxylase. Molecular Cell. 2013;**50**(5):686-698. DOI: 10.1016/j.molcel.2013.05.012

[50] Du J, Jiang H, Lin H. Investigating the ADP-ribosyltransferase activity of sirtuins with NAD analogues and 32p-NAD. Biochemistry. 2009;**48**(13):2878-2890. DOI: 10.1021/bi802093g

[51] Butepage M, Eckei L, Verheugd P, Luscher B. Intracellular mono-ADP-ribosylation in signaling and disease. Cell. 2015;**4**(4):569-595. DOI: 10.3390/cells4040569

[52] Haikarainen T, Lehtiö L. Proximal ADP-ribose hydrolysis in Trypanosomatids is catalyzed by a macrodomain. Scientific Reports. 2016;**6**:24213. DOI: 10.1038/srep24213

[53] Jiang H, Khan S, Wang Y, Charron G, He B, Sebastian C, et al. SIRT6 regulates TNF-α secretion through hydrolysis of long-chain fatty acyl lysine. Nature. 2013;**496**(7443):110-113. DOI: 10.1038/nature12038

[54] Park J, Chen Y, Tishkoff DX, Peng C, Tan M, Dai L, et al. SIRT5-mediated lysine desuccinylation impacts diverse metabolic pathways. Molecular Cell. 2013;**50**(6):919-930. DOI: 10.1016/j.molcel.2013.06.001

[55] Nishida Y, Rardin MJ, Carrico C, He W, Sahu AK, Gut P, et al. SIRT5 regulates both cytosolic and mitochondrial protein malonylation with glycolysis as a major target. Molecular Cell. 2015;**59**(2):321-332. DOI: 10.1016/j.molcel.2015.05.022

[56] Greiss S, Gartner A. Sirtuin/Sir2 phylogeny, evolutionary considerations and structural conservation. Molecules and Cells. 2009;**28**(5):407-415. DOI: 10.1007/s10059-009-0169-x

[57] Chakrabarty SP, Balaram H. Reversible binding of zinc in *Plasmodium falciparum* Sir2: Structure and activity of the apoenzyme. Biochimica et Biophysica Acta. 2010;**1804**(9): 1743-1750. DOI: 10.1016/j.bbapap.2010.06.010

[58] Ritagliati C, Alonso VL, Manarin R, Cribb P, Serra EC. Overexpression of cytoplasmic TcSir2rp1 and mitochondrial TcSir2rp3 impacts on *Trypanosoma cruzi* growth and cell invasion. PLoS Neglected Tropical Diseases. 2015;**9**(4):e0003725. DOI: 10.1371/journal.pntd.0003725

[59] Moretti NS, Augusto LD, Clemente TM, Antunes RP, Yoshida N, Torrecilhas AC, et al. Characterization of *Trypanosoma cruzi* sirtuins as possible drug targets for Chagas disease. Antimicrobial Agents and Chemotherapy. 2015;**59**(8):4669-4679. DOI: 10.1128/AAC.04694-14

[60] Feldman JL, Dittenhafer-Reed KE, Denu JM. Sirtuin catalysis and regulation. The Journal of Biological Chemistry. 2012;**287**(51):42419-42427. DOI: 10.1074/jbc.R112.378877

[61] Shore D, Squire M, Nasmyth KA. Characterization of two genes required for the position-effect control of yeast mating-type genes. The EMBO Journal. 1984;**3**(12):2817-2823

[62] Ivy JM, Klar AJ, Hicks JB. Cloning and characterization of four Sir genes of *Saccharomyces cerevisiae*. Molecular and Cellular Biology. 1986;**6**(2):688-702

[63] Aparicio OM, Billington BL, Gottschling DE. Modifiers of position effect are shared between telomeric and silent mating-type loci in *S. cerevisiae*. Cell. 1991;**66**(6):1279-1287

[64] Bryk M, Banerjee M, Murphy M, Knudsen KE, Garfinkel DJ, Curcio MJ. Transcriptional silencing of Ty1 elements in the Rdn1 locus of yeast. Genes & Development. 1997;**11**(2):255-269

[65] Fritze CE, Verschueren K, Strich R, Easton Esposito R. Direct evidence for Sir2 modulation of chromatin structure in yeast rDNA. The EMBO Journal. 1997;**16**(21):6495-6509. DOI: 10.1093/emboj/16.21.6495

[66] Gottlieb S, Esposito RE. A new role for a yeast transcriptional silencer gene, Sir2, in regulation of recombination in ribosomal DNA. Cell. 1989;**56**(5):771-776

[67] Shou W, Seol JH, Shevchenko A, Baskerville C, Moazed D, Chen ZW, et al. Exit from mitosis is triggered by TEM1-dependent release of the protein phosphatase cdc14 from nucleolar rent complex. Cell. 1999;**97**(2):233-244

[68] Straight AF, Shou W, Dowd GJ, Turck CW, Deshaies RJ, Johnson AD, et al. Net1, a Sir2-associated nucleolar protein required for rDNA silencing and nucleolar integrity. Cell. 1999;**97**(2):245-256

[69] Sinclair DA, Guarente L. Extrachromosomal rDNA circles-a cause of aging in yeast. Cell. 1997;**91**(7):1033-1042

[70] Kaeberlein M, McVey M, Guarente L. The sir2/3/4 complex and sir2 alone promote longevity in saccharomyces cerevisiae by two different mechanisms. Genes & Development. 1999;**13**(19):2570-2580

[71] Muth V, Nadaud S, Grummt I, Voit R. Acetylation of TAF($_i$)68, a subunit of tif-ib/sl1, activates RNA polymerase I transcription. The EMBO Journal. 2001;**20**(6):1353-1362. DOI: 10.1093/emboj/20.6.1353

[72] Brooks CL, Gu W. Ubiquitination, phosphorylation and acetylation: The molecular basis for p53 regulation. Current Opinion in Cell Biology. 2003;**15**(2):164-171

[73] Cheng HL, Mostoslavsky R, Saito S, Manis JP, Gu Y, Patel P, et al. Developmental defects and p53 hyperacetylation in Sir2 homolog (SIRT1)-deficient mice. Proceedings of the National Academy of Sciences of the United States of America. 2003;**100**(19):10794-10799. DOI: 10.1073/pnas.1934713100

[74] Wang RH, Sengupta K, Li C, Kim HS, Cao L, Xiao C, et al. Impaired DNA damage response, genome instability, and tumorigenesis in SIRT1 mutant mice. Cancer Cell. 2008;**14**(4):312-323. DOI: 10.1016/j.ccr.2008.09.001

[75] Canto C, Auwerx J. Caloric restriction, SIRT1 and longevity. Trends in Endocrinology and Metabolism. 2009;**20**(7):325-331. DOI: 10.1016/j.tem.2009.03.008

[76] Hu Y, Liu J, Wang J, Liu Q. The controversial links among calorie restriction, SIRT1, and resveratrol. Free Radical Biology & Medicine. 2011;**51**(2):250-256. DOI: 10.1016/j.freeradbiomed.2011.04.034

[77] Wang Y. Molecular links between caloric restriction and Sir2/SIRT1 activation. Diabetes and Metabolism Journal. 2014;**38**(5):321-329. DOI: 10.4093/dmj.2014.38.5.321

[78] Kenyon CJ. The genetics of ageing. Nature. 2010;**464**(7288):504-512. DOI: 10.1038/nature08980

[79] Fontana L, Partridge L, Longo VD. Extending healthy life span-from yeast to humans. Science. 2010;**328**(5976):321-326. DOI: 10.1126/science.1172539

[80] Rodgers JT, Lerin C, Haas W, Gygi SP, Spiegelman BM, Puigserver P. Nutrient control of glucose homeostasis through a complex of PGC-1alpha and SIRT1. Nature. 2005; **434**(7029):113-118. DOI: 10.1038/nature03354

[81] Cohen HY, Miller C, Bitterman KJ, Wall NR, Hekking B, Kessler B, et al. Calorie restriction promotes mammalian cell survival by inducing the SIRT1 deacetylase. Science. 2004; **305**(5682):390-392. DOI: 10.1126/science.1099196

[82] Civitarese AE, Carling S, Heilbronn LK, Hulver MH, Ukropcova B, Deutsch WA, et al. Calorie restriction increases muscle mitochondrial biogenesis in healthy humans. PLoS Medicine. 2007;**4**(3):485-494. DOI: 10.1371/journal.pmed.0040076

[83] Boily G, Seifert EL, Bevilacqua L, He XH, Sabourin G, Estey C, et al. SIRT1 regulates energy metabolism and response to caloric restriction in mice. PLoS One. 2008;**3**(3):e1759. DOI: 10.1371/journal.pone.0001759

[84] North BJ, Verdin E. Mitotic regulation of SIRT2 by cyclin-dependent kinase 1-dependent phosphorylation. The Journal of Biological Chemistry. 2007;**282**(27):19546-19555. DOI: 10.1074/jbc.M702990200

[85] Vaquero A, Scher MB, Lee DH, Sutton A, Cheng HL, Alt FW, et al. SIRT2 is a histone deacetylase with preference for histone h4 lys 16 during mitosis. Genes & Development. 2006;**20**(10):1256-1261. DOI: 10.1101/gad.1412706

[86] Dryden SC, Nahhas FA, Nowak JE, Goustin AS, Tainsky MA. Role for human SIRT2 NAD-dependent deacetylase activity in control of mitotic exit in the cell cycle. Molecular and Cellular Biology. 2003;**23**(9):3173-3185

[87] Suzuki K, Koike T. Mammalian Sir2-related protein (SIRT) 2-mediated modulation of resistance to axonal degeneration in slow wallerian degeneration mice: A crucial role of tubulin deacetylation. Neuroscience. 2007;**147**(3):599-612. DOI: 10.1016/j.neuroscience.2007.04.059

[88] Luthi-Carter R, Taylor DM, Pallos J, Lambert E, Amore A, Parker A, et al. SIRT2 inhibition achieves neuroprotection by decreasing sterol biosynthesis. Proceedings of the National Academy of Sciences of the United States of America. 2010;**107**(17):7927-7932. DOI: 10.1073/pnas.1002924107

[89] Outeiro TF, Kontopoulos E, Altmann SM, Kufareva I, Strathearn KE, Amore AM, et al. Sirtuin 2 inhibitors rescue alpha-synuclein-mediated toxicity in models of parkinson's disease. Science. 2007;**317**(5837):516-519. DOI: 10.1126/science.1143780

[90] Kim HS, Vassilopoulos A, Wang RH, Lahusen T, Xiao Z, Xu X, et al. SIRT2 maintains genome integrity and suppresses tumorigenesis through regulating apc/c activity. Cancer Cell. 2011;**20**(4):487-499. DOI: 10.1016/j.ccr.2011.09.004

[91] Hiratsuka M, Inoue T, Toda T, Kimura N, Shirayoshi Y, Kamitani H, et al. Proteomics-based identification of differentially expressed genes in human gliomas: Down-regulation of SIRT2 gene. Biochemical and Biophysical Research Communications. 2003;**309**(3):558-566

[92] Ahn BH, Kim HS, Song S, Lee IH, Liu J, Vassilopoulos A, et al. A role for the mitochondrial deacetylase SIRT3 in regulating energy homeostasis. Proceedings of the National Academy of Sciences of the United States of America. 2008;**105**(38):14447-14452. DOI: 10.1073/pnas.0803790105

[93] Lombard DB, Alt FW, Cheng HL, Bunkenborg J, Streeper RS, Mostoslavsky R, et al. Mammalian Sir2 homolog SIRT3 regulates global mitochondrial lysine acetylation. Molecular and Cellular Biology. 2007;**27**(24):8807-8814. DOI: 10.1128/MCB.01636-07

[94] Hirschey MD, Shimazu T, Goetzman E, Jing E, Schwer B, Lombard DB, et al. SIRT3 regulates mitochondrial fatty-acid oxidation by reversible enzyme deacetylation. Nature. 2010;**464**(7285):121-125. DOI: 10.1038/nature08778

[95] Shimazu T, Hirschey MD, Hua L, Dittenhafer-Reed KE, Schwer B, Lombard DB, et al. SIRT3 deacetylates mitochondrial 3-hydroxy-3-methylglutaryl COA synthase 2 and regulates ketone body production. Cell Metabolism. 2010;**12**(6):654-661. DOI: 10.1016/j.cmet.2010.11.003

[96] Onyango P, Celic I, McCaffery JM, Boeke JD, Feinberg AP. SIRT3, a human sir2 homologue, is an NAD-dependent deacetylase localized to mitochondria. Proceedings of the National Academy of Sciences of the United States of America. 2002;**99**(21):13653-13658. DOI: 10.1073/pnas.222538099

[97] Schwer B, North BJ, Frye RA, Ott M, Verdin E. The human silent information regulator (Sir)2 homologue hSIRT3 is a mitochondrial nicotinamide adenine dinucleotide-dependent deacetylase. The Journal of Cell Biology. 2002;**158**(4):647-657. DOI: 10.1083/jcb.200205057

[98] Shi T, Wang F, Stieren E, Tong Q. SIRT3, a mitochondrial sirtuin deacetylase, regulates mitochondrial function and thermogenesis in brown adipocytes. The Journal of Biological Chemistry. 2005;**280**(14):13560-13567. DOI: 10.1074/jbc.M414670200

[99] He W, Newman JC, Wang MZ, Ho L, Verdin E. Mitochondrial sirtuins: Regulators of protein acylation and metabolism. Trends in Endocrinology and Metabolism. 2012;**23**(9):467-476. DOI: 10.1016/j.tem.2012.07.004

[100] Kincaid B, Bossy-Wetzel E. Forever young: SIRT3 a shield against mitochondrial meltdown, aging, and neurodegeneration. Frontiers in Aging Neuroscience. 2013;**5**:48-61. DOI: 10.3389/fnagi.2013.00048

[101] Haigis MC, Mostoslavsky R, Haigis KM, Fahie K, Christodoulou DC, Murphy AJ, et al. SIRT4 inhibits glutamate dehydrogenase and opposes the effects of calorie restriction in pancreatic beta cells. Cell. 2006;**126**(5):941-954. DOI: 10.1016/j.cell.2006.06.057

[102] Jeong SM, Xiao C, Finley LW, Lahusen T, Souza AL, Pierce K, et al. SIRT4 has tumor-suppressive activity and regulates the cellular metabolic response to DNA damage by inhibiting mitochondrial glutamine metabolism. Cancer Cell. 2013;**23**(4):450-463. DOI: 10.1016/j.ccr.2013.02.024

[103] Csibi A, Fendt SM, Li C, Poulogiannis G, Choo AY, Chapski DJ, et al. The mTORc1 pathway stimulates glutamine metabolism and cell proliferation by repressing SIRT4. Cell. 2013;**153**(4):840-854. DOI: 10.1016/j.cell.2013.04.023

[104] Du J, Zhou Y, Su X, Yu JJ, Khan S, Jiang H, et al. SIRT5 is a NAD-dependent protein lysine demalonylase and desuccinylase. Science. 2011;**334**(6057):806-809. DOI: 10.1126/science.1207861

[105] Tan M, Peng C, Anderson KA, Chhoy P, Xie Z, Dai L, et al. Lysine glutarylation is a protein posttranslational modification regulated by SIRT5. Cell Metabolism. 2014;**19**(4):605-617. DOI: 10.1016/j.cmet.2014.03.014

[106] Nakamura Y, Ogura M, Ogura K, Tanaka D, Inagaki N. SIRT5 deacetylates and activates urate oxidase in liver mitochondria of mice. FEBS Letters. 2012;**586**(23):4076-4081. DOI: 10.1016/j.febslet.2012.10.009

[107] Yu J, Sadhukhan S, Noriega LG, Moullan N, He B, Weiss RS, et al. Metabolic characterization of a SIRT5 deficient mouse model. Scientific Reports. 2013;**3**:2806-2813. DOI: 10.1038/srep02806

[108] Kanfi Y, Peshti V, Gil R, Naiman S, Nahum L, Levin E, et al. SIRT6 protects against pathological damage caused by diet-induced obesity. Aging Cell. 2010;**9**(2):162-173. DOI: 10.1111/j.1474-9726.2009.00544.x

[109] Mostoslavsky R, Chua KF, Lombard DB, Pang WW, Fischer MR, Gellon L, et al. Genomic instability and aging-like phenotype in the absence of mammalian SIRT6. Cell. 2006;**124**(2):315-329. DOI: 10.1016/j.cell.2005.11.044

[110] Liszt G, Ford E, Kurtev M, Guarente L. Mouse Sir2 homolog SIRT6 is a nuclear ADP-ribosyltransferase. The Journal of Biological Chemistry. 2005;**280**(22):21313-21320. DOI: 10.1074/jbc.M413296200

[111] Michishita E, McCord RA, Berber E, Kioi M, Padilla-Nash H, Damian M, et al. SIRT6 is a histone H3 lysine 9 deacetylase that modulates telomeric chromatin. Nature. 2008;**452**(7186):492-496. DOI: 10.1038/nature06736

[112] Michishita E, McCord RA, Boxer LD, Barber MF, Hong T, Gozani O, et al. Cell cycle-dependent deacetylation of telomeric histone h3 lysine k56 by human SIRT6. Cell Cycle. 2009;**8**(16):2664-2666. DOI: 10.4161/cc.8.16.9367

[113] Yang B, Zwaans BM, Eckersdorff M, Lombard DB. The sirtuin SIRT6 deacetylates H3 K56Ac *in vivo* to promote genomic stability. Cell Cycle. 2009;**8**(16):2662-2663. DOI: 10.4161/cc.8.16.9329

[114] Mao Z, Hine C, Tian X, Van Meter M, Au M, Vaidya A, et al. SIRT6 promotes DNA repair under stress by activating PARP1. Science. 2011;**332**(6036):1443-1446. DOI: 10.1126/science.1202723

[115] Mao Z, Tian X, Van Meter M, Ke Z, Gorbunova V, Seluanov A. Sirtuin 6 (SIRT6) rescues the decline of homologous recombination repair during replicative senescence. Proceedings of the National Academy of Sciences of the United States of America. 2012;**109**(29):11800-11805. DOI: 10.1073/pnas.1200583109

[116] Zhong L, D'Urso A, Toiber D, Sebastian C, Henry RE, Vadysirisack DD, et al. The histone deacetylase SIRT6 regulates glucose homeostasis via HIF1alpha. Cell. 2010;**140**(2):280-293. DOI: 10.1016/j.cell.2009.12.041

[117] Dominy JE Jr, Lee Y, Jedrychowski MP, Chim H, Jurczak MJ, Camporez JP, et al. The deacetylase SIRT6 activates the acetyltransferase GCN5 and suppresses hepatic gluconeogenesis. Molecular Cell. 2012;**48**(6):900-913. DOI: 10.1016/j.molcel.2012.09.030

[118] Puigserver P, Rhee J, Donovan J, Walkey CJ, Yoon JC, Oriente F, et al. Insulin-regulated hepatic gluconeogenesis through FOXO1-PGC-1α interaction. Nature. 2003;**423**(6939): 550-555. DOI: 10.1038/nature01667

[119] Kim HS, Xiao C, Wang RH, Lahusen T, Xu X, Vassilopoulos A, et al. Hepatic-specific disruption of SIRT6 in mice results in fatty liver formation due to enhanced glycolysis and triglyceride synthesis. Cell Metabolism. 2010;**12**(3):224-236. DOI: 10.1016/j.cmet.2010.06.009

[120] Etchegaray JP, Zhong L, Mostoslavsky R. The histone deacetylase SIRT6: At the crossroads between epigenetics, metabolism and disease. Current Topics in Medicinal Chemistry. 2013;**13**(23):2991-3000

[121] Michishita E, Park JY, Burneskis JM, Barrett JC, Horikawa I. Evolutionarily conserved and nonconserved cellular localizations and functions of human SIRT proteins. Molecular Biology of the Cell. 2005;**16**(10):4623-4635. DOI: 10.1091/mbc.E05-01-0033

[122] Ford E, Voit R, Liszt G, Magin C, Grummt I, Guarente L. Mammalian Sir2 homolog SIRT7 is an activator of RNAa polymerase I transcription. Genes & Development. 2006; **20**(9):1075-1080. DOI: 10.1101/gad.1399706

[123] Tsai YC, Greco TM, Cristea IM. Sirtuin 7 plays a role in ribosome biogenesis and protein synthesis. Molecular & Cellular Proteomics. 2014;**13**(1):73-83. DOI: 10.1074/mcp.M113.031377

[124] Karim MF, Yoshizawa T, Sato Y, Sawa T, Tomizawa K, Akaike T, et al. Inhibition of H3K18 deacetylation of SIRT7 by MYB-binding protein 1a (MYBBP1a). Biochemical and Biophysical Research Communications. 2013;**441**(1):157-163. DOI: 10.1016/j.bbrc.2013.10.020

[125] Tsai YC, Greco TM, Boonmee A, Miteva Y, Cristea IM. Functional proteomics establishes the interaction of SIRT7 with chromatin remodeling complexes and expands its role in regulation of RNA polymerase i transcription. Molecular & Cellular Proteomics. 2012; **11**(5):60-76. DOI: 10.1074/mcp.A111.015156

[126] Kim JK, Noh JH, Jung KH, Eun JW, Bae HJ, Kim MG, et al. Sirtuin7 oncogenic potential in human hepatocellular carcinoma and its regulation by the tumor suppressors mir-125a-5p and mir-125b. Hepatology. 2013;**57**(3):1055-1067. DOI: 10.1002/hep.26101

[127] Vakhrusheva O, Braeuer D, Liu Z, Braun T, Bober E. SIRT7-dependent inhibition of cell growth and proliferation might be instrumental to mediate tissue integrity during aging. Journal of Physiology and Pharmacology. 2008;**59**(Suppl 9):201-212

[128] Kiran S, Oddi V, Ramakrishna G. Sirtuin 7 promotes cellular survival following genomic stress by attenuation of DNA damage, sapk activation and p53 response. Experimental Cell Research. 2015;**331**(1):123-141. DOI: 10.1016/j.yexcr.2014.11.001

[129] Chen S, Seiler J, Santiago-Reichelt M, Felbel K, Grummt I, Voit R. Repression of RNA polymerase I upon stress is caused by inhibition of RNA-dependent deacetylation of PAF53 by SIRT7. Molecular Cell. 2013;**52**(3):303-313. DOI: 10.1016/j.molcel.2013.10.010

[130] Hubbi ME, Hu H, Kshitiz, Gilkes DM, Semenza GL. Sirtuin-7 inhibits the activity of hypoxia-inducible factors. The Journal of Biological Chemistry. 2013;**288**(29):20768-20775. DOI: 10.1074/jbc.M113.476903

[131] Ashraf N, Zino S, Macintyre A, Kingsmore D, Payne AP, George WD, et al. Altered sirtuin expression is associated with node-positive breast cancer. British Journal of Cancer. 2006;**95**(8):1056-1061. DOI: 10.1038/sj.bjc.6603384

[132] Han Y, Liu Y, Zhang H, Wang T, Diao R, Jiang Z, et al. Hsa-mir-125b suppresses bladder cancer development by down-regulating oncogene SIRT7 and oncogenic long noncoding RNA malat1. FEBS Letter. 2013; S0014-5793(13)00780-1. DOI: 10.1016/j.febslet.2013.10.023

[133] Freitas-Junior LH, Hernandez-Rivas R, Ralph SA, Montiel-Condado D, Ruvalcaba-Salazar OK, Rojas-Meza AP, et al. Telomeric heterochromatin propagation and histone acetylation control mutually exclusive expression of antigenic variation genes in malaria parasites. Cell. 2005;**121**(1):25-36. DOI: 10.1016/j.cell.2005.01.037

[134] Issar N, Roux E, Mattei D, Scherf A. Identification of a novel post-translational modification in *Plasmodium falciparum*: Protein sumoylation in different cellular compartments. Cellular Microbiology. 2008;**10**(10):1999-2011. DOI: 10.1111/j.1462-5822.2008.01183.x

[135] Duraisingh MT, Voss TS, Marty AJ, Duffy MF, Good RT, Thompson JK, et al. Heterochromatin silencing and locus repositioning linked to regulation of virulence genes in *Plasmodium falciparum*. Cell. 2005;**121**(1):13-24. DOI: 10.1016/j.cell.2005.01.036

[136] Hviid L, Jensen AT. Pfemp1—A parasite protein family of key importance in *Plasmodium falciparum* malaria immunity and pathogenesis. Advances in Parasitology. 2015;**88**:51-84. DOI: 10.1016/bs.apar.2015.02.004

[137] Scherf A, Hernandez-Rivas R, Buffet P, Bottius E, Benatar C, Pouvelle B, et al. Antigenic variation in malaria: *In situ* switching, relaxed and mutually exclusive transcription of var genes during intra-erythrocytic development in *Plasmodium falciparum*. The EMBO Journal. 1998;**17**(18):5418-5426. DOI: 10.1093/emboj/17.18.5418

[138] Chookajorn T, Ponsuwanna P, Cui L. Mutually exclusive var gene expression in the malaria parasite: Multiple layers of regulation. Trends in Parasitology. 2008;**24**(10): 455-461. DOI: 10.1016/j.pt.2008.07.005

[139] Deitsch KW, del Pinal A, Wellems TE. Intra-cluster recombination and var transcription switches in the antigenic variation of *Plasmodium falciparum*. Molecular and Biochemical Parasitology. 1999;**101**(1–2):107-116

[140] Tonkin CJ, Carret CK, Duraisingh MT, Voss TS, Ralph SA, Hommel M, et al. Sir2 paralogues cooperate to regulate virulence genes and antigenic variation in *Plasmodium falciparum*. PLoS Biology. 2009;**7**(4):e84. DOI: 10.1371/journal.pbio.1000084

[141] Yahiaoui B, Taibi A, Ouaissi A. A *Leishmania major* protein with extensive homology to silent information regulator 2 of saccharomyces cerevisiae. Gene. 1996;**169**(1):115-118

[142] Zemzoumi K, Sereno D, Francois C, Guilvard E, Lemesre JL, Ouaissi A. *Leishmania* major: Cell type dependent distribution of a 43 KDa antigen related to silent information regulatory-2 protein family. Biology of the Cell. 1998;**90**(3):239-245. DOI: 10.1016/S0248-4900(98)80020-8

[143] Vergnes B, Sereno D, Madjidian-Sereno N, Lemesre JL, Ouaissi A. Cytoplasmic Sir2 homologue overexpression promotes survival of *Leishmania* parasites by preventing programmed cell death. Gene. 2002;**296**(1–2):139-150

[144] Sereno D, Vanhille L, Vergnes B, Monte-Allegre A, Ouaissi A. Experimental study of the function of the excreted/secreted *Leishmania* LmSir2 protein by heterologous expression in eukaryotic cell line. Kinetoplastid Biology and Disease. 2005;**4**(1):1-9. DOI: 10.1186/1475-9292-4-1

[145] Vergnes B, Sereno D, Tavares J, Cordeiro-da-Silva A, Vanhille L, Madjidian-Sereno N, et al. Targeted disruption of cytosolic Sir2 deacetylase discloses its essential role in *Leishmania* survival and proliferation. Gene. 2005;**363**:85-96. DOI: 10.1016/j.gene.2005.06.047

[146] Tavares J, Ouaissi A, Santarem N, Sereno D, Vergnes B, Sampaio P, et al. The *Leishmania infantum* cytosolic Sir2-related protein 1 (lisir2rp1) is an NAD^+-dependent deacetylase and ADP-ribosyltransferase. The Biochemical Journal. 2008;**415**(3):377-386. DOI: 10.1042/BJ20080666

[147] Adriano MA, Vergnes B, Poncet J, Mathieu-Daude F, da Silva AC, Ouaissi A, et al. Proof of interaction between *Leishmania* Sir2rp1 deacetylase and chaperone hsp83. Parasitology Research 2007;**100**(4):811-818. DOI: 10.1007/s00436-006-0352-3

[148] Matsuyama A, Shimazu T, Sumida Y, Saito A, Yoshimatsu Y, Seigneurin-Berny D, et al. *In vivo* destabilization of dynamic microtubules by HDAC6-mediated deacetylation. The EMBO Journal. 2002;**21**(24):6820-6831. DOI: 10.1093/emboj/cdf682

[149] Fessel MR, Lira CB, Giorgio S, Ramos CH, Cano MI. Sir2-related protein 1 from *Leishmania amazonensis* is a glycosylated NAD^+-dependent deacetylase. Parasitology. 2011;**138**(10):1245-1258. DOI: 10.1017/S0031182011001077

[150] Purkait B, Singh R, Wasnik K, Das S, Kumar A, Paine M, et al. Up-regulation of silent information regulator 2 (Sir2) is associated with amphotericin B resistance in clinical isolates of *Leishmania donovani*. The Journal of Antimicrobial Chemotherapy. 2015;**70**(5):1343-1356. DOI: 10.1093/jac/dku534

[151] Mishra J, Singh S. Miltefosine resistance in *Leishmania donovani* involves suppression of oxidative stress-induced programmed cell death. Experimental Parasitology. 2013;**135**(2):397-406. DOI: 10.1016/j.exppara.2013.08.004

[152] Silvestre R, Cordeiro-Da-Silva A, Santarem N, Vergnes B, Sereno D, Ouaissi A. Sir2-deficient *Leishmania infantum* induces a defined IFN-gamma/IL-10 pattern that correlates with protection. Journal of Immunology. 2007;**179**(5):3161-3170

[153] Baharia RK, Tandon R, Sharma T, Suthar MK, Das S, Siddiqi MI, et al. Recombinant NAD-dependent sir-2 protein of *Leishmania donovani*: Immunobiochemical characterization as a potential vaccine against visceral *Leishmania*sis. PLoS Neglected Tropical Diseases. 2015;**9**(3):e0003557. DOI: 10.1371/journal.pntd.0003557

[154] Vergnes B, Gazanion E, Grentzinger T. Functional divergence of Sir2 orthologs between Trypanosomatid parasites. Molecular and Biochemical Parasitology. 2016;**207**(2):96-101. DOI: 10.1016/j.molbiopara.2016.06.004

[155] Garcia-Salcedo JA, Gijon P, Nolan DP, Tebabi P, Pays E. A chromosomal Sir2 homologue with both histone NAD-dependent ADP-ribosyltransferase and deacetylase activities is involved in DNA repair in *Trypanosoma brucei*. The EMBO Journal. 2003;**22**(21):5851-5862. DOI: 10.1093/emboj/cdg553

[156] Brachmann CB, Sherman JM, Devine SE, Cameron EE, Pillus L, Boeke JD. The Sir2 gene family, conserved from bacteria to humans, functions in silencing, cell cycle progression, and chromosome stability. Genes & Development. 1995;**9**(23):2888-2902

[157] Landry J, Sutton A, Tafrov ST, Heller RC, Stebbins J, Pillus L, et al. The silencing protein Sir2 and its homologs are NAD-dependent protein deacetylases. Proceedings of the National Academy of Sciences of the United States of America. 2000;**97**(11):5807-5811. DOI: 10.1073/pnas.110148297

[158] Perrod S, Cockell MM, Laroche T, Renauld H, Ducrest AL, Bonnard C, et al. A cytosolic NAD-dependent deacetylase, HST2p, can modulate nucleolar and telomeric silencing in yeast. The EMBO Journal. 2001;**20**(1–2):197-209. DOI: 10.1093/emboj/20.1.197

[159] Tanner KG, Landry J, Sternglanz R, Denu JM. Silent information regulator 2 family of NAD-dependent histone/protein deacetylases generates a unique product, 1-O-acetyl--ADP-ribose. Proceedings of the National Academy of Sciences of the United States of America. 2000;**97**(26):14178-14182. DOI: 10.1073/pnas.250422697

[160] Alsford S, Kawahara T, Isamah C, Horn D. A sirtuin in the african trypanosome is involved in both DNA repair and telomeric gene silencing but is not required for antigenic variation. Molecular Microbiology. 2007;**63**(3):724-736. DOI: 10.1111/j.1365-2958.2006.05553.x

[161] Rusche LN, Kirchmaier AL, Rine J. The establishment, inheritance, and function of silenced chromatin in *Saccharomyces cerevisiae*. Annual Review of Biochemistry. 2003;**72**:481-516. DOI: 10.1146/annurev.biochem.72.121801.161547

[162] Figueiredo L, Scherf A. *Plasmodium* telomeres and telomerase: The usual actors in an unusual scenario. Chromosome Research. 2005;**13**(5):517-524. DOI: 10.1007/s10577-005-0996-3

[163] Kowieski TM, Lee S, Denu JM. Acetylation-dependent ADP-ribosylation by *Trypanosoma brucei* Sir2. The Journal of Biological Chemistry. 2008;**283**(9):5317-5326. DOI: 10.1074/jbc.M707613200

[164] Fahie K, Hu P, Swatkoski S, Cotter RJ, Zhang Y, Wolberger C. Side chain specificity of ADP-ribosylation by a sirtuin. The FEBS Journal. 2009;**276**(23):7159-7176. DOI: 10.1111/j.1742-4658.2009.07427.x

[165] Hailu GS, Robaa D, Forgione M, Sippl W, Rotili D, Mai A. Lysine deacetylase inhibitors in parasites: Past, present, and future perspectives. Journal of Medicinal Chemistry. 2017;**60**(12):4780-4804. DOI: 10.1021/acs.jmedchem.6b01595

[166] Morselli E, Maiuri MC, Markaki M, Megalou E, Pasparaki A, Palikaras K, et al. Caloric restriction and resveratrol promote longevity through the sirtuin-1-dependent induction of autophagy. Cell Death & Disease. 2010;**1**:e10. DOI: 10.1038/cddis.2009.8

[167] Guarente L, Picard F. Calorie restriction-the Sir2 connection. Cell. 2005;**120**(4):473-482. DOI: 10.1016/j.cell.2005.01.029

[168] Lara E, Mai A, Calvanese V, Altucci L, Lopez-Nieva P, Martinez-Chantar ML, et al. Salermide, a sirtuin inhibitor with a strong cancer-specific proapoptotic effect. Oncogene. 2009;**28**(6):781-791. DOI: 10.1038/onc.2008.436

[169] Zheng W. Sirtuins as emerging anti-parasitic targets. European Journal of Medicinal Chemistry. 2013;**59**:132-140. DOI: 10.1016/j.ejmech.2012.11.014

[170] Religa AA, Waters AP. Sirtuins of parasitic protozoa: In search of function(s). Molecular and Biochemical Parasitology. 2012;**185**(2):71-88. DOI: 10.1016/j.molbiopara.2012.08.003

[171] Rogina B, Helfand SL, Frankel S. Longevity regulation by D*rosophila* RPD3 deacetylase and caloric restriction. Science. 2002;**298**(5599):1745. DOI: 10.1126/science.1078986

[172] Tissenbaum HA, Guarente L. Increased dosage of a Sir-2 gene extends lifespan in *Caenorhabditis elegans*. Nature. 2001;**410**(6825):227-230. DOI: 10.1038/35065638

[173] Eddy SR. Where did the BLOSUM62 alignment score matrix come from? Nature Biotechnology. 2004;**22**(8):1035-1036. DOI: 10.1038/nbt0804-1035

[174] Hajduk PJ, Huth JR, Tse C. Predicting protein druggability. Drug Discovery Today. 2005;**10**(23–24):1675-1682. DOI: 10.1016/S1359-6446(05)03624-X

[175] Tavares J, Ouaissi A, Kong Thoo Lin P, Loureiro I, Kaur S, Roy N, et al. Bisnaphthalimidopropyl derivatives as inhibitors of *Leishmania* Sir2 related protein 1. ChemMedChem. 2010;**5**(1):140-147. DOI: 10.1002/cmdc.200900367

[176] Schlicker C, Boanca G, Lakshminarasimhan M, Steegborn C. Structure-based development of novel sirtuin inhibitors. Aging (Albany NY). 2011;**3**(9):852-872

[177] Rumpf T, Schiedel M, Karaman B, Roessler C, North BJ, Lehotzky A, et al. Selective SIRT2 inhibition by ligand-induced rearrangement of the active site. Nature Communications. 2015;**6**:6263-6276. DOI: 10.1038/ncomms7263

[178] Avalos JL, Bever KM, Wolberger C. Mechanism of sirtuin inhibition by nicotinamide: Altering the NAD(+) cosubstrate specificity of a Sir2 enzyme. Molecular Cell. 2005;**17**(6): 855-868. DOI: 10.1016/j.molcel.2005.02.022

[179] Soares MB, Silva CV, Bastos TM, Guimaraes ET, Figueira CP, Smirlis D, et al. Anti-*Trypanosoma cruzi* activity of nicotinamide. Acta Tropica. 2012;**122**(2):224-229. DOI: 10.1016/j.actatropica.2012.01.001

[180] Prusty D, Mehra P, Srivastava S, Shivange AV, Gupta A, Roy N, et al. Nicotinamide inhibits *Plasmodium falciparum* Sir2 activity *in vitro* and parasite growth. FEMS Microbiology Letters. 2008;**282**(2):266-272. DOI: 10.1111/j.1574-6968.2008.01135.x

[181] Sereno D, Alegre AM, Silvestre R, Vergnes B, Ouaissi A. *In vitro* antiLeishmanial activity of nicotinamide. Antimicrobial Agents and Chemotherapy. 2005;**49**(2):808-812. DOI: 10.11 28/AAC.49.2.808-812.2005

[182] Unciti-Broceta JD, Maceira J, Morales S, Garcia-Perez A, Munoz-Torres ME, Garcia-Salcedo JA. Nicotinamide inhibits the lysosomal cathepsin b-like protease and kills African trypanosomes. The Journal of Biological Chemistry. 2013;**288**(15):10548-10557. DOI: 10.1074/jbc.M112.449207

[183] Corda D, Di Girolamo M. Functional aspects of protein mono-ADP-ribosylation. The EMBO Journal. 2003;**22**(9):1953-1958. DOI: 10.1093/emboj/cdg209

[184] Ludden PW. Reversible ADP-ribosylation as a mechanism of enzyme regulation in procaryotes. Molecular and Cellular Biochemistry. 1994;**138**(1–2):123-129

[185] Hemphill A, Lawson D, Seebeck T. The cytoskeletal architecture of *Trypanosoma brucei*. The Journal of Parasitology. 1991;**77**(4):603-612

[186] Inoue T, Hiratsuka M, Osaki M, Yamada H, Kishimoto I, Yamaguchi S, et al. SIRT2, a tubulin deacetylase, acts to block the entry to chromosome condensation in response to mitotic stress. Oncogene. 2007;**26**(7):945-957. DOI: 10.1038/sj.onc.1209857

[187] Pandithage R, Lilischkis R, Harting K, Wolf A, Jedamzik B, Luscher-Firzlaff J, et al. The regulation of SIRT2 function by cyclin-dependent kinases affects cell motility. The Journal of Cell Biology. 2008;**180**(5):915-929. DOI: 10.1083/jcb.200707126

[188] Tanno M, Sakamoto J, Miura T, Shimamoto K, Horio Y. Nucleocytoplasmic shuttling of the NAD^+-dependent histone deacetylase SIRT1. The Journal of Biological Chemistry. 2007;**282**(9):6823-6832. DOI: 10.1074/jbc.M609554200

[189] Cho Y, Sloutsky R, Naegle KM, Cavalli V. Injury-induced HDAC5 nuclear export is essential for axon regeneration. Cell. 2013;**155**(4):894-908. DOI: 10.1016/j.cell.2013.10.004

[190] North BJ, Verdin E. Interphase nucleo-cytoplasmic shuttling and localization of SIRT2 during mitosis. PLoS One. 2007;**2**(8):e784. DOI: 10.1371/journal.pone.0000784

[191] Prieto G, Fullaondo A, Rodriguez JA. Prediction of nuclear export signals using weighted regular expressions (Wregex). Bioinformatics. 2014;**30**(9):1220-1227. DOI: 10.1093/bioin formatics/btu016

[192] Kosugi S, Hasebe M, Tomita M, Yanagawa H. Systematic identification of cell cycle-dependent yeast nucleocytoplasmic shuttling proteins by prediction of composite motifs. Proceedings of the National Academy of Sciences of the United States of America. 2009; **106**(25):10171-10176. DOI: 10.1073/pnas.0900604106

[193] Kamal A, Bolla NR, Srikanth PS, Srivastava AK. Naphthalimide derivatives with therapeutic characteristics: A patent review. Expert Opinion on Therapeutic Patents. 2013; **23**(3):299-317. DOI: 10.1517/13543776.2013.746313

[194] Filosa R, Peduto A, Micco SD, Caprariis P, Festa M, Petrella A, et al. Molecular modelling studies, synthesis and biological activity of a series of novel bisnaphthalimides and their development as new DNA topoisomerase II inhibitors. Bioorganic & Medicinal Chemistry. 2009;**17**(1):13-24. DOI: 10.1016/j.bmc.2008.11.024

[195] Seliga R, Pilatova M, Sarissky M, Viglasky V, Walko M, Mojzis J. Novel naphthalimide polyamine derivatives as potential antitumor agents. Molecular Biology Reports. 2013; **40**(6):4129-4137. DOI: 10.1007/s11033-013-2523-5

[196] Wang X, Chen Z, Tong L, Tan S, Zhou W, Peng T, et al. Naphthalimides exhibit *in vitro* antiproliferative and antiangiogenic activities by inhibiting both topoisomerase II (topo II) and receptor tyrosine kinases (rtks). European Journal of Medicinal Chemistry. 2013; **65**:477-486. DOI: 10.1016/j.ejmech.2013.05.002

[197] Costanza ME, Berry D, Henderson IC, Ratain MJ, Wu K, Shapiro C, et al. Amonafide: An active agent in the treatment of previously untreated advanced breast cancer–a cancer and leukemia group b study (calgb 8642). Clinical Cancer Research. 1995;**1**(7): 699-704

[198] Thompson J, Pratt CB, Stewart CF, Avery L, Bowman L, Zamboni WC, et al. Phase I study of DMP 840 in pediatric patients with refractory solid tumors. Investigational New Drugs. 1998;**16**(1):45-49

[199] Bousquet PF, Brana MF, Conlon D, Fitzgerald KM, Perron D, Cocchiaro C, et al. Preclinical evaluation of LU 79553: A novel bis-naphthalimide with potent antitumor activity. Cancer Research. 1995;**55**(5):1176-1180

[200] Dance AM, Ralton L, Fuller Z, Milne L, Duthie S, Bestwick CS, et al. Synthesis and biological activities of bisnaphthalimido polyamines derivatives: Cytotoxicity, DNA binding, DNA damage and drug localization in breast cancer MCF 7 cells. Biochemical Pharmacology. 2005;**69**(1):19-27. DOI: 10.1016/j.bcp.2004.09.020

[201] Oliveira J, Ralton L, Tavares J, Codeiro-da-Silva A, Bestwick CS, McPherson A, et al. The synthesis and the *in vitro* cytotoxicity studies of bisnaphthalimidopropyl polyamine derivatives against colon cancer cells and parasite *Leishmania infantum*. Bioorganic & Medicinal Chemistry. 2007;**15**(1):541-545. DOI: 10.1016/j.bmc.2006.09.031

[202] Graca NA, Gaspar L, Costa DM, Loureiro I, Thoo-Lin PK, Ramos I, et al. Activity of bisnaphthalimidopropyl derivatives against *Trypanosoma brucei*. Antimicrobial Agents and Chemotherapy. 2016;**60**(4):2532-2536. DOI: 10.1128/aac.02490-15

[203] Ralton L, Bestwick CS, Thoo Lin PK. Polyamine analogues and derivatives as potential anticancer agents. Current Bioactive Compounds. 2007;**3**(3):179-191

[204] Braña MF, Castellano JM, Morán M, Pérez de Vega MJ, Qian XD, Romerdahl CA, et al. Bis-naphthalimides. 2. Synthesis and biological activity of 5,6-acenaphthalimidoalkyl-1,8-naphthalimidoalkyl amines. European Journal of Medicinal Chemistry. 1995;**30**(3): 235-239. DOI: 10.1016/0223-5234(96)88230-4

[205] Roy Chowdhury A, Bakshi R, Wang J, Yildirir G, Liu B, Pappas-Brown V, et al. The killing of african trypanosomes by ethidium bromide. PLoS Pathogens. 2010;**6**(12):e1001226. DOI: 10.1371/journal.ppat.1001226

[206] Terstappen GC, Schlupen C, Raggiaschi R, Gaviraghi G. Target deconvolution strategies in drug discovery. Nature Reviews. Drug Discovery. 2007;**6**(11):891-903. DOI: 10.1038/nrd2410

[207] Hirota T, Lee JW, St John PC, Sawa M, Iwaisako K, Noguchi T, et al. Identification of small molecule activators of cryptochrome. Science. 2012;**337**(6098):1094-1097. DOI: 10.1126/science.1223710

[208] Schenone M, Dancik V, Wagner BK, Clemons PA. Target identification and mechanism of action in chemical biology and drug discovery. Nature Chemical Biology. 2013;**9**(4):232-240. DOI: 10.1038/nchembio.1199

[209] Wyllie S, Oza SL, Patterson S, Spinks D, Thompson S, Fairlamb AH. Dissecting the essentiality of the bifunctional trypanothione synthetase-amidase in *Trypanosoma brucei* using chemical and genetic methods. Molecular Microbiology. 2009;**74**(3):529-540. DOI: 10.1111/j.1365-2958.2009.06761.x

[210] Roberts AJ, Torrie LS, Wyllie S, Fairlamb AH. Biochemical and genetic characterization of *Trypanosoma cruzi* N-myristoyltransferase. The Biochemical Journal. 2014;**459**(2):323-332. DOI: 10.1042/BJ20131033

[211] Jones DC, Foth BJ, Urbaniak MD, Patterson S, Ong HB, Berriman M, et al. Genomic and proteomic studies on the mode of action of oxaboroles against the african trypanosome. PLoS Neglected Tropical Diseases. 2015;**9**(12):e0004299. DOI: 10.1371/journal.pntd.0004299

[212] Jacobs RT, Plattner JJ, Keenan M. Boron-based drugs as antiprotozoals. Current Opinion in Infectious Diseases. 2011;**24**(6):586-592. DOI: 10.1097/QCO.0b013e32834c630e

[213] Bustamante JM, Craft JM, Crowe BD, Ketchie SA, Tarleton RL. New, combined, and reduced dosing treatment protocols cure *Trypanosoma cruzi* infection in mice. The Journal of Infectious Diseases. 2014;**209**(1):150-162. DOI: 10.1093/infdis/jit420

[214] Khare S, Roach SL, Barnes SW, Hoepfner D, Walker JR, Chatterjee AK, et al. Utilizing chemical genomics to identify cytochrome b as a novel drug target for Chagas disease. PLoS Pathogens. 2015;**11**(7):e1005058. DOI: 10.1371/journal.ppat.1005058

2

Eco-Epidemiology of Chagas Disease in Chile

Mauricio Canals Lambarri, Andrea Canals Cifuentes, Salvador Ayala, Valentina Tapia-Garay and Dante Cáceres Lillo

Abstract

There are four vector species of Chagas disease in Chile: *Triatoma infestans*, responsible for the domestic cycle; *Mepraia spinolai*, the main wild vector; and *M. gajardoi* and *M. parapatrica*, two coastal wild species whose importance as vectors is not well known. They are species of dry environments of the central-north region of Chile, whose best predictors of distribution are warm average temperatures and low rainfall. They are found in rock quarries, nests of birds, and small mammals, and *T. infestans* has sylvatic foci associated with a Bromeliaceae species. While human blood represents 70% of the diet of *T. infestans*, in *M. spinolai* this value is 7%, which means that a large part of Chagas disease in Chile is due to *T. infestans*. However, all species have high percentages of *T. cruzi* infection. Chagas disease in Chile follows the distribution of *T. infestans*, and although the cycle of domestic transmission by this vector is interrupted, there is still a constant prevalence and mortality and ascending incidences. Models predict that although climate change will not vary greatly the north-south distribution of vectors, it could increase the reproductive number of the disease, increasing risk areas of Chagas disease.

Keywords: Chagas disease, ecology, vectors, epidemiology, Chile

1. Introduction

American trypanosomiasis or Chagas disease is caused by the flagellated protozoan *Trypanosoma cruzi*, transmitted by several hematophagous insect species (Hemiptera, Reduviidae, and Triatominae) which in Chile are known as vinchucas. This protozoan species undergoes part of its development cycle (epimastigotes and trypomastigotes) in the insect vector, and when it ingests blood of a vertebrate host, the infectious trypomastigotes are eliminated with the dejections on the host; these are able to enter the bloodstream through the small wound or scratch lesions. Inside the *T. cruzi* continues its development with intracellular forms (amastigotes) and extracellular forms (trypomastigotes), producing damage which may be manifested in an acute form, although it generally does so after many years as a chronic form that compromises the digestive tract (megacolon or megaesophagus) and/or heart disease.

Two cycles of vector transmission in Chagas disease are described: (1) the domestic cycle maintained by domestic vectors, in Chile *Triatoma infestans*, which includes a man and an animal reservoir constituted by domestic and peridomestic animals such as cats, dogs, cows, horses, and others, and (2) the wild cycle maintained by wild vectors (such as *Mepraia spinolai*) and the wild animal reservoir composed of rodents, small marsupials, rabbits, etc. These cycles are not completely separated, since there are species that transit between the peridomestic and wild environments such as dogs, cats, goats, and other farm animals (**Figure 1**) [1–3]. In addition, wild vectors can penetrate into domestic environments and feed on humans [4], and domestic vectors can form wild colonies [5–7].

Its discovery is due to the Brazilian doctor Dr. Carlos R. J. Chagas, who in 1907 was the director of the Oswaldo Cruz Institute and director of the National Malaria Control Program. Dr. Chagas examined huts, finding a large number of insects that he named *Conorrhinus sanguessuga* (now *Panstrongylus megistus*) that contained "*Crithidia*." After experiments of inoculation

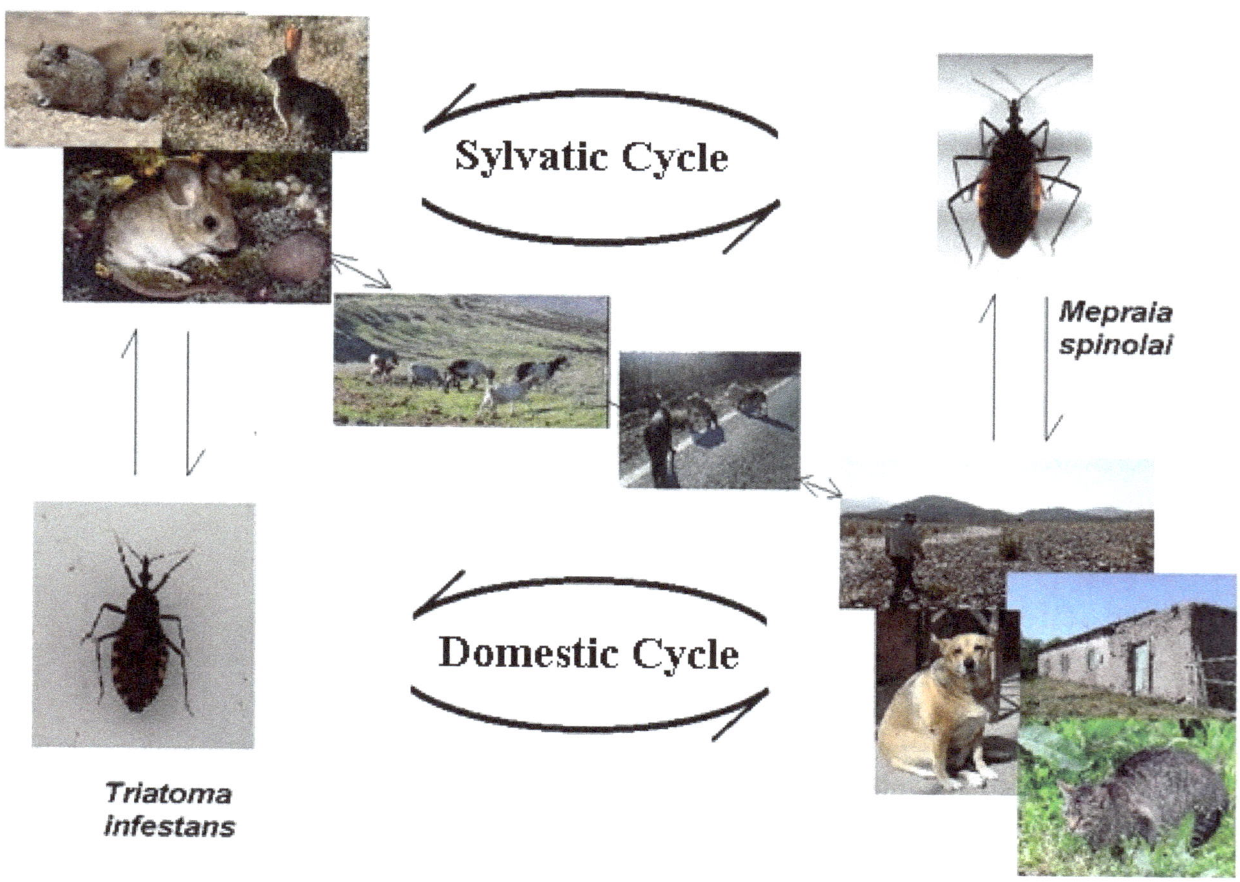

Figure 1. Domestic and wild cycles of Chagas disease.

in monkeys, he found a great quantity of flagellates, calling the new species *Shyzotrypanum cruzi* (today *Trypanosoma cruzi*) in honor of Dr. Oswaldo Cruz. Later, in 1909 he found a naturally infected cat and on April 14 found in the village of Santa Rita a 2-year-old girl named Berenice who lived in a house infested with *P. megistus* with a feverish condition and found in her blood the protozoan *T. cruzi*, describing the disease in 1909 [8]. Later, Carlos Chagas wrote about acute and chronic forms of the disease (1911) and the life cycle of *T. cruzi* (1931) [9], among other topics.

The first studies of Chagas disease in Chile were carried out by Dr. Juan Noé in 1921, with appreciation of *T. cruzi* in the vector *Triatoma infestans* around Santiago. Subsequently, the Argentine Dr. Salvador Massa, led by Noé, demonstrated the specificity of *T. cruzi* in cardiac fibers in experimental animals. With the creation of the Department of Parasitology of the State Health Office in 1937, systematic investigations led to the demonstration of the first case in Chile [10].

Knowledge of this disease has been progressively increasing in Chile thanks to the contribution of numerous researchers. Schenone, in 1980, [11] recognized three stages in the investigation of this disease. In the first stage, from 1937 to 1943, research focused on detecting the disease and tried to determine the endemic areas, detecting vector species and reservoirs. Important studies in this stage included those of Drs. G. Gasic, V. Bertín, *S. Massa*, and R. Gajardo Tobar. In the second stage, from 1944 to 1952, there was a more systematic study, determining the magnitude of the problem and conducting systematic surveys to determine the epidemiology better. The remarkable work of Dr. Amador Neghme was published in this period. The third stage can be established from 1953 to 1994 where there was a fruitful work of many researchers who have helped to clarify clinical aspects, congenital transmission, blood banks, epidemiology, distribution of endemic areas, the reservoir, natural history, ecology, physiology, and behavior of vectors. In this stage, the contributions of Drs. H. Schenone, W. Apt, and A. Atías and their teams stand out in epidemiological and clinical aspects. The fourth stage subsequent to 1995 had been added in which the investigation has focused more on specifying aspects not revealed in the previous periods and that has been marked by the acknowledgment of the interruption of the home transmission chain by *Triatoma infestans* which occurred in 1999. Research was focused mainly on laboratory and diagnostic improvement, on congenital and transfusion treatment and transmission, and on the study of the ecology of Chagas disease vectors and *T. cruzi*. There were important improvements in the detection of the disease, the control of blood banks and the success of domiciliary disinfestation carried out by the vector control area of the Ministry of Health. A negative effect of the declaration of the interruption of the vector transmission chain has been less interesting and resources for the study and control of this disease contributes to perpetuate it as an unattended disease.

2. Eco-epidemiology of vectors

Four species of insect vectors of Chagas disease have been described in Chile. The species responsible for the domestic cycle is *Triatoma infestans*, and the species involved in the wild cycle are *Mepraia spinolai* (**Figure 2**), *M. gajardoi*, and *M. parapatrica*.

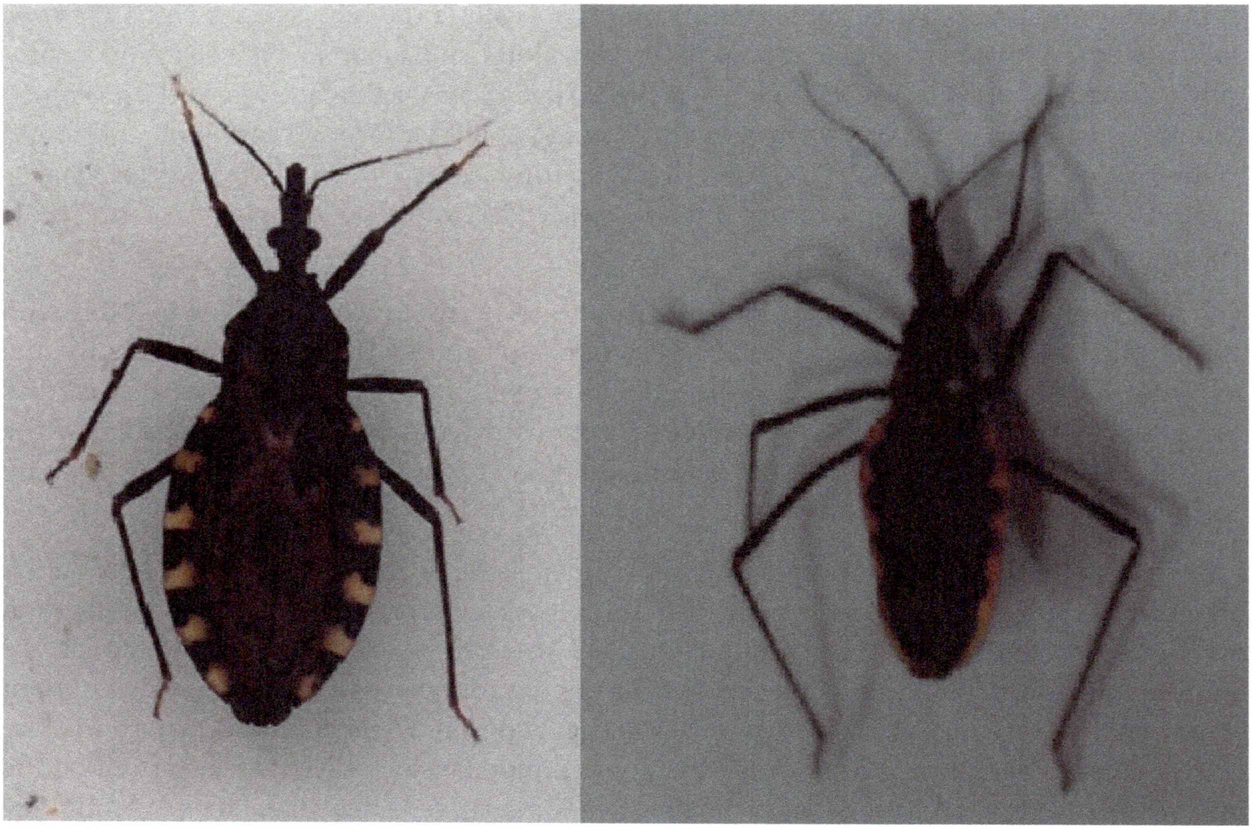

Figure 2. *Triatoma infestans* and *Mepraia spinolai*, the main vectors of Chagas disease in Chile.

2.1. Distribution and niche

The vector *T. infestans*, a bug with characteristic yellow spots in the connexivum, has the widest distribution in Chile, between 18 and 34°S (**Figure 3**). It is found in domestic habitats, but foci of reproductive populations have also been detected in wild habitats [5–7]. In the domestic habitats, it is found in cracks of adobe walls or in "quincha" (wooden branches covered with mud), roofs of branches, and dwellings and chicken coops of the peridomiciliary zone. In sylvatic habitats it has been found forming colonies associated with plants of *Puya chilensis* (Bromeliaceae).

Mepraia spinolai is a wild species endemic to Chile with high polymorphism, with apterous females, and apterous, winged, and brachypterous males with red spots in the connexivum [12–14]. It is found between 26 and 34°S, from the sea level to 3000 m (**Figure 3**) [11]. Their habitat is made up of rocky areas such as quarries and cracks, bird nests, and animal caves [15] and sometimes peridomiciliary pens and walls and in human dwellings [16, 17].

Mepraia gajardoi is a coastal, wild species that lives between latitudes 18 and 26°S, feeding on small reptiles and mammals in the area. The males have generally blackish coloration with small reddish lateral spots in the dorsal part of connexivum. Male brachypterous and female micropterous.

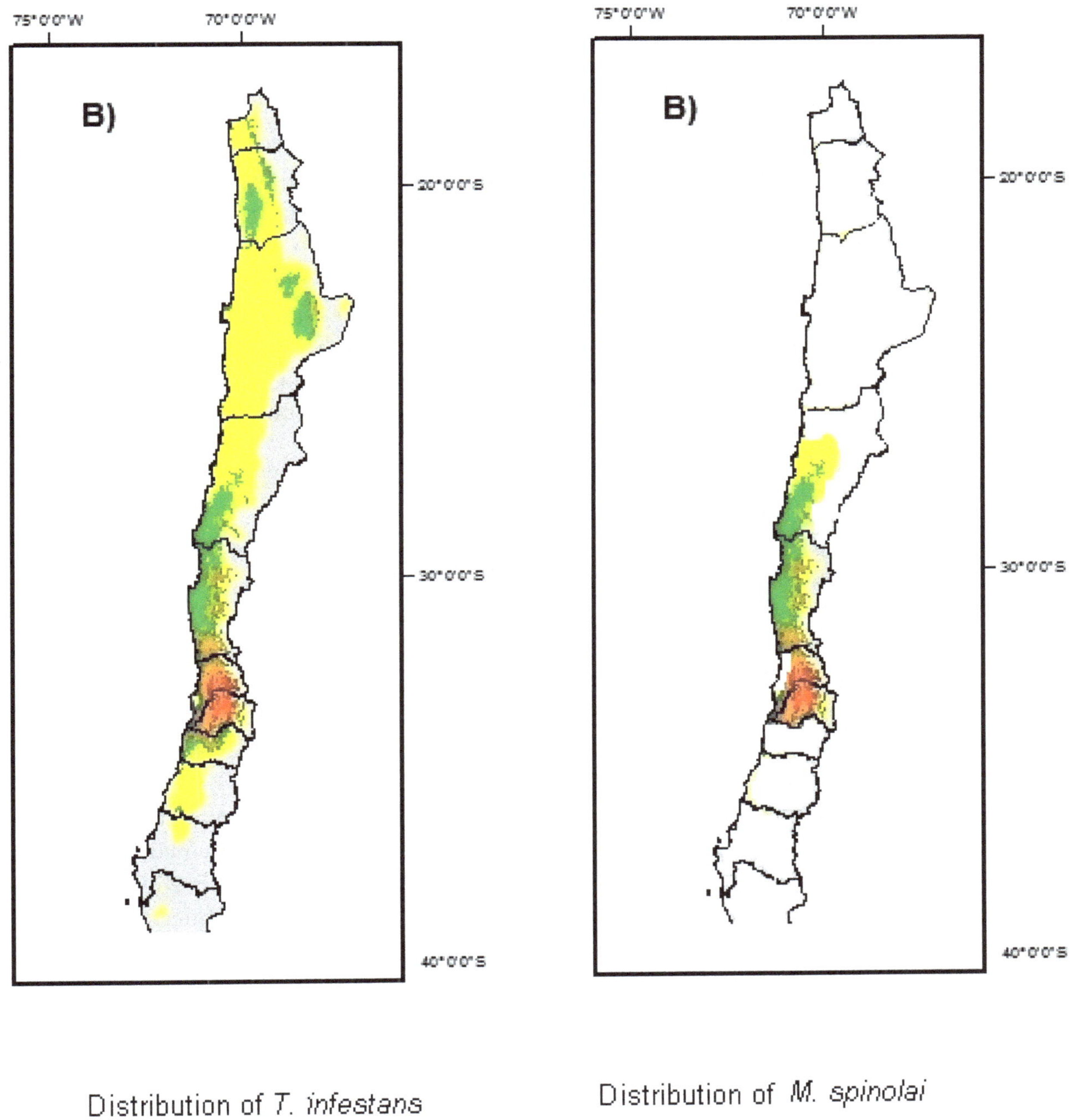

Figure 3. Approximate distribution of the two main vectors of Chagas disease (modified from [18] and [19]).

Mepraia parapatrica is a blackish species with red-orange spots in the connexivum, which only lives at 25°S. The females are micropterous, while the males are brachypterous and macropterous. It also lives on the coast, feeding on rodents and reptiles in the area.

Climate change predictions in Chile include an increase in temperature, with a gradient of higher to lower temperatures from north to south and from the Andes to the Pacific Ocean. During the 2011–2030 period, the temperature increase would be about 0.5°C in the southern zone and 1.5°C for the north and the Chilean altiplano. A decrease in precipitation of 5–15% is expected during the same period. The distribution of *T. infestans* and Chagas disease is associated with maximum temperature and the precipitation during the driest month [18]; thus, the distribution of *T. infestans* would be little affected by climate change. This is consistent with the decrease in suitable areas proposed for *M. spinolai* in the same area and is in contrast to the high impact on the distribution of *M. gajardoi*, a species with a small distribution on the coast of northern Chile [19]. Under the assumption of niche conservatism, the latter species would suffer disappearance of its habitat, while *M. spinolai*, a species with distribution similar to *T. infestans* from 25°S southward and with similar preferred environmental conditions, would decrease its distribution area in the interior valleys while increasing its distribution on the coast [19]. Since *T. infestans* is a species residing in arid and semiarid habitats, its distribution area would not be affected significantly. However, the transmission risk of Chagas disease in this zone could be increased because of changes in metabolism, survival, reproduction, biting rates, or densities of the insects.

2.2. Ecology and population dynamics

There are very few attempts to estimate the population density of vectors. A useful measure is the so-called triatomine index used for domestic vectors such as *T. infestans*, which is defined as the number of insects captured by a person in a house in 1 hour. Schenone estimated in these species indices of 54.5 for the Antofagasta Region in 1980, 19.8 for the Atacama Region, 26.7 for the Coquimbo Region, 37.0 for Valparaíso Region, 50.5 for the Metropolitan Region, and 17.2 for the O'Higgins Region. Later, Canals et al. [20] estimated the densities of vinchucas per human in high endemic rural areas, calculating for these zones an average of 25.3 individuals/humans, with a maximum in the Coquimbo Region of 39.1 individuals/human. For the case of *M. spinolai*, the maximum triatomine index in peridomiciliary zones was 64 vinchucas/person/hour, and the estimated maximum density was 4.59 vinchucas/human [21]. The density per square meter has been estimated in this species between 15 and 364 vinchucas/m^2, with an average of 79 vinchucas/m^2 in areas of rock walls in Colina [22]. This species can be found in high densities [22–26], even in mixed colonies with *T. infestans*, and has been found in human habitations [14, 17, 27, 28]. For example, Schenone et al. [27] reported the presence of 288 specimens in 50 rural dwellings in regions III, IV, V, and Metropolitan. In this sense *M. spinolai* is a potentially dangerous species, especially in areas where the usual contact with humans occurs, as in quarry areas, and in some areas around Santiago where it is currently being urbanized, such as Colina, Lampa, and Til-Til. Also, from the perspective of its food sources, *M. spinolai* is in the phase of domiciliation [4, 29, 30], with 7.4% human blood in its diet [29, 31].

Another approximation to get an idea of the density can be obtained from the number of specimens referred to the Institute of Public Health of Chile; these come in greater proportion from the regions of Antofagasta, Atacama, Coquimbo, Valparaiso, and Metropolitan (Santiago). A recent study [32] reported that 8331 triatomines have been received between 2005 and 2016. A 73.7% correspond to *T. infestans*, 24.0% to *M. spinolai*, and 2.3% to *M. gajardoi*. Their numbers increased over this period. This high proportion of *T. infestans* could be explained because this species, once eliminated from human habitations, has been able to recolonize wild habitats with several foci whose magnitude has not been completely clarified. From the first description of a wild focus in Chile in 2006 [5] in Calera de Tango, and in Til-Til, the new outbreaks in Sahondé, Putaendo [6] to the reports of wild foci in the cities of Valparaiso 2009, Atacama 2014, and Coquimbo 2015 [7].

The data reported by the Ministry of Health show the proportion of infested dwellings (home infestation) in 1999 and annual data since 2010 and divide the information into the percentage of colonized houses, that is, colonies with evidence of active reproduction, the individual visits to houses that receive adult individuals but without colonization, and the total (the sum of both). Household infestation has clearly decreased in this period, but the proportion of houses with individual visitors has increased. Currently, domiciliary infestation is estimated at 0.05% [32].

The vinchucas in Chile are long-lived species, surviving around 18 months in the laboratory [12, 13, 24, 33]. Their development is strongly affected by temperature and relative humidity like all triatomines [34]. The development of *T. infestans* completely ceases at temperatures below 16°C, and temperatures above 40°C are lethal [35]. The effect of relative humidity (RH) and its importance in molt periods has been discussed [36]. Combinations of variable ranges of low temperature and RH affect the maturation of *T. infestans* and *M. spinolai* (**Table 1**). While at constant temperature and humidity, the pre-imago period consisting of five nymph states (N1–N5) is 6.1 months in *T. infestans* [37]; this increases to 14.3 months in variable

	T. infestans	EC	*M. spinolai*	EC
Fecundity (eggs/female/week)	1.9	(15–32/40–90)	0.25	(28/70)
	1.0	(25/75)		
	5.4	(26/60)		
Egg viability (%)	74.6	(17/70)	27.7	(24/73)
	93.7	(24/73)		
Mortality rate (death/individual/day)	0.0083	(25/75)	0.0055	(24/73)
	0.0070	(15–32/40–90)		
Reproductive number (Ro)	1.36	(15–32/40–90)	22.9	(28/70)
	25.04	(26/60)		
Generation time (months)	14.7	(15–32/40–90)	13.2	(28/70)
	7.1	(26/60)		
Intrinsic rate of growth (r)	0.021	(15–32/40–90)	0.24	(28/70)
	0.45	(26/60)		

(EC: Temperature (°C)/Relative humidity (%)). References. Canals et al. [20].

Table 1. Some population parameters of *T. infestans* and *M. spinolai* in different environmental conditions.

environments [24, 38, 39]. In the main wild vector, *M. spinolai,* this period is between 9 and 10 months under constant conditions [12, 33], while in environments with RH and T variability, only nymphs are obtained up to N5 status. With greater restriction at low temperature and humidity, they only reach the N2 status in 12 months [24]. The arrest of secondary development in unfavorable conditions (induced diapause) has been observed in both species [24, 33, 40]. Also, some parameters like the net reproductive rate (R_0) are strongly affected. Both species present survival curves with exponential decays and similar mortality rates [24, 28, 33, 41]. The mortality and fertility rates in *T. infestans* present periodic variations during the year even under relatively constant environmental conditions. For example, under laboratory conditions the mean fecundity of *T. infestans* varied from 0.39 eggs/female/week in autumn to 1.63 eggs/female/week in spring, with maximum values of 7.59 eggs/female/week in spring and 5.83 eggs/female/week in summer. Maximum mean mortality and fertility rates were in spring and summer [42].

2.3. Ecophysiology and behavior

Triatoma infestans is a diurnal insect, while all species of the genus *Mepraia* are diurnal. In the laboratory *M. spinolai* moves between 15 and 42°C with a preferred temperature of 24.8°C [43]. *T. infestans* moves between 18 and 42°C with a preferred temperature of 24.2°C [43]. Other authors have found that *T. infestans* preferred temperatures between 26 and 27°C [44] and variations from 28 to 29°C at the beginning of the night, immediately after the ingestion of blood, but 25°C 12 days later [45, 46]. The synchronization of activity patterns to the L/D cycle is similar to other triatomines [47–51]. Other activities synchronous to the L/D cycles are the rhythms of oviposition [52], molt [53], hatching [46], and aggregation [54]. The stimulus for orientation and approach to a potential prey is temperature, displaying the classic pattern of antennal movements-locomotor movement and extension of the proboscis [55, 56]. *T. infestans* decreases the frequency of antennal movements when it is within 30 to 15 cm of its prey, whereas *M. spinolai* always maintains a low frequency, which may be due to a greater distance of perception in this species [57]. Once in contact with its prey, *T. infestans* introduces its proboscis, sucking blood, being able to increase its weight from four to six times in a single ingestion [38, 39, 57]. The volume of blood ingested is estimated between 30 and 70 ml when fed on a species such as *Mesocricetus auratus* [58]. The bite frequency in *T. infestans* has been estimated at 0.0754 bites/day [21]. The bite frequency of *M. spinolai* has been estimated at 0.155 bites/day, with volumes of blood ingestion between 20 and 160 mg. The intake volume has been found to be inversely correlated with the weight prior to intake, which is an indicator of nutritional status. Thus, the volume of the intake is related to the time elapsed since the last feeding and to the degree of distension of the abdomen [59].

T. infestans emits its dejections during the feeding act [60], which takes on average 19.5 min [38, 39, 57], usually between 3 and 4 min from the start of feeding, while in *M. spinolai* this latency is 24.4 min and not necessarily on the prey, which decreases the probability of transmission [38, 39, 57]. The bite rate and the latency between the start of the bite and the dejection are affected by the presence of the *T. cruzi* parasite in the vector; *M. spinolai* showed a higher frequency of bite and a lower latency of dejection in infected individuals [59].

The feeding spectrum of *T. infestans* in Chile was obtained by means of ag-ac reactions and double gel diffusion [60]. The diet of this species is made up of humans 68.4%, cats 6.1%, dogs 3.2%, rabbits 5.9%, rodents 1.6%, Artiodactyla 0.3%, birds 7.2%, and amphibians 0.5%. The proportions for *M. spinolai* are humans 7.4%, cats 3.7%, dogs 12.3%, rabbits 53.1%, rodents 9.9%, Artiodactyla 12.3%, and birds 1.2% [29]. The amplitude of the trophic niche of *M. spinolai* is greater than that of *T. infestans*, and they have a niche overlap of 0.229 [29]. An increase in the amplitude of the niche in times of greater heat has also been demonstrated [29]. Introducing the information of the food profile of 15 species of triatomines with multivariate analysis techniques has shown a clear separation between species of domiciliary habits and peridomiciliary, wild, and stenophagous specialists; *M. spinolai* is among the peridomiciliary species [4]. In a later study, this species was located between wild and peridomiciliary [30].

The average percentages of *T. cruzi* infection in the vectors (trypano-triatomine indices) are *M. gajardoi* 16.92 ± 17.77%, *M. spinolai* 20.88 ± 11.51%, and *T. infestans* 41.83 ± 13.23% [32]. The trypano-triatomine indices of *M. gajardoi* have remained stable over time, although based on a small number of individuals. The same occurs with the *M. spinolai* indices, but *T. infestans* shows an increasing trend.

The high trypano-triatomine indices in *T. infestans* are interesting, since a decrease of these indices was expected once these insects were removed from human habitats. Thus, for example, in Uruguay, the indices were drastically reduced as a result of vector control actions [61]. An explanation for the lack of a decline in these indices in Chile could be that despite the change in diet that involves the elimination of the human environment, *T. infestans* can find rodents and other species with high infection rates that make high trypano-triatomine indices persist. This may be true, since there is a great diversity of infected wild, domestic, and peridomestic mammals, some reaching levels of infection higher than 10% [15, 62], but this is also probably true in Uruguay.

3. *Trypanosoma cruzi* lineages

Lineages of *T. cruzi* have been recognized for a long time. Initially, isoenzymes that differ in gel electrophoresis were classified as zymodemes Z1 and Z2, the first one mainly associated with the wild cycle and the second one with the domestic cycle [63]. Subsequently, biochemical and genetic differentiation was carried out, and two lineages, TcI corresponding to Z1 and TcII corresponding to Z2, were proposed. However, the first TcII was divided into five subgroups a, b, c, d, and e, where TcIIb corresponded to Z2, TcIIa to the new zymodeme Z3 and TcIIc, and d and e to hybrids [64]. Subsequently, subgroups were also recognized in TcI: a, b, c, and d [63, 65]. Currently, it has been simplified into six subgroups, from TcI to TcVI, where TcI corresponds to Z1, TcII to TcIIb (Z2), TcIII to TcIIc, TcIV to TcIIa (Z3), TcV to TcIId, and TcVI to TcIIe.

Only TcII and TcVI have been found in *M. gajardoi* in Chile [66, 67], TcI and TcII in *M. spinolai* [66] and subsequently TcI, TcII, TcV, and TcVI [68], while in *T. infestans*, the most important lineage is TcI circulating in wild (93.3%) and domiciliary (100%) individuals. TcII, TcV, and TcVI have also been detected mainly in nymphs, suggesting differential adaptation of *T. cruzi* lineages between nymph states [69].

It has been proposed that in small wild mammals TcI and TcII would be associated with marsupials and placental mammals, respectively. However, the TcI, TcII, TcV, and TcVI lineages have been detected in the rodent *Octodon degus* in Chile [26, 70]. The same lineages have been detected in wild *Oryctolagus cuniculus* [71], and in 117 individuals of different infected species, TcI, TcII (TcIIb), TcV (TcIId), and TcVI (TcIIe) have been detected with frequencies of 38, 41, 26 and 9%, respectively, in wild mammals. In peridomestic mammals the frequencies of these lineages were 29, 33, 43, and 14%, respectively. More than one lineage was found in 31% of the individuals analyzed, without specific association with marsupials [72, 73]. Thus, it seems that the information on the wild mammal reservoir and the vectors *T. infestans* and *M. spinolai* is quite consistent in pointing to TcI, TcII, TcV, and TcVI as the main circulating lineages, although more studies are still missing in the other wild vectors of the genus *Mepraia*.

4. Reservoir

The animal reservoir is very extensive; it is constituted by mammals of the peridomestic environment such as dogs, cats, goats, rabbits, sheep, horses, donkeys, and cattle, some carnivores, numerous rodents, and some small marsupials. Infection in mammals by *T. cruzi* has been described in around 150 species in America [74] and is widespread in numerous orders; the most important reservoirs are dogs, cats, and goats, due both to high infection rates and to their mobility which establishes a bridge between domestic and wild cycles. Proportions of infection by *T. cruzi* have been reported 14.5% in dogs, 10.7% in cats, 9.4% in goats, 12.1% in rabbits, and 4.8% in sheep [75]. Current studies with PCR in wild mammals have reported percentages of infection between 26 and 59% in the species *Capra hircus* (goat), *Thylamys elegans* (marsupial), *O. degus*, *Phyllotis darwini*, and *Abrothrix olivaceus* (rodents) [72] and large increases in interannual infection rates from 300–400%, which could be explained by a delayed response to the El Niño weather phenomenon after the emergence of small rodents [25].

5. Distribution of the disease

Chagas disease extends in America from the Southern United States at parallel 35°N to southern South America at parallel 34°S on the Chilean side and 45°S on the Argentine side. In this zone, 21 countries report active transmission, with current prevalence very difficult to assess since most of the studies refer to the prevalence in endemic rural areas [15]. The median prevalence in these areas is approximately 8.15%. The lower extreme values probably represent Chagas disease in controlled or urban areas and the maximum Chagas disease prevalence in hyperendemic areas without protection of health systems. Currently, emergence of Chagas disease in Europe has been reported through immigrants and subsequent congenital

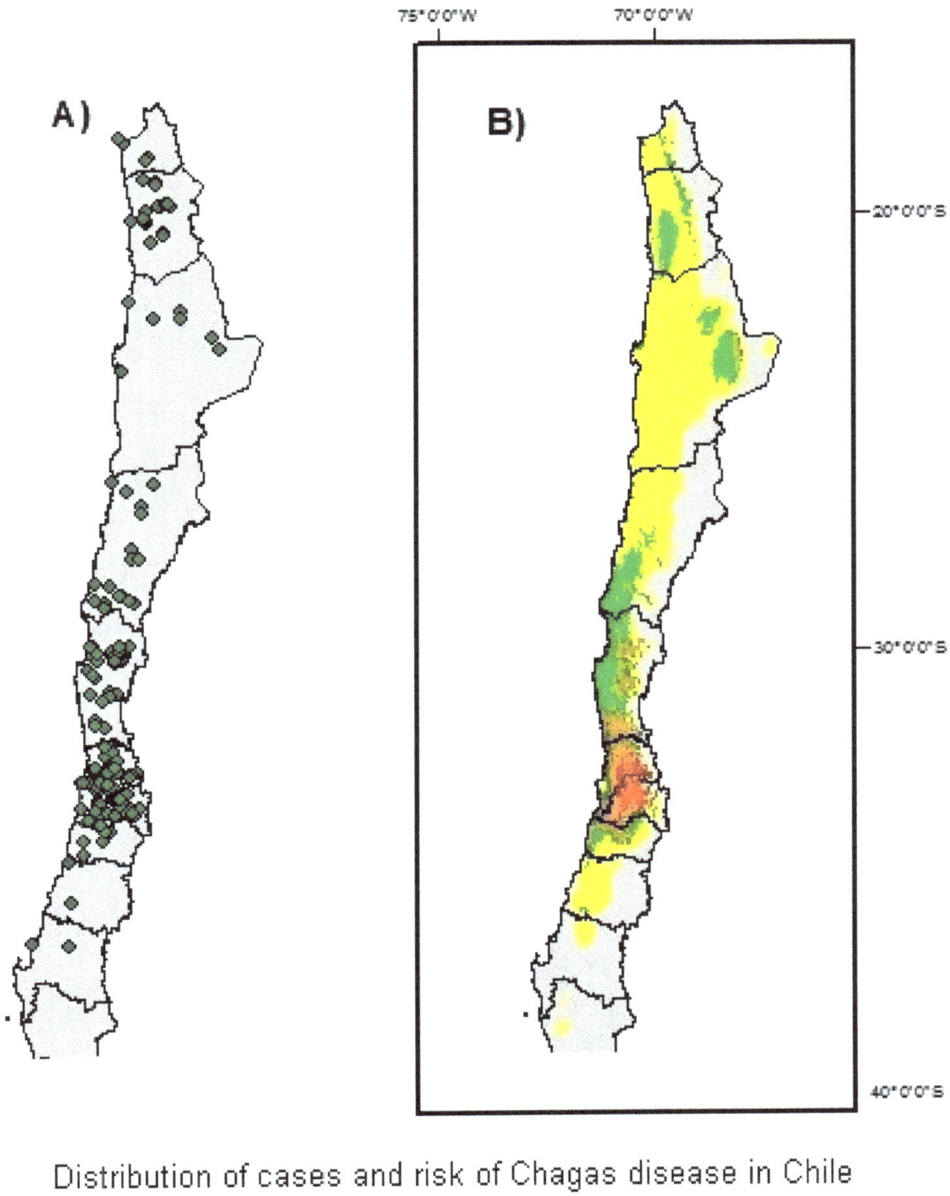

Figure 4. Distribution of cases and the risk of Chagas disease in Chile (modified from [18]).

transmission. For example, Basile et al. [76] reported more than 4000 cases diagnosed in different countries, with the highest number of cases in Spain, but Strasen et al. [77] proposed around 95% underreporting. These latter authors indicated that there could be between 14,000 and 180,000 cases in this continent.

In Chile, Chagas disease is distributed between the Arica and Parinacota Region (18°30'S) and the O'Higgins Region (34°36'S) (**Figure 4**), coinciding in large part with the distribution of the vector domestic *T. infestans* [18]. The highest incidence rates are recorded between Antofagasta and Coquimbo, with Antofagasta, Coquimbo, and Metropolitan Regions concentrating approximately two-thirds of the reported cases (**Table 2**).

Administrative region	Cases	Incidence rate (cases × 10^{-5})
Arica and Parinacota	57	23.8
Tarapacá	64	19.0
Antofagasta	223	35.8
Atacama	67	21.4
Coquimbo	292	37.9
Valparaiso	210	11.5
Metropolitan	313	4.3
O'Higgins	20	2.2
Maule	2	0.2
Bío Bío	11	0.5
Araucanía	1	0.1
Los Ríos	2	0.5
Los Lagos	0	0.0
Aisén	0	0.0
Magallanes	0	0.0
Total country	**1262**	**7.0**

Table 2. Cases and incidence rates of Chagas disease in Chile (2015) (health ministry).

6. Prevalence and incidence

Chagas disease is one of the main neglected diseases that affects the Americas and has now become an emerging disease in some parts of America and Europe [78–81], which has even been compared to the early stage of the HIV/AIDS epidemic [79]. The annual incidence varies between 28,000 and 56,000 people and between 10,000 and 14,000 deaths per year [79], affecting 6–11 million individuals [82] with 65–100 million people at risk in the world [78–80, 83]. The population at risk in Chile is 873,415 people [80, 81]. The latest national health survey (ENS) reports a prevalence of *T. cruzi* infection of 0.7% of the population, with a prevalence of 1.5% in rural areas and 0.6% in urban areas [81], and ministerial reports indicate that home infestation by *T. infestans* is practically nonexistent [80], which contrasts sharply with the data reported in the 1980s and 1990s. For example, between 1937 and 1980, a general prevalence of 16.7% was reported in endemic areas, with a maximum of 43.6% in the Coquimbo Region [11], which did not vary significantly between 1982 and 1985 [84], whereas between 1982 and1989 differences were already reported between rural areas with prevalence of 16.7% and urban areas with prevalence of 1.9% [16]. The same occurs with domiciliary infestation, in which previous reports indicated infestations between 26.8 and 33.2% of dwellings in endemic areas between Arica and the O'Higgins Regions [11, 80].

A study covering 60 years of the disease in Chile of patients referred to the University of Chile and studied through xenodiagnosis revealed an average prevalence of 9.35 ± 0.1% [32]. This prevalence value of 9.35% should be considered as the level for highly endemic zones. It is in the range between 8 and 12% reported by Apt and Reyes in 1986, also based on xenodiagnosis, and is similar to the estimated value for Latin America. This value does not present any variation in the 65 years of study, regardless of the changes in the health systems or interruption of the chain of transmission. Accurate estimation of the prevalence of Chagas disease is a difficult task since it depends not only on the sampling characteristics (random, stratified, etc.), sample size, and bias but also on the screening method used, which in the case of Chagas disease can be by xenodiagnosis, ELISA, immunofluorescence, and/or Western blot.

The values reported by the 2009–2010 ENS based on 4650 volunteers using IgG ELISA show 0.7% average prevalence, with 1.5% in the rural population and 0.6% in the urban population. These values are surprisingly similar to those reported for the urban population in 1982–1989 [85]. In this sense, the prevalence shows an evolution toward the values of an urbanized population.

The incidence in Chile shows a progressive rise from 1985 onward (**Figure 5**), without a slope change attributable to the interruption of the vector transmission chain. On the other hand, there is no appreciable effect attributable to the improvement in detection. For example, supreme decree 158 of 2004 in Chile declares Chagas disease as a notifiable disease, which is not reflected in the trend curve; later in 2008 circular four instructs blood banks to investigate the presence of *T cruzi*; law 1839 of 2009 stipulates the national policy of blood services; and in 2011 in circular B51, number 17 stipulates the surveillance of Chagas disease and establishes ways to record and inform the health authority [80, 81]. The incidence before 2009 had an average value of 2.7 ± 1.29 per 100,000 inhabitants, whereas after 2009 the average is 7.3 ± 2.02

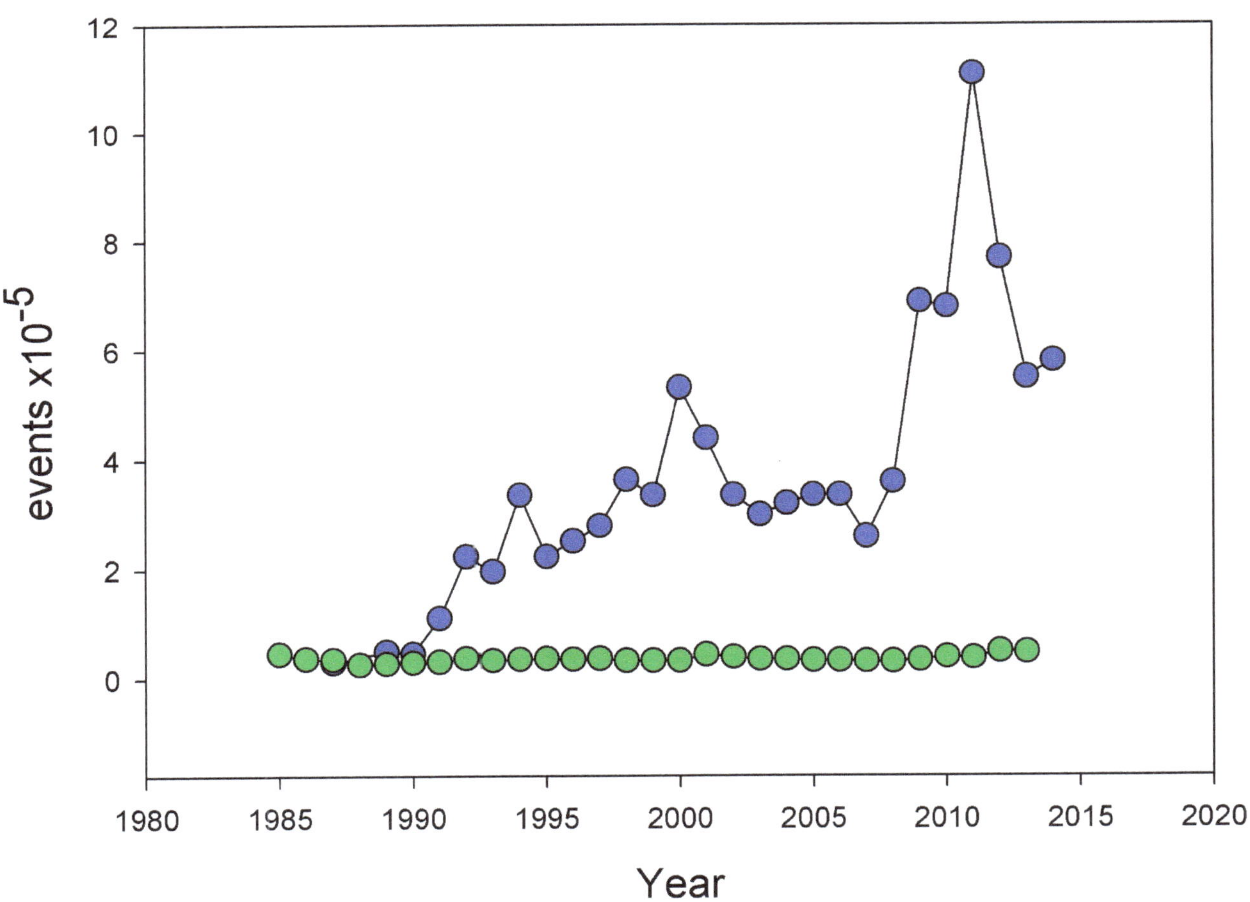

Figure 5. Incidence (blue) and mortality rates (green) of Chagas disease in Chile (Health Ministry).

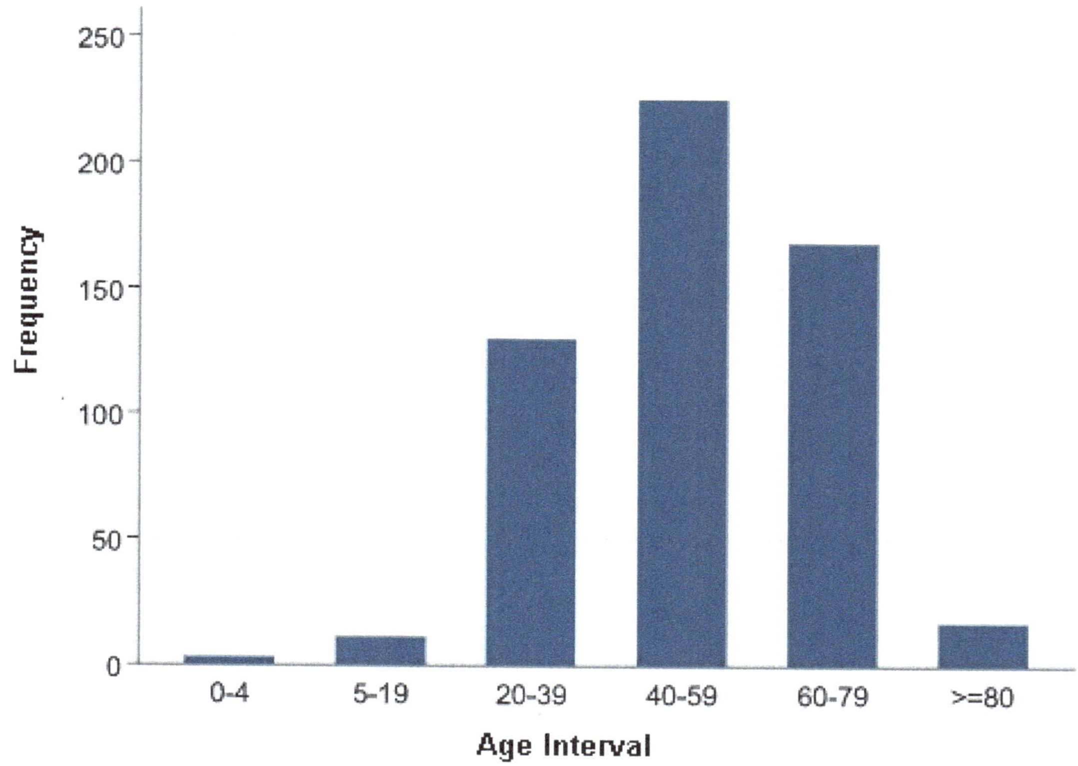

Figure 6. Age distribution of Chagas disease in 2010 (Health inistry).

per 100,000 inhabitants [32], staying relatively stable. One explanation for this temporal dynamics is that the progressive increase was not explained by a particular milestone but by a progressive improvement in the notification attributable to better staff preparation and a better notification system. Another possibility that cannot be ruled out is that this increase is real, and in this case, it should have an impact on mortality rates in the long run, a fact that is not yet evident. If the relative stability detected since 2009 persists, it would indicate that it would be reaching an adequate estimation of the endemic equilibrium, as the models predict [23, 86].

Mortality shows stability over the years (**Figure 5**). The average mortality rate is 0.36 ± 0.55 per 100,000 inhabitants [32]. Chagas disease affects the entire population in Chile, especially people of working age, with the highest rates between 30 and 65 years of age (**Figure 6**) [81].

7. Transfusion and congenital Chagas disease

The seroprevalence of *T. cruzi* in blood donors has been studied in Chile since the 1960s, with a national average of 3.7% reported between 1962 and 1988 [15]. Subsequently, this value has decreased; it was estimated between 0.5 and 1.6% according to information from the ISP between 2000 and 2005, estimated with the ELISA IgG method, and confirmed with IFI [87]. Currently, the seroprevalence of *T. cruzi* in blood donors is estimated at approximately 0.6%. The latest studies in the blood bank of the Clinical Hospital of the University of Chile were 0.4% positive out of a total of 24,568 [87].

A meta-analytic study that considered 13 case studies and 51 observational studies in ten countries estimated the rate of congenital infection was 4.7% with a CI of 3.4–5.7%. This means that in a population of mothers infected with *T. cruzi*, 4.7% of newborns are congenitally infected [88]. In this study it is proposed that in endemic areas the rate is 5% in endemic countries but lower in non-endemic countries (2.7%) and proposes a rate of 2.5% for Chile. In the same year, in a study conducted in Choapa, a highly endemic area, this rate was estimated at 4.7% [89].

8. The reproductive number (R_0)

The transmission of Chagas disease depends mainly on vector and congenital transmission. Accidental and transfusion transmissions are very rare and oral transmission only occurs in particular areas where the contact between man and nature is very close. The reproductive number of an infectious disease (R_0) corresponds to the average number of secondary infections produced by an infected individual. Thus, if R_0 is greater than 1, the disease is established in the population, and if R_0 is less than 1, the disease disappears. In the case of Chagas disease, the main component of the reproductive number is given by vector transmission, and when this is cut off, congenital transmission alone is incapable of perpetuating the disease [86, 90]. There are very few attempts to estimate the R_0 of this disease, an exception being the study by Massad [91], who estimated it at $R_0 = 1.25$ for a region of Brazil. Other estimates based on plausible approximations of many parameters obtained values of $R_0 = 7$ in Colombia [92] and $R_0 = 2.86$ [23] and $R_0 = 1.52$ in Chile [86]. However, recently in a spatial approach, a median value of $R_0 = 1.02$ has been proposed, with an approximate spatial variability between 0 and 5. The reproductive number could vary in different climate change scenarios as consequence of changes in entomological parameters such as biting rate, density, and mortality rate, increasing the Chagas risk area between 13 and 18% [93].

9. Conclusion and the way forward

Chile is in a privileged situation. It has only one domestic vector and probably only one wild vector of epidemiological importance, and the chain of domestic vector transmission by *T. infestans* is cut off. The wild reservoir is made up of small rodents, and the circulating lineages of *T. cruzi* are similar to the rest of America. However, there are some problems that persist: (1) The peri-anthropic reservoir is diverse and has bridging animals between the wild and domestic cycles that facilitate the spread of Chagas disease, such as dogs and goats; (2) housing and education conditions in Northern Chile are limited; (3) there are no control or education campaigns on wild vectors, and human dwellings are built on their territory. In addition there are wild foci of *T. infestans* and vector home intrusion; (4) prevalence, incidence, and trypano-triatomine indices still do not decrease; and (5) climate could change the epidemiological situation.

Given the obvious opportunity to eradicate Chagas disease in two generations, as predicted by the models, the way forward should be focused on (1) strengthening education campaigns of the population; (2) strengthening the monitoring of housing and peridomestic animals; (3) detection, study, and control of wild foci; and (4) reinforcing the study of the effect of climate change on the epidemiology of Chagas disease.

Acknowledgements

The authors acknowledge the financial support of Fondecyt (1150514 to MCL) and the revision of English language to Lafayette Eaton.

Author details

Mauricio Canals Lambarri[1,2]*, Andrea Canals Cifuentes[3,4], Salvador Ayala[5], Valentina Tapia-Garay[1] and Dante Cáceres Lillo[1]

*Address all correspondence to: mcanals@uchile.cl

1 Programa de Salud Ambiental, Escuela de Salud Pública, Facultad de Medicina, Universidad de Chile, Chile

2 Departamento de Medicina, Facultad de Medicina, Universidad de Chile, Chile

3 Programa de Bioestadística, Escuela de Salud Pública, Facultad de Medicina, Universidad de Chile, Chile

4 Dirección Académica, Clínica santa María, Chile

5 Departamento de Asuntos Científicos, Instituto de Salud Pública, Chile

References

[1] Rojas A, Sotelo JM, Villarroel F, Contreras MC. La importancia del perro y el gato en la epidemiología de la enfermedad de Chagas. Boletin Chileno De Parasitología. 1973;**28**:42-43

[2] Alcaino H, Ríos A, Apt W, Arrau S. Enfermedad de Chagas en animales sinantrópicos de un área hiperendémica de Chile. Parasitología al Día. 1981;**4**:88

[3] Alcaino H, Arrau S, Apt W, Ríos A. Enfermedad de Chagas en caprinos sinantrópicos de la provincia de Limarí, Chile. Revista Medica De Chile. 1982;**110**:328

[4] Canals M, Ehrenfeld M, Cattan PE. Situación de *Mepraia Spinolai*, vector silvestre de la enfermedad de Chagas en Chile, en relación con otros vectores, desde la perspectiva de sus fuentes de alimentación. Revista Medica De Chile. 2000;**128**:1108-1112

[5] Bacigalupo A, Segura JA, Garcia A, Hidalgo J, Galuppo S, Cattan PE. Primer hallazgo de vectores de la enfermedad de Chagas asociados a matorrales silvestres en la Region Metropolitana, Chile. Revista Médica de Chile. 2006;**134**:1230-1236

[6] Bacigalupo A, Torres-Perez F, Segovia V, Garcia A, Correa JP, Moreno L, et al. Sylvatic foci of the Chagas disease vector *Triatoma infestans* in Chile: Description of a new focus and challenges for control programs. Memórias do Instituto Oswaldo Cruz. 2010;**105**(5): 633-641

[7] Bacigalupo A, Correa JP, García A, Cattan PE. Focos silvestres de *Triatoma infestans* en Latinoamérica: análisis y perspectivas para Chile. Parasitología latinoamericana. 2015; **64**(3):33-42

[8] Chagas C. Nova trypanosomíase humana. Estudo sobre a morfología e o ciclo evolutivo do *Schizotrypanum cruzi* n. gen Sp, ajente etiológico de nova entidade mórbida do homen. Memórias do Instituto Oswaldo Cruz. 1909;**1**:159-218

[9] Coura JR. The discovery of Chagas disease (1908-1909): Great successes and certain misunderstandings and challenges. Revista da Sociedade Brasileira de Medicina Tropical. 2013;**46**(4):389-390

[10] Gasic G, Bertín V. Epidemiología de la enfermedad de Chagas en Chile. Revista Chilena de Pediatría. 1940;**11**(8):561-584

[11] Schenone H, Villarroel F, Rojas A, Alfaro E. Factores biológicos y ecológicos en la epidemiología de la enfermedad de Chagas en Chile. Boletín Chileno de Parasitología. 1980;**35**:42-54

[12] Lent H, Jurberg J. Algunas informacoes sobre *T. spinolai*, com um estudo sobre as genitalias externas. Revista Brasileira de Biologia. 1967;**27**:273-288

[13] Frías D, Martinez H, Wallace A. Algunos aspectos taxonómicos de *T. spinolai*. Acta Entomológica Chilena. 1987:155-170

[14] Frías-Lasserre D. A new species and karyotype variation in the bordering distribution of *Mepraia spinolai* (Porter) and *Mepraia gajardoi* Frías *et al* (Hemiptera: Reduviidae: Triatominae) in Chile and its parapatric model of speciation. Neotropical Entomology. 2010;**39**(4):572-583

[15] Apt W, Reyes H. Algunos aspectos de la enfermedad de Chagas en Latinoamérica. Parasitología al Día. 1990;**14**:23-40

[16] Schenone H, Rojas A. Algunos datos y observaciones pragmáticas en relación a la epidemiologia de la enfermedad de Chagas. Boletín Chileno de Parasitología. 1989;**44**: 66-86

[17] Frías-Lasserre D, González C, Reyes C, de Carvalho DB, Oliveira J, Canals M, da Rosa JA. Wing polymorphism and *Trypanosoma cruzi* infection in wild, peridomestic and domestic collections of *Mepraia spinolai* (Hemiptera: Reduviidae) from Chile. Journal of Medical Entomology. 2017;**54**(4):1061-1066

[18] Tapia-Garay V, Figueroa DP, Maldonado A, Frías-Laserre D, Gonzalez CR, Parra A, Canals L, Apt W, Alvarado S, Cáceres D, Canals M. Assessing the risk zones of Chagas′ disease in Chile in a world marked by global climatic change. Memórias do Instituto Oswaldo Cruz. 2018;**113**(1):24-29

[19] Garrido R. Impacto del cambio climático en la distribución geográfica de dos vectores silvestres de la enfermedad de Chagas en Chile, *Mepraia spinolai* y *Mepraia gajardoi* (Hemiptera: Reduviidae) [Tesis Magister en Ciencias Biológicas]. Santiago: Universidad de Chile; 2017. p. 54

[20] Canals M, Cattan PE, Ehrenfeld M. Algunas estimaciones numéricas de la importancia epidemiológica de los vectores de la enfermedad de Chagas en Chile. Parasitología al Día. 1993;**17**:79-86

[21] Canals M, Bustamante RO, Ehrenfeld M, Cattan PE. Assesing the impact of insect vectors on animal populations. Acta Biotheoretica. 1999;**46**:337-345

[22] Cattan PE, Pinochet C, Botto-Mahan C, Acuña MI, Canals M. Abundance of *Mepraia spinolai* in a periurban zone of Chile. Memórias do Instituto Oswaldo Cruz. 2002;**97**(3):285-287

[23] Canals M, Cattan PE. Dinamica de transmisión de la infección de la infección chagásica en Chile: Modelo y simulación. Revista Medica De Chile. 1992;**120**(12):1359-1365

[24] Canals M, Cattan PE, Ehrenfeld M, Torres P. Poblaciones experimentales de *T. infestans*: efectos de condiciones ambientales variables. Parasitología al Día. 1992;**16**(3-4):72-77

[25] Botto-Mahan C, Campos R, Acuna-Retamar M, Coronado X, Cattan PE, et al. Temporal variation of *Trypanosoma cruzi* infection in native mammals in Chile. Vector-Borne and Zoonotic Diseases. 2010;**10**:317-319

[26] Botto-Mahan C, Rojo G, Sandoval-Rodríguez A, Peña F, Ortiz S, Solari A. Temporal variation in *Trypanosoma cruzi* lineages from the native rodent *Octodon degus* in semiarid Chile. Acta Tropica. 2015;**151**:178-181

[27] Schenone H, Contreras MC, Salinas P, Sandoval L, Rojas A, Villarroel F. Epidemiología de la enfermedad de Chagas en chile. Frecuencia de infección humana por *Trypanosoma cruzi* por grupos de edad y regiones. Boletín Chileno de Parasitología. 1995;**50**:84-86

[28] Canals M, Cattan PE, Ehrenfeld M. Sobrevivencia de *Triatoma spinolai* en ambiente habitacional. Parasitología al Día. 1994;**18**(3):82-87

[29] Canals M, Cruzat L, Ehrenfeld M, Molina MC, Ferreira A, Cattan PE. Blood sources of *Mepraia spinolai* (Hemiptera Reduviidae), wild vector of Chagas's disease in Chile. Journal of Medical Entomology. 2001;**38**(2):303-307

[30] Rabinovich JE, Dan Kitron U, Obed Y, Yoshioka M, Gottdenker N, Chaves LF. Ecological patterns of blood-feeding by kissing-bugs. Memórias do Instituto Oswaldo Cruz. 2011;**106**(4):479-494

[31] Molina MC, Cattan PE, Canals M, Cruzat L, Aguillon JC, Ferreira A. A simple immunometric assay to assess the feeding habits of *Mepraia spinolai*, a *Trypanosoma cruzi* vector. Parasitology Research. 2004;**92**:375-379

[32] Canals M, Gonzalez C, Canals L, Canals A, Cáceres D, Alvarado D, et al. Que dicen los números de la evolución temporal de la enfermedad de Chagas? Revista Chilena De Infectologia. 2017;**34**(2):120-127

[33] Ehrenfeld M, Canals M, Cattan PE. Population parameters of *Triatoma spinolai* under different environmental conditions and densities. Journal of Medical Entomology. 1998; **35**(5):740-744

[34] Lehane MJ. Biology of Blood Sucking Insects. Cambridge: Cambridge University Press; 2005

[35] Schofield CJ. Triatominae. Biologia y Control. UK: Eurocomunica Pub; 1994

[36] Wood SF. The laboratory culture of *Triatoma*. Bulletin of the World Health Organization. 1964;**31**:579-581

[37] Rabinovich J, Rossel O. Mathematical models and ecology of Chagas disease. PAHO Pan American Journal of Public Health. 1978;**318**:359-369

[38] Canals M. Thermal ecology of small animals. Biological Research. 1998;**31**:367-374

[39] Canals M, Ehrenfeld M, Solís R, Cruzat L, Pinochet A, Tapia C, Cattan PE. Biología comparada de *Mepraia spinolai* en condiciones de laboratorio y terreno: cinco años de estudio. Parasitología al Día. 1998;**22**:72-78

[40] Jorg ME. Influencia de temperaturas fijas en periodos anuales sobre metamorfosis y fertilidad de *T. infestans*. Boletin Chileno De Parasitologia. 1962;**17**:17-19

[41] Canals M, Cattan PE, Ehrenfeld M. Dinámica comparada de cohortes de *T. infestans* en ambiente habitacional. Revista Medica De Chile 1994;**122**(9):993-997

[42] Canals M, Alvarado S, Cáceres D, Cattan PE. Twenty years of monitoring of mortality and fecundity of *Triatoma infestans* in the laboratory. Parasitología latinoamericana. 2016;**65**(2):54-60

[43] Canals M, Solís R, Valderas J, Ehrenfeld M, Cattan PE. Preliminary studies on temperature selection and activity cycles of *Triatoma infestans* and *T. spinolai*, Chilean vectors of Chagas disease. Journal of Medical Entomology. 1997;**34**:11-17

[44] Di Luciano VS. Orientation of *Triatoma infestans* to environmental temperatures. Journal of Medical Entomology. 1983;**20**:446-454

[45] Lazzari C. Temperature preference in *Triatoma infestans*. Bulletin of Entomological Research. 1991;**81**:273-276

[46] Lazzari C. Circadian rhythm of egg hatching in *T. infestans*. Journal of Medical Entomology. 1991;**28**:740-741

[47] Wiesinger D. Die Bedeutung der Umweltkartoren fur der Saugakt von *T. infestans*. Acta Tropica. 1956;**13**:97-141

[48] Nuñez JA. Food source orientation and activity in *R. prolixus*. Bulletin of Entomological Research. 1982;**72**:252-262

[49] Settembrini BP. Circadian rhythms of locomotion activity in the hematophagous bug *T. infestans*. Journal of Medical Entomology. 1984;**21**:204-212

[50] Lazzari C. Circadian organization of locomotor activity in the hematophagous bug. *T. infestans*. Journal of Insect Physiology. 1992;**38**:895-903

[51] Lazzari CR, Nuñez JA. The response to radiant heat and the estimation of the temperature of different sources in *Triatoma infestans*. Journal of Insect Physiology. 1989;**35**(6):525-529

[52] Ampleford E, Davey K. Egg laying in the insect *R. prolixus* is timed in a circadian fashion. Journal of Insect Physiology. 1989;**35**:183-187

[53] Ampleford E, Steel C. Circadian control of ecdysis in *R. prolixus*. Journal of Comparative Physiology.1982;**147**:281-286

[54] Lorenzo AN, Kenigsten A, Lazzari C. Daily dynamics and factors affecting aggregation in *T. infestans*. Memórias do Instituto Oswaldo Cruz. 1991;**86**:246

[55] Wigglesworth VB, Gillet JD. The function of the antennae in *R. prolixus* and the mechanism of orientation of the host. The Journal of Experimental Biology. 1934;**11**:120-138

[56] Guerenstein PG, Lazzari CR. Host-seeking: How triatomines acquire and make use of information to find blood. Acta Tropica. 2009;**110**(2-3):148-158

[57] Canals M, Solís R, Tapia C, Ehrenfeld M, Cattan PE. Comparison of some behavioural and physiological parameters of the feeding of *Triatoma infestans* KLUG, 1834 and *Mepraia spinolai* PORTER, 1934; vectors of the Chagas's disease in Chile. Memórias do Instituto Oswaldo Cruz. 1999;**94**(5):687-692

[58] Schofield CJ. Population dynamics and control of *T. infestans*. Annales de la Societe Belge de Medicine Tropicale. 1985;**65**:149-164

[59] Friend WG, Smith JB. Factors affecting feeding by blood sucking insects. Annual Review of Entomology. 1977;**22**:309-331

[60] Schenone H, Christensen HA, De Vasquez AM. Fuentes de alimentación de triatomas domésticos y su implicancia epidemiológica en relación a la enfermedad de Chagas en áreas rurales de siete regiones de Chile. Boletín Chileno de Parasitología. 1985;**40**:34-38

[61] Salvatella R. Evolución del índice de infección tripanosómica en *Tríatoma infestans* (KlugJ834) con las acciones de control antivectorial, en dos áreas endémico chagásicas de Uruguay. Revista Médica del Uruguay. 1995;**11**:105-110

[62] Apt W, Reyes H. Aspectos epidemiológicos de la enfermedad de Chagas en Chile. II: Infección en animales, algunas características especiales del problema, el control. Parasitología al Día. 1986;**10**:129-133

[63] Stevens JR, Gibson W. Molecular evolution of trypanosomes. Parasitology Today. 1999; **15**:432-437

[64] -Brisse S, Verhoef J, Tibayrenc M. Characterization of large and small subunit rRNA and mini-exon genes further supports the distinction of six *Trypanosoma cruzi* lineages. International Journal for Parasitology. 2001;**31**:1218-1226

[65] Zingales B, Andrade S, Briones RS, Campbell DA, Chiari E, Fernandes O, et al. A new consensus for *Trypanosoma cruzi* intraspecific nomenclature: Second revision meeting recommends TcI to TcVI. Memórias do Instituto Oswaldo Cruz. 2009;**104**(7):1051-1054

[66] Botto-Mahan C, Sepúlveda M, Vidal M, Acuña-Retamar M, Ortiz S, Solari A. *Trypanosoma cruzi* infection in the sylvatic kissing bug *Mepraia gajardoi* from the Chilean southern pacific ocean coast. Acta Tropica. 2008;**105**:166-169

[67] Toledo A, Vergara F, Campos R, Botto-Mahan C, Ortiz S, Coronado X, Solari A. *Trypanosoma cruzi* genotypes in *Mepraia gajardoi* from wild ecotopes in Northern Chile. The American Journal of Tropical Medicine and Hygiene 2012;**88**(2):285-288

[68] Coronado X, Rozas M, Botto-Mahan C, Ortiz S, Cattan PE, Solari A. Molecular epidemiology of Chagas disease in the wild transmission cycle: The evaluation in the sylvatic vector *Mepraia spinolai* from an endemic area of Chile. The American Journal of Tropical Medicine and Hygiene. 2009;**81**(4):656-659

[69] Bacigalupo A, Segovia V, García A, Botto-Mahan C, Ortiz S, Solari A, Acuña-Retamar M, Torres-Pérez F, Cattan PE. Differential pattern of infection of sylvatic nymphs and domiciliary adults of *Triatoma infestans* with *Trypanosoma cruzi* genotypes in Chile. The American Journal of Tropical Medicine and Hygiene. 2012;**87**(3):473-480

[70] Campos R, Botto-Mahan C, Ortiz S, Coronado X, Solari A. Temporal fluctuation of infection with different *Trypanosoma cruzi* genotypes in the wild rodent *Octodon degus*. The American Journal of Tropical Medicine and Hygiene. 2010;**83**(2):380-381

[71] Botto-Mahan C, Acuña-Retamar M, Campos R, Cattan PE, Solari A. European rabbits (*Oryctolagus cuniculus*) are naturally infected with different *Trypanosoma cruzi* genotypes. The American Journal of Tropical Medicine and Hygiene. 2009;**80**(6):944-946

[72] Rozas M, Botto-Mahan C, Coronado X, Ortiz S, Cattan PE, Solari A. *Trypanosoma cruzi* infection in wild mammals from a chagasic area of Chile. The American Journal of Tropical Medicine and Hygiene. 2005;**73**(3):517-519

[73] Rozas M, Botto-Mahan C, Coronado X, Ortiz S, Cattan PE, Solari A. Coexistence of *Trypanosoma cruzi* genotypes in wild and peridomestic mammals in Chile. The American Journal of Tropical Medicine and Hygiene 2007;**77**(4):647-653

[74] Durán JC, Videla MI, Apt W. Enfermedad de Chagas en una comunidad de pequeños mamíferos simpátricos de la reserva nacional de las chinchillas. Parasitol al Día. 1989;**13**:15-20

[75] Correa V, Zuñiga J, Contreras MC, Valdes JC, Rojas A, Villarroel F, Schenone H. Epidemiología de la enfermedad de Chagas en Chile. Sectores rurales. Infestación domiciliaria por triatominos, tasas de infección de estos por *Trypanosoma cruzi* y nuevos aportes al conocimiento de la infección chagásica en mamíferos domésticos de la IV Región (1982-1983). Boletín Chileno de Parasitología. 1984;**39**:24-27

[76] Basile L, Jamsa JL, Carlier Y, Salamanca DD, Angheben A, Bartoloni A, et al. Chagas disease in European countries: The challenge of a surveillance system. Eurosurveillance. 2011;**16**(37):pii:19968

[77] Strasen J, Williams T, Ertl G, Zoller T, Stich A, Ritter O. Epidemiology of Chagas disease in Europe: Many calculations; little knowledge. Clinical Research in Cardiology. 2013;**103**(1):1-10

[78] Hotez PJ, Bottazzi ME, Franco-Paredes C, Ault S, Periago MR. The neglected tropical diseases of Latin America and the Caribbean: A review of disease burden and distribution and a roadmap for control and elimination. PLoS Neglected Tropical Diseases. 2008;**2**:e300. DOI: 10.1371/journal.pntd.0000300

[79] Hotez PJ, Dumonteil E, Woc-Colburn L, Serpa JA, Bezek S, Edwards MS, et al. Chagas disease: "The new HIV/AIDS of the Americas". PLoS Neglected Tropical Diseases. 2012;**6**(5):e1498. DOI: 10.1371/journal.pntd.0001498

[80] MINSAL. Norma general técnica. Control y prevención nacional de la enfermedad de Chagas. Febrero. Ministerio de Salud de Chile. 2014

[81] MINSAL. Informe Programa Nacional Integral de Enfermedad de Chagas, Julio. Disponible en http://epi.minsal.cl/chagas-materiales-relacionados/ Consultado en 9/2016. 2016

[82] Cucunubá ZM, Okuwoga O, Basáñez MG, Nouvellet P. Increased mortality attributed to Chagas disease: A systematic review and meta-analysis. Parasites &Vectors. 2016;**9**:42. DOI: 10.1186/s13071-016-1315-x

[83] Fuentes R, Maturana M, De la Cruz R. Eficacia de Nifurtimox para el tratamiento de pacientes con enfermedad de Chagas crónico. Revista Chilena de Infectología. 2012;**29**(1): 82-86

[84] Apt W, Reyes H. Aspectos epidemiológicos de la enfermedad de Chagas en Chile. I: Distribución geográfica, índices de infección en vectores y en humanos. Parasitología al Día. 1986; 10: 84-10162.-Apt W. Parasitología humana. Mexico: McGraw-Hill; 2013. 800 pp

[85] Schenone H, Villarroel F, Rojas A. Presencia de *Triatoma spinolai* en viviendas humanas. Boletín Chileno de Parasitología. 1995;**50**(3-4):76-80

[86] Canals M, Caceres D, Alvarado S, Canals A, Cattan PE. Modeling the Chagas disease: From the vectorial to congenital transmission. Biosystems. 2017;**156**:63-71

[87] Apt W, Heitmann I, Jersic MI, Jofré L, Muñoz P, Noemí I, et al. Parte III. Enfermedad de Chagas en donantes de bancos de sangre. Revista chilena de infectología. 2008;**25**(4): 285-288

[88] Howard EJ, Xiong X, Carlier Y, Sosa-Estani S, Buekens P. Frequency of the congenital transmission of *Trypanosoma cruzi*: A systematic review and meta-analysis. BJOG: An International Journal of Obstetrics and Gynaecology. 2014;**121**:22-33

[89] Apt W, Zulantay I, Arnello L, Oddó D, González S, Rodriguez J, et al. Congenital infection by *Trypanosoma cruzi* in an endemic area of Chile: A multidisciplinary study. Transactions of the Royal Society of Tropical Medicine and Hygiene. 2013;**107**:98-104

[90] Raimundo SM, Massad E, Yang HM. Modelling congenital transmission of Chagas, disease. Bio Systems. 2010;**99**:215-222

[91] Massad E. The elimination of Chagas disease from Brazil. Epidemiology and Infection. 2008;**136**:1153-1164

[92] Cordovéz JM, Rendon LM, Gonzalez C, Guhl F. Using the basic reproduction number to assess the effects of climate change in the risk of Chagas disease transmission in Colombia. Acta Tropica. 2014;**129**:74-82

[93] Ayala S. Distribución especial del riesgo de transmisión vectorial de la enfermedad de Chagas basada en la estimación del número reproductivo básico (R0). Tesis Magister en Salud Pública. Facultad de Medicina, Universidad de Chile: 2017; 73 pp

3

The Mouse Model as a Tool for Histological, Immunological and Parasitological Studies of *Trypanosoma cruzi* Infection

María Elena Villagran-Herrera,
José Alejandro Martínez-Ibarra,
Manuel Sánchez-Moreno,
Hebert Luis Hernández-Montiel,
Ricardo Francisco Mercado-Curiel,
Nicolás Camacho-Calderón and
José Antonio de Diego-Cabrera

Abstract

The global expansion of Chagas disease is due to the constant migration of individuals from endemic countries with incidence of vector and nonvector transmission of *Trypanosoma cruzi*. The disease is present in its various stages: chronological characteristic signs and symptoms of the infection and its mechanism of immune system and cell and tissue damage. The first stage, which lasts 90 days approximately, is diagnosed by direct methods (blood smears stained with Giemsa, fresh and xenodiagnosis). The indeterminate-chronic stage is asymptomatic, but the growth and intracellular binary multiplication of the trypomastigotes continue promoting cell lysis and allowing parasites to infect other cells, with preferential tropism to organs producing mega syndromes such as cardiomyopathy, myocarditis, meningoencephalitis, megaesophagus and megacolon. Inadvertently, this process is repeated for several years leading to Chagas disease. The mouse inoculation allows checking the parasitemia in vivo and the development of the disease in short time (signs, behavior and tropism), histopathological alterations and detection of antibodies in serum. These parameters may vary when using different strains of *T. cruzi* from different geographical areas; Triatoma species due to their genetic variability are influenced by the environment, nutrition, reservoirs and habitat. The murine model ECA CD-1 has the ability to replicate human findings of Chagas disease.

Keywords: Trypomastigote, Chagas disease, murine model, amastigote, CD-1 strain

1. Introduction

In 1909, the Brazilian doctor and researcher Carlos Ribeiro Justiniano das Chagas discovered the etiological agent of the later called Chagas disease in the triatomine insect (family *Reduviidae*), a flagellate protozoan of the genus *Trypanosoma* and subgenus *Schizotrypanum* and designated the specie adding "cruzi" in honor of his teacher and mentor Oswaldo Cruz, hence the name *Trypanosoma (Schizotrypanum) cruzi*. Later, in 1926, another doctor of Argentine origin, Salvador Mazza described the magnitude of the endemy in Argentina, Bolivia and Paraguay, identifying the hemoflagellate parasite in blood samples, demonstrating in this way, the existence of the trypanosomatida infection, which was given the name of American Trypanosomiasis, since the vectors of *Trypanosoma cruzi* had been found only in America [1].

Chagas disease is a chronic debilitating affectation which impairs the health and the quality of life of infected people all around the world. The estimated number of infected people in the world arose from 30 million in 1990 to 6–8 million in 2010. In the past 20 years, the annual incidence decreased from 700,000 to 28,000 and the burden of Chagas disease decreased between 1990 and 2006 from 2.8 million disability-adjusted life to less than half a million [2]. Chagas disease is in close relation to the socioeconomic status of the population migration between Latin America and the rest of the world, and it currently represents one of the most important public health concerns [3]. The initiatives of the Americas have allowed achieving significant reductions in the number of acute cases and the presence of domiciliary Triatominae vectors in all endemic areas.

Trypanosoma cruzi belongs to the order of the kinetoplastid diseases, a group of parasites that has one or two flagella from a monophyletic group that diverged early from the branch common to all eukaryotic organisms. The morphological feature that distinguishes them is a prominent and paraflagellar structure known as kinetoplast, which corresponds to a condensation of DNA (DNAk), located on the inside of a single mitochondrion, which is branched across the cell. Within the family *Trypanosomatidae*, the *Trypanosoma* genus is most important because it includes a number of human diseases vectors such as *T. cruzi, T. brucei gambiense* and *T. brucei rhodesiense*, causal agents of Chagas and Sleeping sickness disease, respectively. Depending on the behavior of the parasite within the vector, the trypanosome genus has been divided into two groups. The first one called stercoraria, includes the trypanosomes that develop in the digestive tract of the vector, with the release of the infective forms in the stool (*T. cruzi* and *T. lewisi*). The second group called Salivaria includes trypanosomes that are initially developed in the digestive tube then passing through the epithelium and reaching the salivary glands, from where the infective forms are inoculated mechanically by bite or sting of the vector (*T. brucei, T. congolense* and *T. rangeli*) [4].

1.1. Life cycle

T. cruzi displays a digenetic life cycle alternating its multicellular life between the vertebrate host and its invertebrate vector. The cycle starts in the invertebrate arthropod when the insect sucks the blood of an animal carrying trypomastigotes in its blood, which gets to the stomach and are transformed into esferomastigotes and the replicative form epimastigotes. Subsequently, parasites migrate to the intestine where they multiply and eventually are transformed into the infective forms metacyclic trypomastigote, staying in the rectal ampulla until they are excreted with feces and urine. In this point, the life cycle continues in humans where the highly infective metacyclic forms aim to penetrate the skin or mucous membranes; although unable to pass through intact skin, they enter the body through skin or mucous membrane abrasions infecting macrophages, fibroblasts, smooth muscle and striated cells, Schwann cells, glial cells and neurons, excepting eosinophil and neutrophil cells. Once parasites have penetrated the cell, proliferation occurs and the trypomastigotes are released in the interior of a parasitophorous vacuole giving rise to amastigotes forms. The life cycle restarts with the insect feeding from an infected animal (**Figure 1**).

1.2. Routes of transmission

We can distinguish three cycles of vector transmission in *T. cruzi*. The primitive or wild cycle is zoonotic in nature. The protozoan parasite circulates between the insect vectors and the wild reservoirs (mammals of small and medium size). More than a hundred wild reservoirs of *T. cruzi* among marsupials, xenarthrans, bats, carnivores, lagomorphs, rodents and nonhuman primates have been described [6].

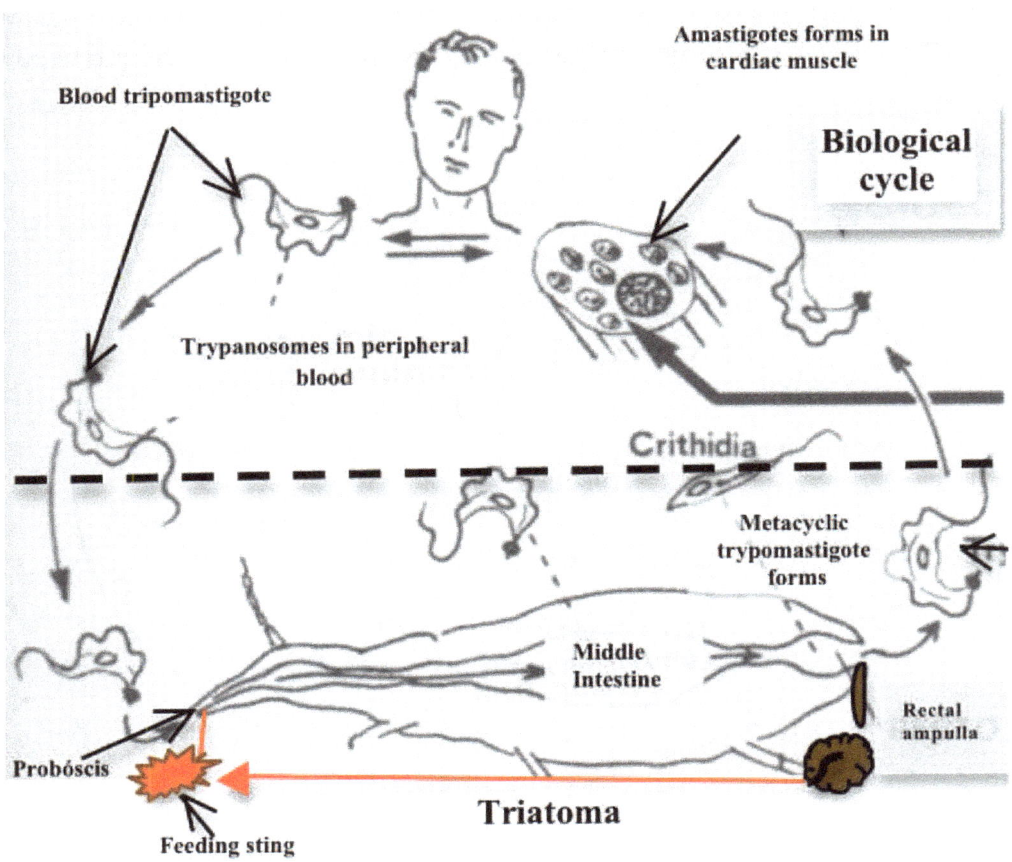

Figure 1. Digenetic biological cycle of *Trypanosoma cruzi*. Adapted by Federico-Mayer Rodolfo† and modified by de Diego-Cabrera José Antonio. Faculty of Medicine. Autonomous University of Madrid [5]. Spain, 1984 [5].

The domestic cycle comprises the infection of humans and the consequent Chagas disease. The domestic cycle is defined by factors in the anthroponotic foci, making people one of the last natural reservoirs of *T. cruzi*. Finally, the peridomestic cycle, comprising peridomestic mammals (rodents, marsupials, cats and dogs), which are in close contact with humans and their residences that have been built invading the habitat of wild triatomas that are attracted by the food and the lights of the houses.

Depending on the eco-epidemiological conditions of the place, both circles can overlap becoming an intradomiciliary cycle, especially when mankind invades the natural habitat of these vectors and builds houses fearing the entrance of reduvids (**Figure 2**).

On the other hand, the infection transmission by blood transfusion has become a serious complication in nonendemic countries, due to the migration of infected individuals from endemic regions [7]. This route is considered the second most important route of transmission in endemic areas [8]. *T. cruzi* resists processes of cryopreservation and thawing and can survive up to 18 days in total blood stored at 4°C. The vertical transmission is also known as a natal or congenital transmission, including prenatal, perinatal and postnatal care. This mechanism of transmission has a variable incidence between 0.1% and 18% according to geographical region [9], and has been regarded as the third in order of importance, next to vector-borne and transfusion transmission. An infected mother can transmit the parasite circulating in her blood during the second half of gestation. Among infected newborns, only 10–30% present symptoms [10].

The infection is not detected until adulthood in the course of the latent or indeterminate phase [11]. Spontaneous abortions have been reported, premature birth, intrauterine growth retardation, stillbirths and various clinical forms that can go from low birth weight, hepatomegaly,

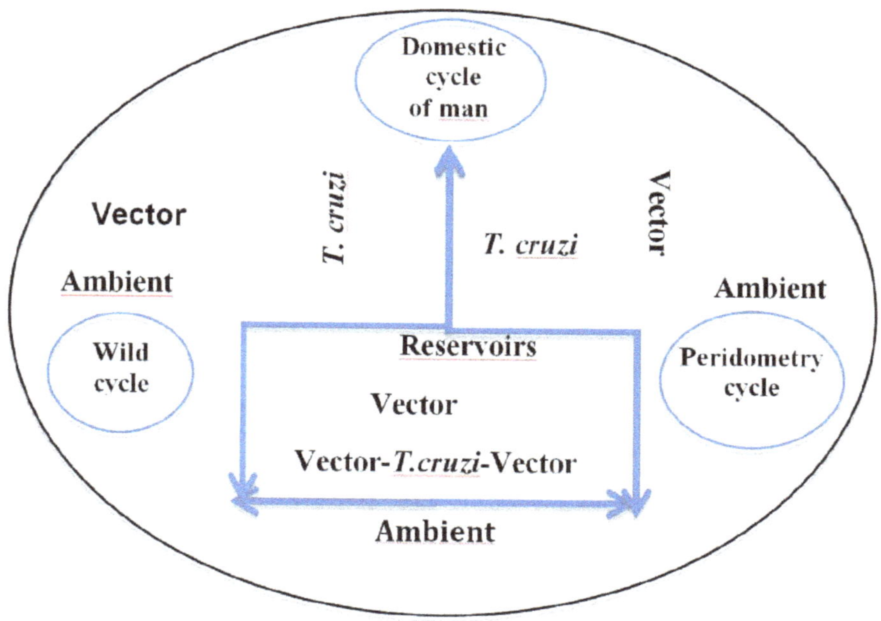

Figure 2. Exchanges between wild, peridomestic and domestic cycles of *T. cruzi* transmission. Adapted from Coura and Pinto Dias [6].

splenomegaly, acute respiratory symptoms, anemia, digestive disorders, Cardiac and Central Nervous System (CNS). The donation of organs has increased the number of infected people in urban areas. It has been informed about the transmission of infection to seronegative heart, bone marrow, liver, pancreas and kidney transplant recipients with variable transmission rates that reach 35% [12]. Patients infected with *T. cruzi* that should receive a transplant also represent a particular challenge, with risk of reactivation of the disease because of the immunosuppression after transplantation. The raw meat from infected rats and rabbit can be induced by the consumption of foods contaminated with triatomines or its feces, or by the ingestion of raw meat from infected mammalian hosts [13]. It must be confirmed by the detection of the parasites in a direct microscopic examination of a blood sample or other biological fluids of the patient. Many cases of numerous outbreaks of acute Chagas Disease are attributed to oral transmission; it has been detected in the Amazon region, due to the consumption of drinks or food contaminated with feces of infected triatomines [14]. It is also important to take into account the laboratory accidents that arise when research animals are handled mainly by postgraduate students, even though they occur in a smaller proportion [15].

1.3. Pathology and mechanism of injury

The disease presents three phases: the acute, chronic asymptomatic (intermediate or dormant) and the chronic symptomatic. The incubation period in the acute phase is 4–10 days and of shorter duration when the route of transmission is blood transfusion. This stage is generally asymptomatic, or it can occur with systemic manifestations that are common to other diseases such as fever, edema, lymphadenopathy, hepatomegaly and splenomegaly. It is accompanied by anorexia, fatigue, myalgia, headache and, occasionally, arthralgia. In some cases, there are signs of inoculation or entrance door, chagomas, lesions that are more frequent in the face and limbs of a forunculoid aspect, pink or violet and indurated borders. A typical sign in children is the bipalpebral edema (sign of Roman-Mazza). In this phase, the trypomastigotes are easily detected in the blood due to the high parasitemia.

In case the acute phase is overcome, there will be an extended period of chronic disease without clinical symptoms that lasts from 5 to 10 years, characterized by low parasitemia and by the presence of anti-*T. cruzi* IgG antibodies. About 30% of seropositive individuals reach the chronic phase, and in a span of 10–30 years, clinical manifestations such as heart disease and digestive megasyndromes show up, which may occur separately or coexist in the same patient. The chronic phase progresses slowly with a predominance of tissue damage. Digestive disorders consist in dilatation of viscera (mainly colon and esophagus, and in two-thirds of cases, the progressive myocarditis leads to the development of chronic Chagas disease heart (CChC). The relative prevalence of the various clinical manifestations varies according to geographic regions. In Argentina, as well as in Venezuela and Central America, the main clinical manifestation is the cardiomyopathy. On the contrary, in Chile and in the central region of Brazil, the mega syndromes are more frequent. This heterogeneous incidence of manifestations in different endemic areas could obey both biological and genetic differences of the circulating parasites [16] and host-related factors (age, gender, ethnicity, exposure to infections, family history of Chagas disease heart) [17], in addition to the introduction by migration of infected people from different countries around the world (**Figure 3**).

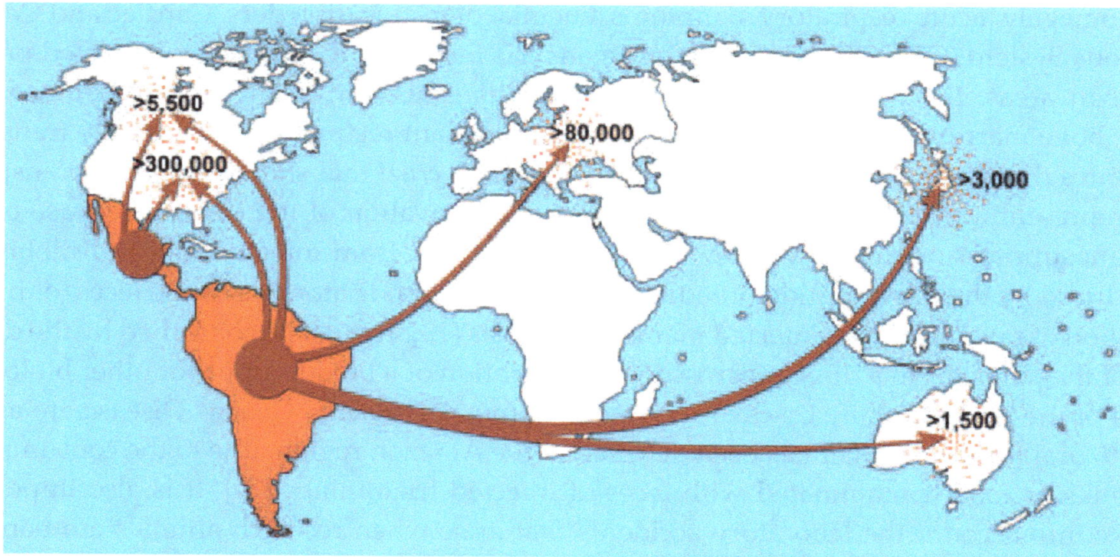

Figure 3. The estimated number of cases of Chagas disease in nonendemic countries, driven by constant migration. (ISGlobal, 2015).

In this last Chagas disease's phase, histological lesions are disseminated in the heart muscle, intestines and nervous system, inflammatory infiltrates composed mainly of CD8+ cells, in addition to nests (pseudocysts) full of parasites in their form of amastigotes [18].

Regarding the treatment, there are currently only two drugs available, benznidazole and nifurtimox. The therapeutic success is closely related to the stage of infection at the time of starting the treatment. Patients in acute phase (regardless of the route of infection), neonates and children, have better therapeutic prognosis [12, 15]. On the other hand, the success of such drugs is discussed in individuals with chronic infection and so far, there is no established therapeutic regimen [19]. The adverse effects are much more important among the adult patients; cases of photosensitivity and skin rashes, nausea, anorexia, weight loss and abdominal pain have been reported.

Recently, a group of biomedical and clinical scientists members of the network NHEPACHA (New Tools for the diagnosis and evaluation of the patient with Chagas disease), based on clinical and immunological evidence, have suggested new paradigms regarding the medicines for the Chagas disease in order to provide better treatment for patients in chronic phase [20].

On the other hand, the study of biochemical and biological characteristics of the hemoflagellate parasite has enabled the identification of new targets for chemotherapeutic agents; an example would be the drug trials with inhibitors of the biosynthesis of Ergosterol, Posaconazole and Ravuconazole, respectively, in patients with chronic Chagas disease.

1.4. Diagnosis of infection

Parasitological methods for detection of the acute phase have great sensitivity (direct methods) [21].

In the same way, these methods are used for the diagnosis of congenital infection in newborns and in children under the age of 6 months. The lack of maturation of the immune system and the presence of maternal IgG antibodies make, in the latter, the use of the serology for the infection diagnosis impossible [22]. The protozoan *Trypanosoma cruzi* is a powerful antigen and a few months after the initial inoculation, there is a humoral immune response that is effective is controlling the increase of parasitemia, which is mediated by antibodies and enzymes of the complement system. There are antibodies to various antigens of *T. cruzi* (surface, somatic and excretion), which belong to different classes (IgG, IgA, IgM) and subclasses [23–25]. The serologic test for the selection of blood donors must conform to the Official Mexican Standard for Epidemiological Surveillance, Prevention and Control of Vector-borne Diseases [26–28], citing that it must analyze the serum of each donor with two conventional immunological tests; if one of them is reactive, a third one will be carried on in such a way so as to qualify the donor as either positive or negative, with two reactive or two negative tests. In all cases, the laboratory diagnosis should be accompanied with epidemiological and clinical history of the patient, as the current and past source, the type of housing where it is found, the trips that could have been made to endemic areas and the history of blood transfusions and the infected mother.

1.5. Origin of the discrete units (UDTs) typing of *Trypanosoma cruzi*

The evolutionary history of *T. cruzi* infection is closely related to its vertebrate host [29]. The mammal fauna of South America in the cretaceous period mainly consisted of marsupials and

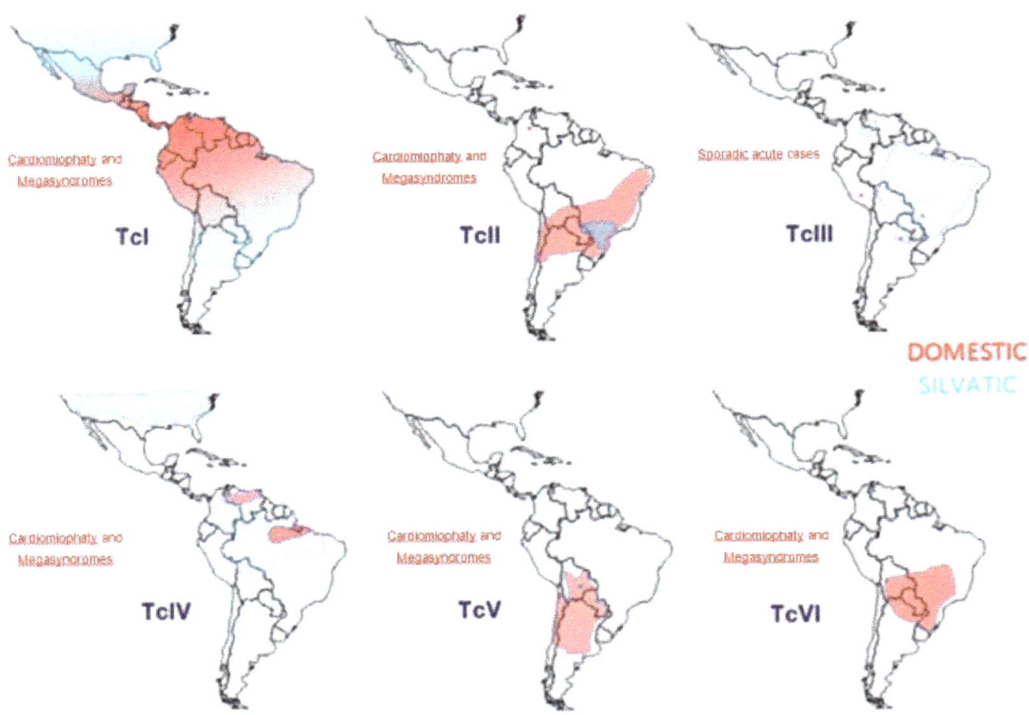

Figure 4. Geographic distribution of *Trypanosoma cruzi*, subpopulations disease phases with the corresponding primary clinical manifestations.

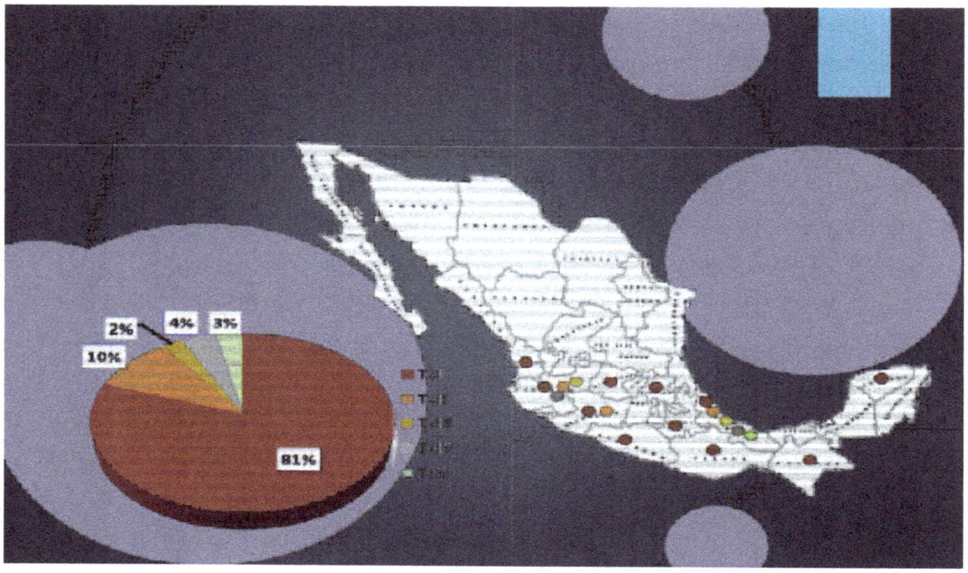

Figure 5. Distribution of *Trypanosoma cruzi* strains in México [35, 36].

placentals, the ancestral of the order Xenarthra (armadillos, anteaters and sloths), which were the natural reservoirs of the parasite at the time. The various ecotopes in whom were these two groups of hosts would have made possible the evolution by clonal propagation of two groups of parasites, which gave rise to the ancestral UDTs, TcI and TcII. It has been suggested that 1Cwi, evolved in association with the marsupial mammals of the genus *Didelphis* (weasels) and *T. cruzi* II, did in relation to the terrestrial mammals, such as armadillos [30]. *Trypanosoma cruzi* is a species composed of heterogeneous populations that circulate in nature between human beings, arthropod vectors, domestic animals, and wild reservoirs [31]. Currently, it is generally accepted that *T. cruzi* is a paradigmatic pattern of clonal evolution with low rate of gene recombination. A constant pattern of *T. cruzi*, behavior cannot be expected since different strains (subpopulations) circulate in nature. Extensive polymorphism promotes variation in infecting capacity, behavior in different hosts (virulence, histotropism, curves of parasitemia), adaptation to different vectors, immune response, stimulation, susceptibility to different chemical compounds, capacity of replication and differentiation, among others. Subpopulations are currently identified in the laboratory by biochemical, immunological and molecular biology assays [32, 33] (**Figure 4**).

Studies in murine experimental models have shown that both the parasite and host genotypes are crucial for tissue distribution and pathophysiology of infection by *T. cruzi* [34]. It has been previously reported that 81% of the Mexican strains of *T. cruzi* belong to lineage TcI and have different capabilities of infection, virulence and processing capacity in vitro, when compared to the other lineages [35, 36] (**Figure 5**).

2. Importance of the murine model in research American trypanosomiasis

2.1. The murine model in biomedical research

Animal models are very useful for studying human diseases because there are hundreds of pathogens that affect both humans and animals. The use of experimental animals in biomedical research represents a key element for development of new prevention approaches and treatment of transmissible and nontransmissible diseases. Suffice it to recall the rabies vaccines, smallpox, tetanus, diphtheria, whooping cough and polio, the development of several antibiotics, insulin, and the knowledge of the genetic bases of inheritance [37]. No doubt that mice are the most commonly used animal for in vivo assays among experimental animal models in biology and medicine. The use of mice allows the study of mammal's reactions against aggressions like poisoning or infection (viral, bacterial, or parasitic), the study of immune responses and disorders and many others in several different fields like oncology, teratology and embryology [38] (**Figure 6**).

Herein, we present a comparative cross-sectional study involving four *Trypanosoma cruzi* strains obtained from three different species of triatomas captured in endemic areas of the states of Jalisco (*T. longipennis*), Morelos (*T. palidipennis*), Nayarit(*T. longipennis*) and Queretaro (T. Mexicana)

2.2. Collection sites

Several communities from different States of México were included in the present study: San Pablo, Tolimán in Querétaro State, Milpillas of Talpa de Allende in Jalisco State, Sant Catarina in Morelos State and Jala in Nayarit State (**Figure 7**).

2.3. Triatoma collection and maintenance

Cages covered with adhesive tape were used, with the glue facing outward. A live Wistar rat was placed inside the cage. Cages were placed at late night in strategic areas under the loose stones of poultry and farm animal fences, fallen leaves and wooden logs. Cages were collected the next day, early in the morning (**Figure 8**).

Triatomas glued to the surface of the gummed paper were carefully detached, with the aid of entomological tweezers and placed in jars covered with mosquito mesh. A piece of filter paper in accordion shape was placed inside the bottle to facilitate the movement of the triatomas and the collection of urine or feces deposited on its surface.

The triatomas are maintained inside the bottles at 25–26°C and 60% humidity (RH) in bacteriological incubator. Triatomas were blood fed directly from a shaved rabbit every 2 weeks allowing them to feed for 20–25 m and then they were placed back in the incubator (**Figure 9**).

2.4. Study of the intestinal content in the triatomine

We use two techniques for collecting intestinal content from triatomine after blood feeding. In the first one, the triatomine is introduced in a 10 x 20 mm tube; normally the bug deposits

Figure 6. The laboratory animal is "any specie of animal that is kept under certain conditions and is used for scientific purposes" [37, 39].

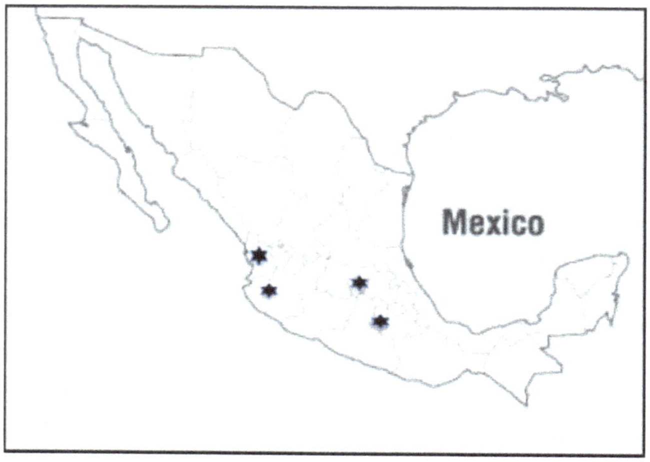

Figure 7. Map of the Mexican Republic. The black stars indicate the capture zones of the triatomas, used in our investigation.

stool or urine in the bottom of the tube and then it is collected with saline solution. The second technique consists in pressing gently the triatomine abdomen, inducing that the rectal blister freely releases the stool (semi-separated blood). Intestinal content is collected in a watch glass and saline solution is added at 37°C. In both techniques, the metacyclic trypomastigote and epimastigote forms are observed fresh, using a microscope with 400 magnifications. The trypomastigotes are counted in a Neubauer chamber. If the count is above 10,000 parasites per cubic centimeter, mice are inoculated as mentioned below.

The same procedure is performed with each one of the strains of species of triatomas captured (**Figure 10**).

2.5. *Trypanosoma cruzi*, inoculation in mice

Male mice of CD-1 strain are used since estrogen in females can stimulate the activity of macrophage phagocytes and, the localized immune response [38].

Using an insulin syringe four groups of 10 mice were inoculated intraperitoneally with $3x10^3$ epimastigote and/or trypomastigote forms of *Trypanosoma cruzi*, isolated from four species of

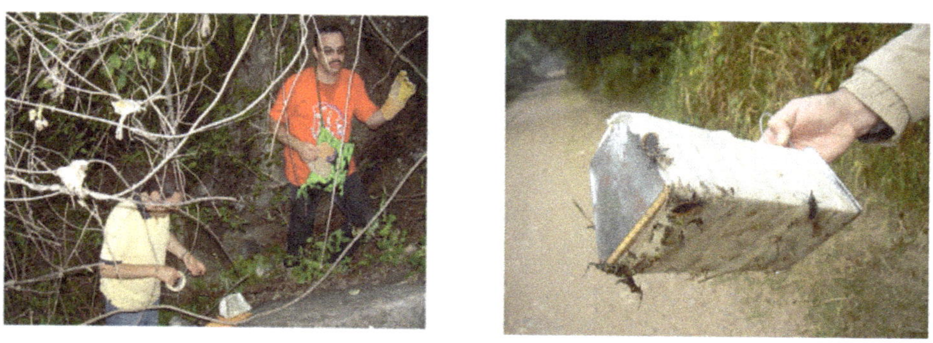

Figure 8. Traps are placed in the collection site (A). Cage with triatomas stuck to the adhesive tape (B) Photos. Villagrán-Herrera.

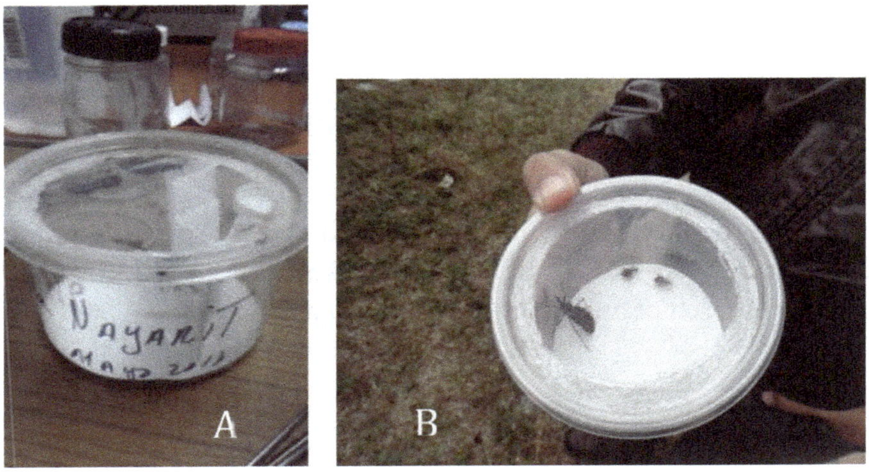

Figure 9. A and B. Transportation and storage of collected triatomas. Photos Villagrán Herrera.

triatomas (*T. mexicana, T. pallidipennis, T. longipennis* and *T. dimidiata*). Mice from the control group were inoculated with saline solution.

2.6. Study of behavior (signs)

After the first day of inoculation, the behavior of the infected murine model was observed, comparing it with an uninfected control.

2.7. Study of the parasitemia

Parasitemia levels are determined in infected mice 5,10,15,20,25 and 30 days post *T. cruzi* inoculation. Blood is obtained from the distal part of the queue 1:4000 EDTA is used as anti-coagulant, in a pipette of leukocyte count. Numbers of parasites per milliliter are calculated from sample observations in Neubauer chamber [37, 38].

2.8. Histopathological analysis

Histological sections of 10 microns are obtained from mouse dissected organs (brain, heart, intestines and skeletal muscle) and stained with H/E. Microscope slide preparations are

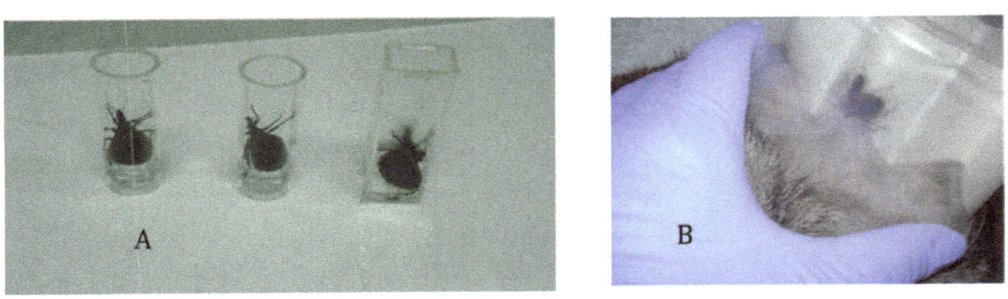

Figure 10. Tube techniques to obtain stool from the Triatoma (10A). Fourth stage Triatoma nymphs feeding on a rabbit. Photos Villagrán-Herrera.

observed at 40X [39]. Tissues from infected mice and the respective control animals are included in the analysis.

2.9. Detection of antibodies in serum (detection of anti-*Trypanosoma cruzi* antibodies in serum)

Blood is obtained by cardiac puncture and centrifuged at 5000 rpm to separate the clot from the serum and maintained at −20°C until it is used to carry out an ELISA (Accutrack Chagas Microelisa Test) in the search of anti-*Trypanosoma cruzi* antibodies.

3. Results

The mice inoculated with all the studied *T. cruzi* strains showed an altered behavior when compared to control animals. The signs presented 24 h post *T. cruzi* inoculation, the mice exhibited hyperactivity, the hair was dull and bristled, the hind legs became intertwined, and it began to drag them away, with great difficulty in moving forward.

However, it was possible to observe some differences in the virulence of each strain according to the geographic area geographic area where they came from (**Figure 11**).

The inoculant obtained from triatomines from Talpa de Allende in Jalisco state and Santa Catarina in Morelos state generated in the corresponding mice a parasitemia of 3: 4 trypanosomes per field, at 14 and 16 days postinoculation, respectively. In both cases, altered movements and physical shape of the mice began at about the same time. By day 20 and 23, respectively, the parasitemia reached the peak, so it was proceeded to sample fresh blood and dissect organs in order to perform the serological and histopathological assays

Parasitemia in mice inoculated with the *Trypanosoma cruzi* from triatomines caught in Jala, in Nayarit State reached the peak 30 days post inoculation. It was possible to detect anti-*T. cruzi* antibodies in 2 mice out of 10 by conventional ELISA test.

Blood parasitemia was undetectable in mice inoculated with *T. cruzi* strains obtained from triatomines collected in San Pablo and Tolimán in Querétaro State. The animal behavior was

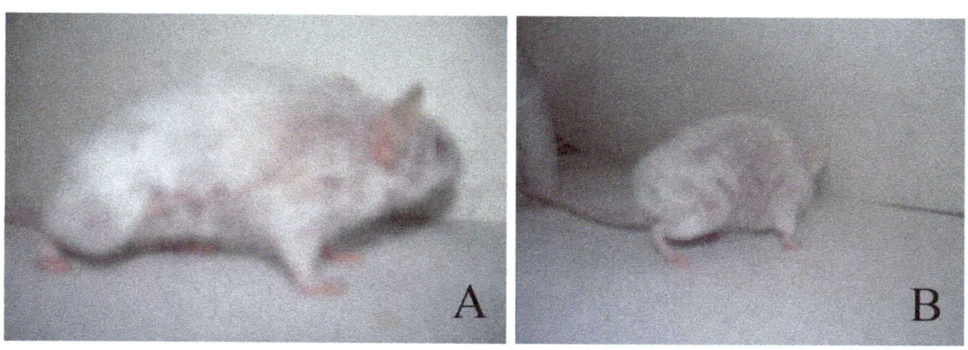

Figure 11. *T. cruzi* infected mice exhibiting hyperactivity, dull and bristled hair and intertwined hind legs. (11A and 11B). Photos Villagran Herrera.

Geographic area	Species of Triatoma	Days in which presents parasitemia	Frizz hair	Difficulty walking	ELISA test	Brain	Heart	Skeletal muscle	Intestine
Talpa de Allende. Jalisco	*T. longipennis*	14	Positive	Positive	Reactive	Negative	Positive	Positive +++	Negative
Jala Nayarit	*T. dimidiata*	30	Positive	Negative	Reactive	Negative	Negative	Positive ++	Negative
San Pablo Tolimán Qro.	*T. mexicana*	It was presented in 90 days	Negative	Negative	Reactive	Negative	Negative	Negative	Negative
Sta. Catarina Morelos	*T. pallidipennis*	16	Positive	Positive	Reactive	Negative	Positive	Positive++	Negative

Table 1. Results of the behavior, parasitemia, serology and histology in the murine model, infected with inoculum of four strains of *Trypanosoma cruzi*, isolated from triatomas captured in different geographical areas.

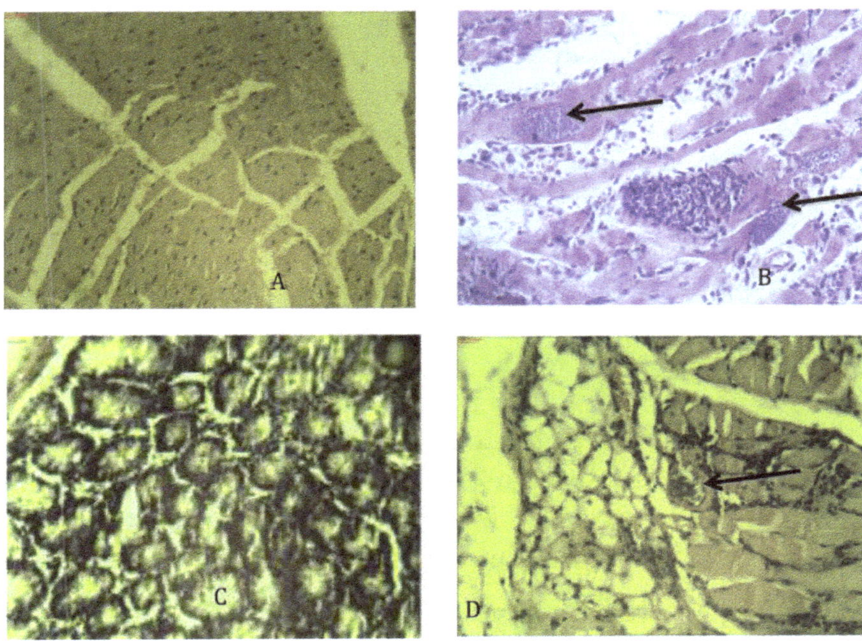

Figure 12. Histopathological analysis of cardiac (A, B) and intestine muscle (C, D) tissues. A and C, control groups. B, cardiac tissue with pseudocysts with high parasitemia and formation of new agglomerations of amastigotes, Jalisco strain. D, intestine muscle tissue with a mild *T. cruzi* parasitemia, Nayarit strain. Photos Villagran-Herrera.

completely normal when comparing to control group. Organs looked slightly bigger, mainly the intestines and heart. It was possible to detect anti-*T. cruzi* antibodies in the serum. Results are summarized in **Table 1**.

Presence of amastigote nests and histopathological damage in heart and intestine muscle showed direct relationship with parasitemia level, which indicates that trypanosomes are installed and recognize different tissues where they reproduce rapidly intracellularly, resulting in a greater number of parasites in blood after they differentiate into trypomastigotes. This sequence is only observed in the most virulent strains such as those from the States of Jalisco, Morelos and Nayarit (**Figure 12**).

4. Conclusions

In the present study, assessment of clinical manifestations, parasitemia levels, histological changes and seropositivity in murine model allowed us to know the behavior of different *T. cruzi* strains found in triatomas from different geographic areas in Mexico. This confirms the existence of genetically different strains that produce a complex called "cruzi" from the pathognomonic and morphophysiological point of view, as previously reported [40].

T. cruzi infection depends on genotype of both the parasite and the mammalian host, which in turn influences tissue tropism and the pathophysiology of infection.

We were able to identify two different *T. cruzi* strains (Tc I) from triatomines from two communities from Queretaro State that exhibited mild virulence when compared to other three strains from triatomines from three different States in México. Isozyme characterization waits to be carried out in order to explain if those observed differences might be attributable to the fact that different species of blood-sucking triatomine insects were used [40].

5. Discussion

Mitie-Nisimura et al., in 2014, were able to induce acute phase inoculating mice by intraperitoneal injection trypomastigote forms of *T. cruzi*. Authors observed the microvascular alterations and oxidative stress in the brain and the formation of pseudocysts full of amastigotes in the heart muscle [41]. Espinoza et al., in 2010 inoculated Balb/c mice with two strains of *T. cruzi* I (Tc I) isolated from patients in Mexico in order to study the immune response [35]. The first case of clinical infection with *T. cruzi* was reported in a horse in South Texas in 2015, observing forms of amastigotes in the spinal cord and cardiac tissue.

Espinoza et al., in 2010, observed contrasting differences between two *T. cruzi* strains isolated from *Triatoma barberi* and *Triatoma mexicana*. In the first case, virulence was clearly observed while in the second one, productive infection and morphological alterations were not observed, and only the anti-*T. cruzi* antibodies were detected.

Author details

María Elena Villagran-Herrera[1*], José Alejandro Martínez-Ibarra[2], Manuel Sánchez-Moreno[3], Hebert Luis Hernández-Montiel[1], Ricardo Francisco Mercado-Curiel[1], Nicolás Camacho-Calderón[1] and José Antonio de Diego-Cabrerade[4]

*Address all correspondence to: mevh@uaq.mx

1 Department of Biomedical Research, Faculty of Medicine, Autonomous University of Queretaro, Santiago de Querétaro, Queretaro, Mexico

2 Area of Medical Entomology, University Center of the South, University of Guadalajara, Guadalajara, Jalisco, Mexico

3 Laboratory of Molecular Biology of Parasites, Faculty of Science, University of Granada, Granada, Spain

4 Department of Preventive Medicine, Public Health and Microbiology, Faculty of Medicine, Autonomous University of Madrid, Madrid, Spain

References

[1] Storino R, Milei J. Introducción. Enfermedad de Chagas. In: Storino R, Milei J, editors. Buenos Aires: Mosby-Doyma. 1994;1-7. Chapter 1

[2] OMS. Control of Chagas Disease. Second Report of the WHO Expert Committe. WHO TRS905; 2002

[3] WHO Expert Committee. Control of Chagas Disease-Second Report of the WHO Expert Committee;2003

[4] Azambuja P, Ratcliffe-Norman A, García-Eloi S. Towards an understanding of the interactions of *Trypanosoma cruzi* and *Trypanosoma rangeli* within the reduviid insect host *Rhodnius prolixus*. Anais da Academia Brasileira de Ciencias. 2005;**77**(3):397-404

[5] Peña-Yañez J, Mayer RF, de D, Cabrera JA. Practicas en Parasitología y Micología. Editorial Ciencia. 1984:55-56

[6] Coura JR, Pinto-Dias JC. Epidemiology, control and surveillance of Chagas disease 100 years after its discovery. Memórias do Instituto Oswaldo Cruz. 2009:31-40

[7] Gascon J, Bern C, Pinazo MJ. Chagas disease in Spain, the United States and other non-endemic countries. Acta Tropica. 2010;**115**(1-2):22-27

[8] Dias JC, Silveira AC, Schofield CJ. The impact of Chagas disease control in Latin America: A review. Memórias do Instituto Oswaldo Cruz. 2002;**97**(5):603-612

[9] Carlier Y, Truyens C. American Trypanosomiasis: Chagas Disease, One Hundred Years of Research. 2nd ed. Elsevier; 2010. pp. 539-581

[10] Torrico F, Alonso-Vega C, Suarez E, Rodríguez P, Torrico MC, Dramaix M, Truyens C, Carlier Y. Maternal *Trypanosoma cruzi* infection, pregnancy outcome, morbidity, and mortality of congenitally infected and non-infected new-borns in Bolivia. The American Journal of Tropical Medicine and Hygiene. 2004;**70**(2):201-209

[11] Freilij H, Altcheh J. Congenital Chagas' disease: Diagnostic and clinical aspects. Clinical Infectious Diseases. 1995;**21**(3):551-555

[12] Barcán L, Luna C, Clara L, Sinagra A, Valledor A, De Rissio AM, Gadano A, García MM, de Santibañes E, Riarte A. Transmission of *T. cruzi* infection via liver transplantation to a nonreactive recipient for Chagas disease. Liver Transplantation. 2005;**11**(9):1112-1116

[13] Días JC. Notas sobre o *Trypanosoma cruzi* e suas características bio-ecológicas, como agente de enfermidades transmitidas por alimentos. Revista da Sociedade Brasileira de Medicina Tropical. 2006;**39**(370):370-375

[14] Días JP, Bastos C, Araújo E, Mascarenhas AV, Martins-Netto E, Grassi F, Silva M, Tatto E, Mendonça J, Araújo RF, Shikanai-Yasuda MA, Aras R. Acute Chagas disease outbreak associated with oral transmission. Revista da Sociedade Brasileira de Medicina Tropical. 2008;**41**(3):296-300

[15] OMS. Control of Chagas Disease. Second Report of the WHO Expert Committe. WHO TRS905 ed. Ginebra, Suiza;2002

[16] Macedo AM, Machado CR, Oliveira RP, Pena SD. *Trypanosoma cruzi*: Genetic structure of populations and relevance of genetic variability to the pathogenesis of Chagas disease. Memórias do Instituto Oswaldo Cruz. 2004;**99**(1):1-12

[17] Zicker F, Smith PG, Netto JC, Oliveira RM, Zicker EM. Physical activity, opportunity for reinfection, and sibling history of heart disease as risk factors for Chagas cardiopathy. The American Journal of Tropical Medicine and Hygiene. 1990;**3**(5):498-505

[18] Hoff R, Teixeira RS, Carvalho JS. *Trypanosoma cruzi* in the cerebrospinal fluid during the acute stage of Chagas disease. The New England Journal of Medicine. 1978;**298**:604-606

[19] Viotti R, Vigliano C. Etiological treatment of chronic Chagas disease: Neglected evidence' by evidence-based medicine. Expert Review of Anti-Infective Therapy. 2007;**5**(4):717-726

[20] Viotti R, Alarcón de Noya B, Araujo-Jorge T, Grijalva MJ, Guhl F, López MC, Ramsey JM, Ribeiro I, Schijman AG, Sosa-Estani S, Torrico F, Gascon J. Latin American network for Chagas disease, NHEPACHA. Towards a paradigm shift in the treatment of chronic Chagas disease. Antimicrobial Agents and Chemotherapy. 2014;**58**(2):635-639

[21] Freilij H, Muller L, González Cappa AS. Direct diagnostic micromethod for acute and congenital Chagas disease. Journal of Clinical Microbiology 1983;**18**:277-290

[22] Rottenberg ME, de Titto EH, Cardoni RL, Segura EL. Immune response in *Trypanosoma cruzi* infection. Revista Argentina de Microbiología. 1991;**23**(2):101-121

[23] Gomes YM, Lorena VM, Luquetti AO. Diagnosis of Chagas disease: What has been achieved? What remains to be done with regard to diagnosis and follow up studies? Memórias do Instituto Oswaldo Cruz. 2009;**104**(1):115-121

[24] Vexenat Ade C, Santana JM, Teixeira AR. Cross-reactivity of antibodies in human infections by the kinetoplastid protozoa *Trypanosoma cruzi, Leishmania chagasi* and *Leishmania (viannia) braziliensis*. Revista do Instituto de Medicina Tropical de São Paulo. 1996;**38**(3):177-185

[25] Schechter M, Stevens AF, Luquetti AO, Snary D, Allen AK, Miles MA. Prevalence of antibodies to 72-kilodalton glycoprotein (GP72) in patients with Chagas' disease and further evidence of zymodeme-associated expression of GP72 carbohydrate epitopes. Infection and Immunity. 1986;**53**(3):547-552

[26] Umezawa ES, Silveira JF. Serological diagnosis of Chagas disease with purified and defined *Trypanosoma cruzi* antigens. Memórias do Instituto Oswaldo Cruz. 1999; **94**(1):285-288

[27] Hernández P, Heimann M, Riera C, Solano M, Santalla J, Luquetti AO, Beck E. Highly effective serodiagnosis for Chagas disease. Clinical and Vaccine Immunology. 2010; **17**(10):1598-1604

[28] Norma Oficial Mexicana NOM-032-SSA2-2002. Para la vigilancia epidemiológica, prevención y control de enfermedades transmitidas por vector [Internet]. 2002. Available from: http://www.salud.gob.mx/unidades/cdi/nom/032ssa202.html [Accessed: August 2017]

[29] Briones MR, Souto RP, Stolf BS, Zingales B. The evolution of two *Trypanosoma cruzi* subgroups inferred from rRNA genes can be correlated with the interchange of American mammalian faunas in the Cenozoic and has implications to pathogenicity and host specificity. Molecular and Biochemical Parasitology. 1999;**104**(2):219-232

[30] Marcili A, Lima L, Valente VC, Valente SA, Batista JS, Junqueira ACV, Souza AI, da Rosa JA, Campaner M, Lewis MD, Llewellyn MS, Miles MA, Teixeira MMG. Comparative phylogeography of *Trypanosoma cruzi* (TcII): New hosts, association with terrestrial ecotopes, and spatial clustering. Infection, Genetics and Evolution. 2009;**9**(6):1265-1274

[31] Fernandes CD, Murta SM, Cerávolo IP, Krug LP, Vidigal PG, Steindel M, Nardi N, Romanha AJ. Characterization of *Trypanosoma cruzi* strains isolated from chronic chagasic patients, triatomines and opossums naturally infected from the state of Rio Grande do Sul, Brazil. Memórias do Instituto Oswaldo Cruz. 1997;**92**(3):343-351

[32] Tibayrenc M, Ayala FJ. The clonal theory of parasitic protozoa: 12 years on. Trends in Parasitology. 2002;**18**(9):405-410

[33] Zingales B, Miles MA, Campbell DA, Tibayrenc M, Macedo AM, Teixeira MM, Schijman AG, Llewellyn MS, Lages-Silva E, Machado CR, Andrade SG, Sturm NR. The revised *Trypanosoma cruzi* subspecific nomenclature: Rationale, epidemiological relevance and research applications. Infection, Genetics and Evolution. 2012;**12**(2):240-253

[34] Marinho CR, Bucci DZ, Dagli ML, Bastos KR, Grisotto MG, Sardinha LR, Baptista CR, Gonçalves CP, Lima MR, Alvarez JM. Pathology affects different organs in two mouse strains chronically infected by a *Trypanosoma cruzi* clone: A model for genetic studies of Chagas' disease. Infection and Immunity. 2004;**72**(4):2350-2357

[35] Espinoza B, Rico T, Sosa S, Oaxaca E, Vizcaino-Castillo A, Caballero ML, Martínez I. Mexican *Trypanosoma cruzi* (Tc-I) strains with different degrees of virulence induce diverse humoral and cellular immune responses in a murine experimental infection model. Journal of Biomedicine and Biotechnology. 2010;**2010**:1-10. DOI: 10.1155/2010/890672

[36] López-Olmos V, Pérez-Naser N, Piñero D, Ortega E, Hernández R, Espinoza B. Biological characterization and genetic diversity of Mexican isolates of *Trypanosoma cruzi*. Acta Tropica. 1998;**69**:239-254

[37] Zuñiga J, Tur M, Milocco S, Piñeiro R. Ciencia y tecnología en protección y experiment-ación animal. 1st ed. Vol. 682. McGraw-Hill Interamericana: Mexico; 2001

[38] Benavides F, Guénet J. Manual de genética de roedores de laboratorio: principios básicos y aplicaciones. Sociedad Española para las Ciencias del Animal de Laboratorio (SECAL) ed. Universidad de Alcalá; 2003. 312 p

[39] Institute of laboratory animals National Research Council. Guía para el cuidado y uso de animales de laboratorio. Academia Nacional de Medicina. 2002;**39**:148 p

[40] Andrade LO, Machado CR, Chiari E, Pena SD, Macedo AM. Differential tissue distribution of diverse clones of *Trypanosoma cruzi* in infected mice. Molecular and Biochemical Parasitology. 1999;**100**(2):163-172

[41] Nisimura LM, Estato V, de Souza EM, Reis PA, Lessa MA, et al. Acute Chagas Disease Induces Cerebral Microvasculopathy in Mice. Public Library of Science Negl Trop Dis 2014;**8**(7):e2998. DOI: 10.1371/journal.pntd.0002998

4

Chagas Cardiomyopathy: Role of Sustained Host-Parasite Interaction in Systemic Inflammatory Burden

Rodolfo A Kölliker-Frers, Matilde Otero-Losada, Gabriela Razzitte, Mariela Calvo, Justo Carbajales and Francisco Capani

Abstract

The economic and social burden associated with Chagas disease morbidity and mortality is regrettably large in Latin America causing more deaths than does any other parasitic disease. Inflammatory dilated cardiomyopathy is, by far, the most important clinical consequence of *Trypanosoma cruzi* infection. The insidious persistence of this parasite determines chronic myocarditis progression. The clinical outcome is multifactorial and depends on the particular parasite strain and virulence factors, the infective load and route of infection, the parasite ability to by-pass the protective immune response, the intensity and type of immune response during the acute infective phase, and the host genetic background. From the immunological viewpoint, host control of *T. cruzi* has been shown to depend on both humoral and cell-mediated adaptive responses and from the innate immune system. In this review, we discuss the most relevant literature conveying information on the relevance of identifying a subset of systemic inflammatory molecules as potential markers of cardiovascular risk morbidity and mortality in patients with Chagas disease. Concurrently, a direct role for the parasite in the perpetuation of myocardial inflammation is substantiated. Ultimately, host-parasite interactions determine the course of the ongoing systemic inflammation and the perpetuation of myocardial inflammation in genetically predisposed patients.

Keywords: Chagas disease, myocarditis, cardiomyopathy, inflammation, immune system, cardiovascular risk

1. Introduction

Chagas disease is a parasitic disease caused by the *Trypanosoma cruzi* that affects over 12 million people in Central and South America, causing more deaths than any other disease of its kind. Large migrations of infected people from the endemic areas are usually observed mainly in the United States of America and Europe. The most frequent cardiac complications of chronic Chagas disease are left ventricular dilation and dysfunction, aneurysm, congestive heart failure, thromboembolism, ventricular arrhythmias, and sudden cardiac death. Chagas disease diagnosis is based on serology, namely immunopositivity for immunoglobulin G antibodies to *T. cruzi.*

Inflammatory dilated cardiomyopathy is, by far, the most important clinical consequence of *T. cruzi* infection. The chronic chagasic cardiomyopathy (CCC) is roughly progressive, and its treatment does not differ from that of any other non-chagasic cardiomyopathy in the absence of strong evidence. Clinical symptoms usually include dyspnea, palpitations, precordial pain, syncope and eventually, sudden death.

Epidemiological data show high mortality and morbidity resulting from the cardiovascular disease in chagasic patients. However, there are no hints to suspect cardiovascular risk in the silent period of the disease (asymptomatic form). Noticeably, inflammatory factors are upraised during the silent period of the Chagas disease. Like atherogenesis, immune-inflammatory-mediated effector mechanisms commanded by Th1/Th17 cells are involved in the pathophysiology of Chagas disease, having a similar histological hallmark which includes Th1/Th17 cells, macrophages, and a characteristic cytokine profile.

Host control of the *T. cruzi* appears to depend on both humoral and cell-mediated adaptive responses, and on the innate immune system as well [1]. The cytokines strongly activate multiple functions relevant to cardiovascular homeostasis. According to the literature on the subject, there is robust evidence of a systemic upraised level of inflammatory mediators in patients with Chagas disease suggesting that the interplay between the parasite aggressiveness and the host immune response might have a key role in the perpetuation of myocardial inflammation.

The role of the parasitemia is more controversial associated with immunosuppression, disease reactivation, and disease severity. Due to the arousal of a strong and specific immune response against the parasite, nearly two-thirds infected people become protected and may stay in an indeterminate stage of the infection characterized by low parasitemia level for 10 or even up to 40 years after the prime infection. The other one-third infected people, however, develop symptoms, entering the symptomatic chronic stage of infection typically characterized by cardiomyopathy.

The antigenic stimulation though persists all over the chronic stage. Then, the clinical outcome depends on multiple factors like parasite persistence, the particular *T. cruzi* strain, the infective load and virulence factors, the route of infection and sidestepping the host immune response by the parasite, the strength of the immune response at any time, and of course, genetic predisposition [2]. In fact, the sustained parasite-host immunity interactions induce systemic inflammatory mediators' upregulation and fibrosis, both crucially involved in myocardial tissue damage and the resulting disturbances in the cardiac conduction system, mainly affecting the autonomic ganglia, nerves, and the microvasculature.

Unlike the study of the classical risk factors, research studies on how inflammatory status affects the development and determines the progression of cardiomyopathy have not yet identified or clinically validated relevant biomarkers [3]. Interestingly, secluded evidence suggests that the inflammatory status might be associated with increased morbidity and mortality. Deepening our understanding of the pathophysiology of Chagas disease, it will make way to identifying new molecular targets for the design of CCC prophylactic vaccines and therapeutic drugs.

2. Cardiomyopathy genes

Dilated cardiomyopathies (DCM) are characteristically defined by the presence of left ventricular dilatation, and contractile dysfunction [4]. Genetic mutations that involve genes encoding the cytoskeleton sarcomere, nuclear envelope proteins and others account for up to 35% of the total cases. Hypertrophic cardiomyopathies (HCM) and dilated (DCM) cardiomyopathies are heart muscle diseases related to genes variants encoding sarcomere proteins [5]. Among these proteins, the most common are the β-myosin heavy chain (MYH7) [6], the cardiac myosin-binding protein C (MYPBC3) while the myosin light chain (MYL3) and the regulatory myosin light chain (MYL2) are rare [7]. Certain variants in sarcomere genes also cause DCM, albeit less frequently. Of note, variant location does not absolutely predict whether it will trigger HCM or DCM.

Heart failure associated with cardiomyopathies is often caused by mutations in sarcomeric genes, resulting in contractile dysfunction and cellular damage. This may stimulate the production of a robust proinflammatory response. Intriguingly, flow cytometry analysis revealed a significant increase in total macrophages and classically activated proinflammatory (M1) macrophages in DCM hearts as compared with normal hearts. Serum cytokine analysis in dilated cardiomyopathy hearts showed a striking increase in interleukin IL-6 in rodents. Furthermore, RNA-seq analysis revealed the upregulation of inflammatory pathways in DCM hearts. Altogether, these data indicate a robust proinflammatory response in DCM hearts, likely in response to cellular damage triggered by an MYBPC3 mutation and the resultant contractile dysfunction [8]. In addition, other genes have been implicated in DCM, particularly the monocyte chemoattractant protein-1 gene polymorphism [9].

The epigenetic factors that contribute to myocarditis include consumption of alcohol or drugs, exposure to toxins, and metabolic and endocrine disturbances. The typically presenting symptoms are related to congestive heart failure, and can also include circulatory collapse, arrhythmias, and thromboembolic events [10].

3. Anatomopathological findings of Chagas cardiomyopathy

Chagas disease is typified in the WHO classification within the group of specific diseases of the myocardium. Alternatively, the denomination of cardioneuropathy has been proposed to express the frequent and severe importance of the autonomic affectation and the consequent dysautonomia associated with the functional and clinical alterations. The observed

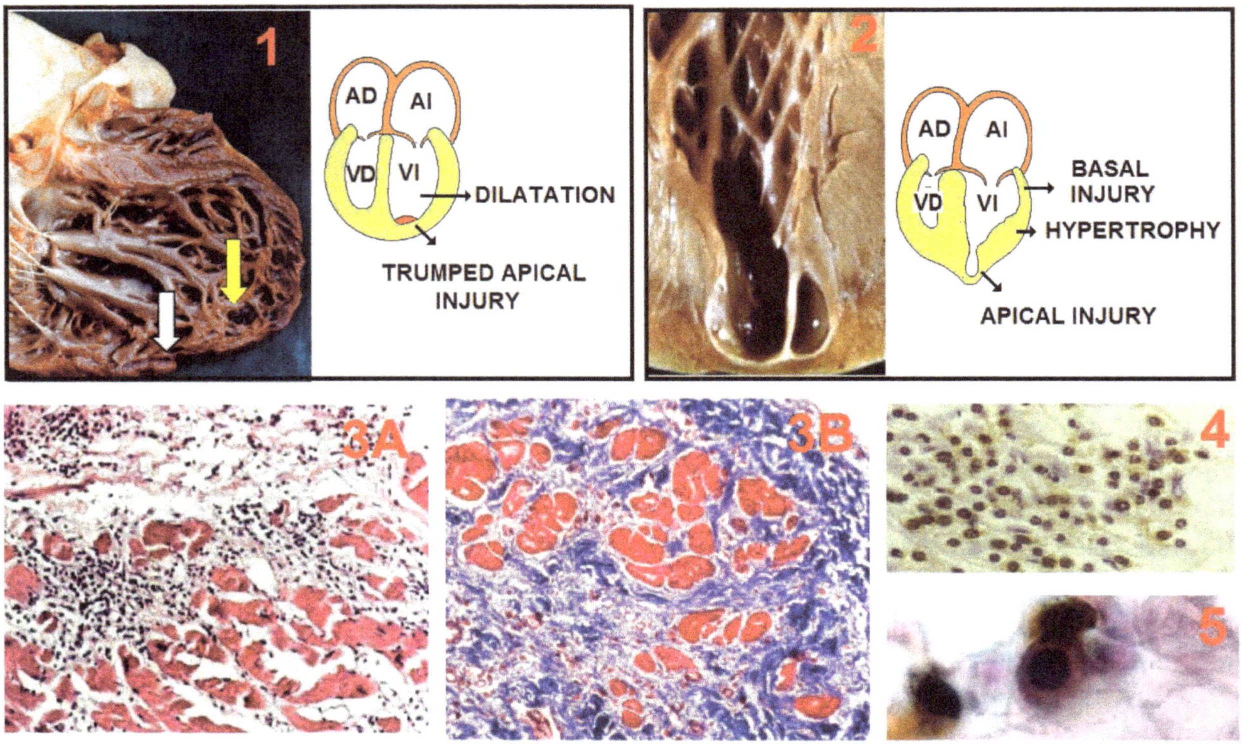

Figure 1. Anatomopathological findings. Figure courtesy of Dr. José Milei. Panel 1, left. High-grade heart dilatation. Thining of the apical wall of the left ventricle (white arrow) and cavitary thrombus (yellow arrow). Panel 1, right. Schematic representation. Panel 2, left. Characteristic apical aneurysm. Panel 2, right. Schematic representation. Panels 3–5. Histological features. Panels 3A and 3B. Microscopically, myocardial lesions consisted of a chronic inflammatory process with fibrotic scars and extensive mononuclear infiltrates. Panel 4. Immunostaining for T lymphocyte. Positive cells express CD45R0 antigen (brown); specialized myocardial cells have almost disappeared. Extensive mononuclear infiltrate, the majority of them being T lymphocytes. X20. Panel 5. Double immunostaining for the simultaneous demonstration of T lymphocytes (CD45RO) and macrophages (CD68). T lymphocytes (brown) in close contact with a macrophage (pinky cytoplasm). X1000.

macroscopic alterations are: (a) cardiomegaly (more than 500 g weight) and (b) characteristic apical lesion associated with localized parietal thinning, rarely presenting as posterior basal or parietal, or an apex aneurysm. Some authors propose two characteristic morphological types of chronic chagasic cardiopathy: "type I" or concentric, is characterized by a predominance of left ventricular hypertrophy with little dilatation or none, and circumscribed closed apical lesion and "type II" or eccentric, characterized by a wide dilatation and opening of the apical zone and frequently associated with thrombosis. Pathological evolution can progress from the concentric to eccentric type (**Figure 1**).

4. Clinical expression of the acute phase of Chagas disease

The Chagas disease presents two phases [10]. The initial acute phase, lasting for about 2 months after the infection and characterized by high parasitemia and parasite invasion to the tissues, is asymptomatic or shows mild unspecific symptoms. In this phase, symptomatic patients usually develop characteristic skin lesions or unilateral purplish swelling of the lids, usually known as the Romana's sign, and can present fever, headache, difficulty in breathing, lymphadenitis, vague myalgia, and abdominal or chest pain. In this phase too, immunosuppression, and the decreased inflammatory response result in increased parasite load in locally infected tissues upon generalized tissue invasion [11].

5. Clinical expression of the chronic phase of Chagas disease

To date, regardless the chronic phase be asymptomatic or symptomatic with cardiological alterations, the prognosis on the eventual development of heart disease in a given patient is not feasible.

5.1. Clinical asymptomatic expression of the chronic phase

The reason most patients with Chagas do not develop heart disease is uncertain. The first studies suggested that asymptomatic patients without clinical and cardiological alterations and the general population had a similar cardiovascular risk, but over time, epidemiological data suggest a higher risk than presumed.

Collectively, the studies highlight the importance of studying the early inflammatory parameters indicative of early cardiovascular damage, evaluating potential implication on morbidity and mortality, and prognostic and therapeutic relevance.

5.2. Clinical symptomatic expression of the chronic phase

The clinical expression of the chronic phase usually manifests as alterations in the cardiac conduction system, mainly arrhythmogenesis and dysrhythmias derived from the fibrotic and atrophic lesions compromising the AV nodule, and the His bundle and branches, and autonomic dysfunction as well. Dysautonomia may affect blood pressure and cardiac frequency, eventually leading to orthostatic hypotension, syncope, and heart failure. Myocardial alterations are associated with chronic inflammation, fibrous hypertrophy, fibrosis, myocytolysis, tissue depletion of neurons, and vascular damage contributing to sudden death or heart failure. Some clinical features may result from upstream molecular mimicry and cardioactive autoantibodies production. Patients with chagasic cardiomyopathy produce anti-ß1 and -ß2 adrenergic, and anti-M2 cholinergic autoantibodies in the heart. These autoantibodies, originally directed against the parasite, would indistinctly recognize similar antigenic determinants in the host, a phenomena known as mimicry.

6. Factors that define blood inflammatory outcome in Chagas disease

The sustained systemic inflammatory burden may result from many host-parasite interactions, whereby the interplay of the natural and adaptive immune host response with the parasite will result in a varying degree of tissue damage, host aggression, and clinical outcome.

Then, the perpetuation of the Chagas disease inflammatory phenotype [10] is critical in understanding the complexity of the clinical outcome given that immunological homeostasis in chronically infected hosts could be spoiled by both parasite and host immune molecules and cells [10].

6.1. Factors that promote parasite evasion and persistence

The presence of the parasite [11] or its products like DNA, and other constitutive molecules in blood, myocardium, and the autonomic tissues lead to sustained immunological stimulation and *T. cruzi* evasive strategies. Today, the DNA amplification by polymerase chain reaction and other sensitive assays allow detecting parasites or their components in chronic symptomatic patients.

6.1.1. Parasitemia and sustained antigen stimulation

There is scarce evidence linking Chagas seropositivity with cardiovascular events in asymptomatic patients [9]. The perpetuation of *T. cruzi* antigens in cardiac tissue and the immune-mediated dysautonomia might be implicated in the cardiovascular pathogenesis [12] being responsible for the asymptomatic-to-the *cardiac* phenotype transition in Chagas disease. Different studies have shown the relevance of effector or memory CD4/CD8 lymphocytes and their effector cytokines not only in controlling parasite multiplication over the course of acute and chronic infection, but also participating in the pathogenesis of chronic Chagas disease [12]. The Th1 lymphocytes are critical in the control of Chagas disease during the acute stage unlike the chronic phase when they could be harmful. The adoptive transfer of *T. cruzi*-specific CD8+ T cells confers mice partial protection from *T. cruzi* inoculation [13], while cardiac damage may still develop. Conversely, the human being develops myocarditis in the presence of $CD4^+$ and $CD8^+$ T cells, and parasite components as well [14].

6.1.2. Cruzi virulence and immunomodulatory factors

Cruzi parasites cause pathology depending on factors like the parasite species and strains, the route of infection [15], and the host genetic background. Different parasite strains coexist in infected patients, and in natural reservoirs in domestic and peridomestic areas. The strain-dependent immunomodulatory effects of the parasite might influence parasite-host interactions [14]. Mucin-like sialic acid-acceptor glycoproteins and other parasite cell membrane products determine *Cruzi* virulence [15]. One of the hallmark parasite-derived molecules are the glycol-inositol-phospholipids (GIPLs) covering the parasite cell surface that alter the B cell compartment, work as TLR4 agonists, and mediate proinflammatory effects [16, 17]. In sum, *T. cruzi* virulence factors actively subvert the host immune system leading to chronic infection [18–21].

6.1.3. White adipose tissue is an immune active endocrine organ

Another survival strategy of *Cruzi* parasites is targeting the adipose tissue (AT) [22], both brown (BAT) and white (WAT), the largest endocrine organ in the body shaped by adipocytes, fibroblasts, macrophages, and endothelial cells. The adipose tissue is involved in many physiologic functions including energy homeostasis and immunity [23], and might warrant long-term parasite persistence by providing a safe reservoir to avoid the host-defense mechanisms. Then, immune system suppression would result in parasite recrudescence and multiple tissue invasion [24]. Besides, the AT might be the major site for parasite reactivation as indicated by the finding of parasite-derived DNA in AT [25] in patients with CCC [25]. Likely, the AT serves as a parasite reservoir favoring opportunistic reinfection upon immunosuppression, as observed in chagasic transplanted or HIV patients, or those under immunosuppressive therapies [26]. As infection increases the level of TLR4 and TLR9, and of the mRNA of cytokines, chemokines, and of their receptors, the adipose tissue appears to be both a target and a sensor of parasitic infection even in the early, latent stage of *T. cruzi* infection. Recently, the *T. cruzi* was detected in the adipose tissue of chronically infected individuals [25].

6.2. Host-protective and pathogenic anti-*T. cruzi* immune-mediated-response

6.2.1. The innate immune system

Innate, nonspecific, immunity involves any pathogen-eliminating mechanism triggered promptly without memory requirement. The acute nonspecific inflammatory molecules serve not only as 'gateway' signals, generating conditions unfavorable for the invading agent, but they are also implicated in chronic inflammatory diseases. Chronic sustained inflammation actually contributes to cardiac hypertrophy.

6.2.1.1. Toll-like receptors agonists expressed by T. cruzi activate inflammatory pathways

Nonspecific immune system cells modify their functional repertoire (phagocytic activity, activation, antigenic presentation, migration, and adhesion) through pathogen-associated molecular pattern recognition receptors (PAMPs) like the toll-like receptors (TLRs), many of which can recognize several types of structurally unrelated PAMPs. These receptors trigger proinflammatory pathways' activation interacting with their pathogen-derived ligands, and even with endogenous molecules, and releasing effector molecules like cytokines. This signal cascade triggers the expression of cytokine genes, where the type of TLRs bound determines the type of response.

Different *T. cruzi*-derived molecules belong to the PAMPs family and act as TLR agonists inducing the secretion of inflammatory cytokines, chemokines, and the production of nitric oxide (NO) by cells of the monocytic lineage. In this regard, the first evidence was the identification of the trypomastigotes-derived glycosylphosphatidylinositol (tGPI) that anchors mucin-like glycoproteins (tGPI-mucins), as a potent agonist of the human TLR2 [27] inducing proinflammatory responses on cells which express normal levels of TLR2 and TLR4 (**Figure 2**).

Another epimastigote-derived GPI family member, the glycoinositolphospholipid characterized by a lipid moiety, induced TLR4-mediated NF-κB activation. Many GIPLs freely anchor at the surface membrane of all the parasite life-cycle stage forms, whether infective metacyclic trypomastigotes or epimastigotes forms and have pleiotropic properties [28]. The variable lipid moiety composition of different GPI anchors determines the TLR type specificity for TLR2 (alkylacylglycerol) or TLR4 (dihydroceramide).

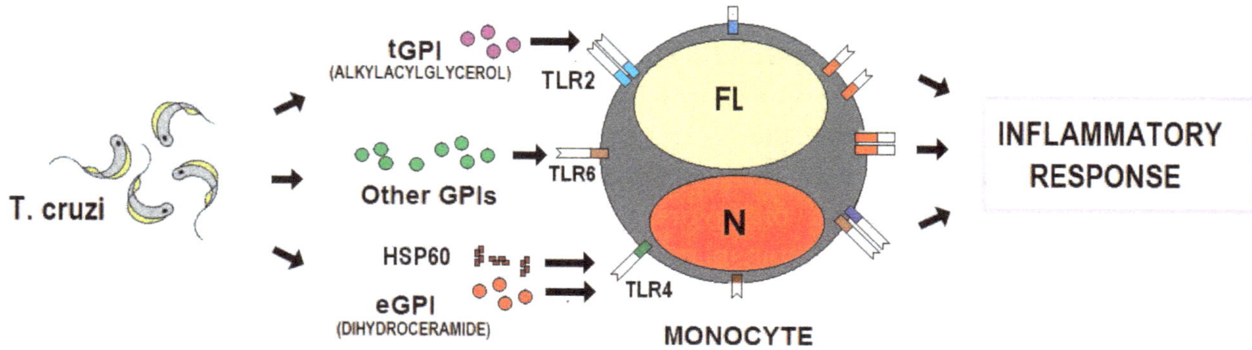

Figure 2. *T. cruzi* molecules PAMPs members are TLR agonists. The variable lipid moiety composition of different GPI determines whether their recognition is mediated by TLR2 (alkylacylglycerol) or TLR4 (dihydroceramide). TLR4 agonist triggers powerful proinflammatory molecules release. FL: Phagolysosome; GPI: Glycosylphosphatidylinositol; tGPI: Trypomastigotes-derived glycosylphosphatidylinositol; eGPI epimastigote-derived glycosylphosphatidylinositol, HSP: Heat shock protein.

6.2.1.2. Toll-like receptors and resistance to infection

Direct testing of the hypothesis that TLR triggering by PAMPs is crucial for host resistance to infection but is currently not possible due to unavailability of *T. cruzi* strains lacking the expression of any TLR agonist. Nevertheless, studying the course of infection in TLR-encoding genes-deficient mice, evaluating mortality, parasitemia, and several parameters of the innate and acquired immune responses have brought an additional understanding of the impact of impairing TLR-mediated recognition of *T. cruzi* in developing host susceptibility to the infection. In this regard, MyD88-deficient mice lacking the transducer of multiple TLR-signaling pathways first evidenced the crucial involvement of TLRs in host resistance to *T. cruzi* [29, 30].

6.2.1.3. Cardiac toll-like receptors increase in ischemia/reperfusion-induced cardiac hypertrophy

The development of cardiac hypertrophy involves TLR signaling so that MyD88 blockage attenuates cardiac hypertrophy and extracellular heat shock protein 70 (HSP70) induces cardiomyocyte inflammation [31, 32].

6.2.2. The adaptive immune system

The immune-mediated-pathology (IMP) links to parasite persistence inducing protective effector and autoimmune response and has been a subject of debate in CCC for years. Immune effector cells along with autoantibodies participate in both protective and pathogenic adaptive responses in CCC. Typically, histopathological examination in chronic myocarditis reveals inflammatory polymorphism with macrophages, eosinophils, mast cells, B and T lymphocytes, and granuloma cells, and a predominance of B cells and plasma cells in the epicardium and T cells in the myocardium, which progresses towards fibrosis. The mononuclear infiltrate and its mediators would be, at least partly, primarily responsible for myocardial damage [33].

6.2.2.1. *Autoimmunity*

At first post-infectious autoimmune myocarditis was proposed to reasonably explain the mismatch between myocardial areas showing parasite invasion and those with myocardial damage revealed by pathology examination that hampered reliably establishing Chagas disease pathogenesis.

- Cardiac epitopes share amino acid sequences with *T. cruzi* epitopes.
- The transfer of lymphocytes to syngeneic recipients produces inflammatory lesions in cardiac and nervous tissue.
- Chronic chagasic patients have autoantibodies in the bloodstream.
- Plasma cells obtained from murine myocardial lesions release anti-cardiac antibodies.
- T-lymphocytes obtained from human biopsies show cardiac muscle reactivity.

6.2.2.1.1. *Evidence derived from the autoreactive immune response*

While activation of autoreactive clones (possibly by polyclonal activation) occurs during the acute primary infection phase, autoantibodies appear to be generated during both the acute and chronic phases of the disease, likely perpetuated due to myocardial reactivity regardless of the etiologic agent. Both humoral and cellular cardiac autoimmunity might develop upon acute *T. cruzi* infection in the genetically susceptible host [34]. Another hypothesis sustained that autoimmunity develops only after sustained low-level stimulation of self-reactive cells over the chronic phase. Altogether, self-reactivity was initially proposed as a mechanism of tissue damage.

Many publications have mentioned the presence of cardiac tissue-parasite cross-reactivity. *T. cruzi* may induce antibodies and T cells also reactive to host antigens causing autoimmune reactions.

Certain antigens might induce nonspecific polyclonal activation, expanding clones that were in the anergic state as the polyclonal B cell activation associated with hypergammaglobulinemia and delayed specific humoral immunity reported in *T. cruzi* experimental infection in mice [35].

All in all, self-reactivity is accepted in Chagas disease though only subsidiarily contributing to myocardial tissue damage and deterioration as argued for the presence of autoantibodies and lymphocytes at the site of the lesion. Actually, immunosuppression not only does not cause improvement but rather aggravation of the course of the disease. Indeed, was self-reactivity relevant to injury, immunosuppression should be beneficial. Immunosuppression during acute infection reduces tissue inflammation while the parasite load increases in the infected tissues in mice. However, immunosuppression results in a generalized tissue invasion aggravating the disease. In chronically infected individuals, parasitemia is undetectable but any induced or acquired immunosuppression condition including pharmacological treatments,

AIDS, a transplant, an autoimmune disease, leukemia or pregnancy, may trigger reactivation. When immunosuppression occurs during the chronic stage, skeletal and cardiac muscle inflammation increases, allegedly explaining why a subset of patients presenting an insufficient or suboptimal immune response develop heart disease [36].

6.2.2.1.2. Evidence derived from molecular mimicry and the formation of cardioactive autoantibodies

Cardioactive substances from sera from chagasic patients. Subsequently they were characterized as antibodies with specificity towards the cardiac β-adrenergic receptors that acting as partial agonists increased mechanical tension and sinus beating frecuency in chagasic patients. The Cardiology Service of the Ramos Mejía Hospital contributed to the characterization of the anti-cardiac receptor reactions, and the results indicated that self-reactivity of this kind was caused by parasite epitopes with low affinity for cardiac receptors, later proved by the identification of anti-*T. cruzi* P ribosomal proteins in chagasic individuals. In *in vitro* or *ex vivo* experiments, IgG-enriched serum fractions obtained from chagasic patients modify baseline heart beating frequency in cultured cardiomyocytes, increase cardiac inotropism, and trigger atrioventricular blockage in isolated hearts. Rabbits immunized with the major immunogenic region of β-adrenergic receptors develop cardiomyopathies and malignant arrhythmias, and cardioactive antibodies have also been observed in other pathologies. Patients with ethiologically different chronic heart diseases like the idiopathic dilated cardiomyopathy or presenting primary electrical alterations produce chagasic IgG-like enriched fractions with antibody activity. Circulating autoantibodies to cardiac beta-adrenergic and muscarinic receptors may affect cardiac function in chagasic patients. The prevalence of anti-autonomic receptors antibodies was higher in patients with chronic chagasic heart disease and other forms of heart disease than in the healthy counterparts [36].

6.2.2.2. Immune origin of the disease and the localized inflammatory response

The 'tissue load of parasites' is associated with the 'severity of the lesion' and might predict not only the characteristics of the immune response in the acute or chronic (reactivation by immunosuppression) stages of the disease of the disease but also of the localized inflammatory response. Accordingly, tissue specificity would result from the local 'parasites persistence' in the site of inflammation. Whole, fractionated, or recombinant parasites immunization triggers inflammatory lesions and electrocardiographic alterations. The spectrum of clinical presentations might result from both the efficacy of the immune response during the acute stage and the parasite strain involved. Individuals infected with less virulent strains and immunocompetent hosts should become asymptomatic over the chronic stage (**Figure 3**). The immune response so results from the net balance of the *T. cruzi* strain immunogenic potency and the regulatory T cells and effector lymphocyte subpopulation Th1/Th17 during the infection. The IL-17 produced during experimental *T. cruzi* infection regulates Th1 cells differentiation and parasite-induced myocarditis. A low regulatory T cell activity and the frequency of IL-17-producing T cells correlate with CCC severity [37], not precluding a minor participation of the self-reactive immune reactions in producing injury.

Induced immunosuppression fails to cause relevant autoimmune-mediated damage for it aggravates rather than ameliorates the disease. Adoptive lymphocytes transfer to syngeneic

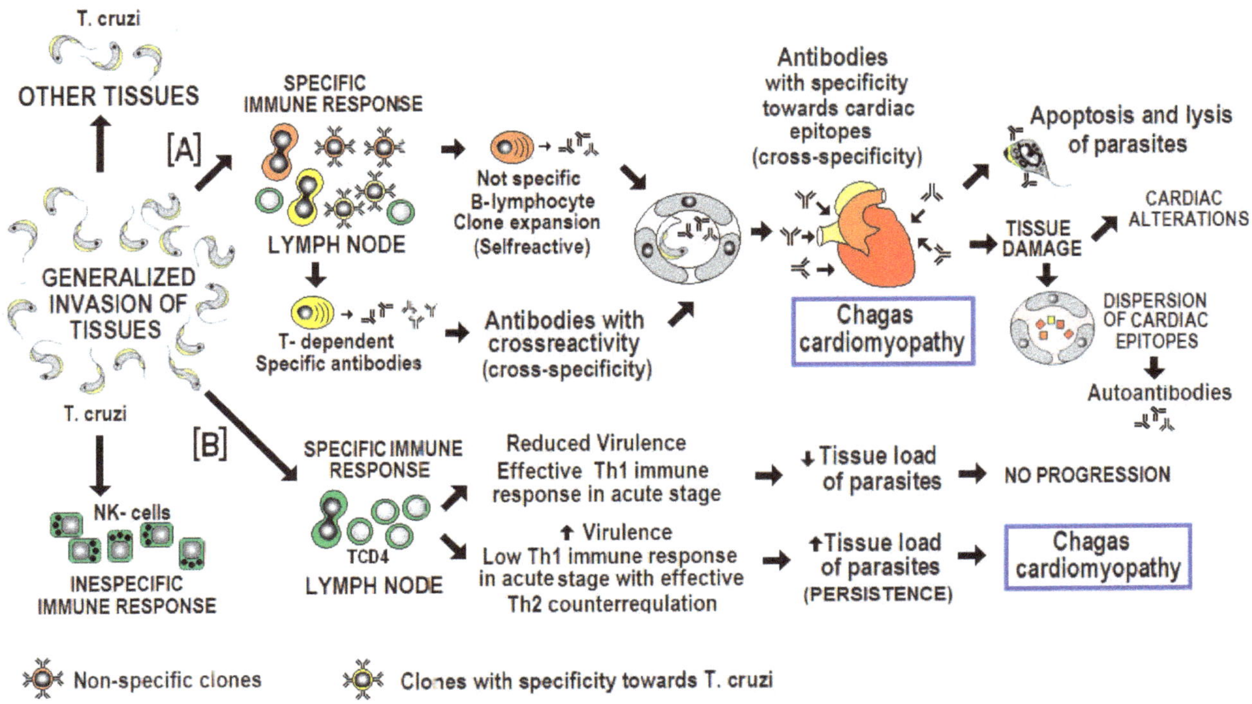

Figure 3. Possible mechanisms involved in the immunopathogenesis of Chagas disease. Although the immune system protects man from massive infection, he is unable to completely eliminate all parasites. (A) The humoral protective and immunopathogenic immune response to *T. cruzi* has been intensely studied. Although many questions remain, the antibody response is always present in infected individuals and many of the antibodies have a protective capacity. Several aspects are related to the presence of autoreactive antibodies in chagasic patients and in experimental chagasic models. The presence of similarities between the epitopes of the parasite and cardiac tissue leads to the expansion of autoreactive clones. Some authors argue that some autoantibodies should be due to the existence of polyclonal activation. Other autoantibodies may be the result of the autoantigen release of damaged tissue (epitopes dispersion epiphenomenon). (B) Th1 lymphocytes have great relevance in the control of the disease. The importance of the T-dependent response is evidenced by the observations recorded in immunosuppressed patients in whom the disease worsens. In vitro studies would indicate that the NK cell-mediated immune response (ADCC and natural cytotoxicity) could participate in the in vivo response. According to some authors the antigenic persistence would be the main mechanism inducing the inflammatory immune response in the chronic stage and IL17 seems to be involved in CCC. This interpretation postulates that the sustained activation of the immunoinflammatory response is the main cause of tissue damage.

recipients produces inflammation indicating that the T-response can effectively control the disease. The cellular immune response is critical in controlling *T. cruzi* infection, and the developed vaccine so far exacerbates damage and progression of the disease. Then, the vaccine either failed in enhancing the adequate response and/or its design requires further adjusting the epitopes. Of note, despite cellular control the infection, immune response persistence and cardiac infiltrated cells may cause injury. Finally, the contribution of autoantibodies is complex as it is likely involved in further enhancing cardiovascular damage.

7. Suppressor of cytokine signaling proteins, immune regulation, and dilated cardiomyopathy

Cell-cell signaling is an essential hallmark of multicellular organisms for communicating different cell populations [38] and is particularly crucial for the immune system function. The 'suppressor of cytokine signaling' (SOCS) plays a critical role in the regulation of all

SOCS type	Factor	Effect	References
SOCS3	G-CSF	Hematopoietic neutrophilia/inflammatory conditions	Chen et al. [35]
	IL-23 (↑IL17), (↑IFN-γ)	Enhance Th1 and Th17 polarization	Chen et al. [35]
	Leptin	Resistance to diet-induced obesity	Yang et al. [39]
	IL-6, (+IL-27)	Reduced CD8+ T cell proliferation	Yang et al. [39]
	TNF-γ, IL1β	Hypertrophy, fibrosis and inflammation	Liongue et al. [33]
	Global action	• Critical role in regulation of cytokine signaling • Control of hyperproduction of IL-10 and TGFβ • Promote Th2 response • Indirect sustained Th1 activity	Kinjyo et al. [34], Chen et al. [35]

Table 1. Main action of SOCS3 as a critical regulator.

crossroads of the cytokine-induced pathogenesis of dilated cardiomyopathy. The SOCS3 transgene induces Th2 responses, and SOCS3 gene deletion did not enhance Th1 polarization as expected but induced a negative regulator of the Treg subset with increased IL-10 and TGFβ production in mice [39, 41]. Not only SOCS3 is essential for G-CSF, IL-6, LIF, and leptin signaling, but is also an indirect regulator of IFNγ signaling and a negative regulator of IL-23 signaling, inducing IL-17-secreting T cells (Th17) polarization (**Table 1**).

The SOCS3 pathways are important, altering cardiac physiology by affecting molecular targets associated with myocardial changes implicated in structural pathologies. The SOCS3 proteins regulate specific cytokine pathways related to cardiac growth and enlargement and seem to be consistent with their roles critical regulators of hypertrophy, contractile dysfunction, and ventricular arrhythmias. They were, as their name suggests, first described as cytokine signaling inhibitors as observed for the Janus kinase/Signal Transducer and Activator of Transcription/Suppressor of Cytokine Signaling (JAK/STAT/SOCS) signaling pathway (JSS-SP). The remodeling by cytokine receptor signaling mediated by the JSS-SP provides a morphological basis explaining the pathogenesis of myocardial hypertrophy, fibrosis, and inflammation [41] in CCC. The inflammatory markers TNFα, and IL1-β represent potential targets in cardioprotection and therapy [42].

The SOCS3 protein is a key negative-feedback regulator of the gp130 receptor involved in signaling pertaining cardiac hypertrophy and survival. Activation of the gp130 without SOCS3 regulation leads to cardiac hypertrophy, in line with their roles as negative regulators of cardiac growth. Also, SOCS3 regulation on cardiac gp130 signaling participates in the pathogenesis of contractile dysfunction and ventricular arrhythmias. Consistently, human CCC is characterized by segmental left ventricular wall motion abnormalities (WMA), mainly in the early stages of the disease.

The failure of the SOCS3 protein, also a major negative regulator of both leptin, and insulin signaling, might participate in the pathogenesis of obesity, and associated metabolic abnormalities as found for diet-induced and genetic obesity, systemic inflammatory burden, and hyperlipidemia. In sum, the SOCS3 may be critically negative regulators of inflammation, cardiac hypertrophy, contractile dysfunction, and ventricular arrhythmias. However, our understanding of the origins of the individual pathway components and their assembly into a functional pathway has remained limited.

8. Long-lasting systemic inflammatory burden and clinical Chagas progression

The immune-inflammatory response plays a key role in cardiovascular damage [40, 41], and *T. cruzi*-derived molecules may sustain the TLR-mediated innate immune response inducing inflammatory cytokines and chemokines secretion. The adaptive immune response to Chagas antigens may protect the host from secondary reinfection, though damaging the CV system due to inflammation, and the associated connective repair (fibrosis).

Crossroads between "natural, and specific immunity effector cells and molecules" and "parasite persistence strategies in blood, adipose tissue, the heart, and other infected tissues" seem to contribute to cardiovascular risk. Tissue damage induces inflammatory reactions. Immune-activated pathways are the main contributors to systemic inflammation in human CCC by active crosstalk between different CVRFs, metabolic and immune-mediated innate and adaptive host-parasite interactions. The contribution of natural and specific immunity against Chagas antigens enhance systemic inflammatory burden (SIB). Certainly, the immune system is not the only source of inflammatory molecules, but other tissues also contribute to enhancing systemic inflammatory burden as the WAT which releases inflammatory cytokines.

In a recent study, the levels of IL1β, IL6, IL10, TGFβ, IL12, IL17, TNFα, and serum IFNα were different in either chronic asymptomatic or cardiac chagasic patients compared with healthy controls. The asymptomatic patients had a higher plasma TNFα concentration (eightfold) and IL10, and lower IFNα than in normal controls, suggesting a process of immune regulation. Neither the interaction with traditional CVRFs and their contribution to CVR nor control-matching for age, sex, weight, or BMI were considered in this study. The advent of noninvasive imaging techniques allows studying the relationship between inflammatory markers in subclinical atherosclerosis development. The association of many systemic diseases with an increase in the prevalence of cardiovascular diseases involves immunoinflammatory mediators related to chronic inflammation and cannot be explained by the classic CVRFs. Unlike the classical CVRFs like the lipid profile, the approaches based on the contribution of the inflammatory milieu to cardiovascular disease development have not yet allowed identifying clinically validated biomarkers regardless the evidence suggesting their association with increased morbidity, and mortality except CRP [43].

Scientific research is encouraged to delve into the important role suggested for the inflammatory response in the metabolism and control of the atherogenic potential [44]. Hypercholesterolemia and inflammation are certainly considered contributive partners in atherosclerosis.

Only lipid-related indicators like LDL- and HDL-cholesterol fractions, and triglycerides are currently recommended in predicting cardiovascular risk. Paradoxically, plasma total cholesterol level is accepted as a marker of relative CVR, though more than 50% of all cardiovascular events can occur in individuals with concentrations below the accepted normal total cholesterol level [56].

With a complete understanding of atherogenesis, the atherothrombotic markers, and the already mentioned inflammatory markers [45] are potentially available for CVR estimation.

Recent data suggest that the measurement of related inflammatory markers may improve cardiovascular risk assessment. Certain markers being evaluated include a group termed as "cellular" cytokines (e.g., IL1, IL2, IL12p40, IL15, IL17, TNF, IFN, and IFN), and "humoral" cytokines (e.g.IL4, IL5, IL6, IL10, and IL13), growth factors and angiogenic [e.g., EGF, VEGF, FGF, granulocyte colony-stimulating factor (G-CSF), granulocyte-macrophage-colony-stimulating factor (GM-CSF)], and chemokines [e.g. CCL2 (MCP1), CCL3 (MIP1), CCL11 (Eotaxin), and CXCL8 (IL8)]. The role of some of them in cardiovascular pathogenesis is described below.

8.1. Soluble ICAM1

Inflammatory stimuli trigger a dramatic increase in ICAM1 expression on the vascular surface. Later on, inflammatory cytokines induce the endothelial expression of VCAM1 which, like ICAM1, interacts with leukocyte integrins promoting the firm adhesion of leukocytes to the surface of the endothelial cells. After proteolytic cleavage, the endothelial ICAM1 molecules can be released into the circulation as soluble molecules (ICAM1s), the level of which correlates with CVRFs like smoking, hypertension, hypercholesterolemia, and hypertriglyceridemia and with acute phase reactants like the PCR, and increases in patients with coronary disease. The circulating level of the soluble forms of ICAM-1, VCAM-1, selectin, and CD44 are remarkably high during the acute *T. cruzi* infection, while the soluble forms of VCAM-1 and P-selectin increase in chronic infection [46–52]. As inflammation markers, the soluble forms of ICAM-1 might be notably higher in patients with DCM [53–55].

8.2. Chemotactic monocyte-1 protein

An important early step in atherosclerosis is the adhesion of monocytes to activated endothelial cells. The endothelium produces several molecules critical in the proatherogenic events like the endothelium-released MCP1 which contributes to increased monocyte recruitment, and activation of nuclear factor kappa B (NF-kB) involved in the transcription of many functional genes in the inflammatory process [64]. Recently, CCL2/MCP-1 has emerged as a critical factor in infectious and autoimmune myocarditis, is largely produced in *T. cruzi*-loaded mice hearts, and it promotes macrophages infiltration and parasite destruction. *T. cruzi*-infected CCL2$^{(-/-)}$ mice developed higher parasitemia, dying prematurely, and showed increased levels of TNF, IFN-gamma, and IL-10 in plasma, clinical signs of systemic inflammatory response. Cardiac density of amastigote nests was associated with leukocytes infiltrates. Other studies demonstrated that CCL2 contributes to the reduction of parasite growth by controlling the distribution, cellular composition, and the status of inflammatory infiltrates in acute *T. cruzi* infection [21]. More recent evidence shows that polymorphisms involved key molecules related to innate immunity, and that cell migration plays a critical role in genetic susceptibility to CCC [56–58].

8.3. Interleukin 10

Within the group of the so-called anti-inflammatory cytokines, the human IL10 is associated with an anti-atherogenic action reducing inflammation. Cytokine knockout of the Th1 inhibitor IL10 increase vascular lesions [59]. IL10 has strong regulatory properties on macrophages and T cells, and negatively regulates many cellular processes involved in atherosclerotic plaque development and stability.

A recent study revealed comparable serum cytokine levels in cardiac chagasic and asymptomatic patients though IL10 level was higher, and IFNγ level was lower in the former suggesting a greater regulatory activity in cardiac patients. Presumably, the IL10 level is ineffective to restore homeostasis. Likewise, circulating IL10 increases in patients with DCM.

8.4. Transforming growth factor beta (TGFβ)

The transforming growth factor beta is produced by different cell types including adipocytes, macrophages, endothelial cells, smooth muscle cells, platelets, and regulatory T cells. The TGFβ1 factor stimulates PAI-1 release and suppresses leptin release from the human adipose tissue. It inhibits atherogenesis modulating T-lymphocyte activity rather than modulating the prothrombotic and fibrinogenic activity, as confirmed in TGF II receptor type-KO models. It is also involved in regulating host tissue fibrosis. The oral administration of GW788388, a novel kinase inhibitor type associated with TGFß I and II receptors, remarkably increased cardiac cells' survival time and decreased cardiac fibrosis, offering a potential alternative to the current asymptomatic Chagas treatment. However, the cost-benefit balance is uncertain since circulating TGFβ modulates the pathogenic effector immune response avoiding immune damage but exacerbating fibrosis. Recent studies indicate that the deep alterations induced by circulating TGFβ increase in patients with DCM with or without cardiac fibrosis [60–62].

8.5. Interleukin-17A

The interleukin-17A cytokine released by Th17 cells is elevated in plasma in atherogenesis mice models. Increased serum levels of IL17 and IFNγ are found in patients with coronary atherosclerosis. The proatherogenicity of IL17A results from the monocytes/macrophages recruitment into the aortic wall [63]. The differentiation of Th17 depends on IL23 and IL6 released by myeloid dendritic cells, IL1, IL6, and IL21 derived from macrophages and T lymphocytes [64]. In humans, TGFα acts as a negative regulator of IL17. For years, Chagas-associated cardiac damage has been attributed to immunological dysregulation, including an imbalance between pro- and anti-inflammatory cytokines, Th1-Th2 immune deflection, and regulatory T cell activity. Recently, IL17 produced during experimental *T. cruzi* infection regulated Th1 differentiation, and parasite-induced myocarditis. The decrease in IL10 and IL17 cytokines' production in association with high levels of IFNγ, and TNFα correlates with the severity of human chagasic cardiomyopathy. This immunological imbalance might be causally related to a poor suppressor activity of the regulating T cells controlling myocardial inflammation. Finally, the derived IL17A-fibroblast and the derived -GM-CSF-macrophage axis are potential targets for the treatment of DCM and related inflammatory cardiac disorders [64].

8.6. C-reactive protein

The CRP marker level is used as a predictor of future cardiovascular events, being a good estimator of mortality risk in different contexts, particularly in metabolic syndrome in the general population. It has also been suggested as a direct stimulator of plaque formation decreasing endothelial nitric oxide synthase (eNOS) activity [65], and implicated in other deleterious effects. *In vitro* studies provide evidence of the proatherogenic direct effects of CRP as found in endothelial dysfunction, Also, an increase CRP serum level in chagasic patients has been associated with a greater progression towards heart failure. High hs-CRP level is associated with a higher incidence of the long-term combined endpoint of all-cause mortality and hospitalization in patients with DCM. Besides, oxidative stress molecules and hs-CRP are both associated with heart failure and damage severity in patients with DCM [66, 67].

8.7. Tumor necrosis factor alpha (TNFα)

The pleiotropic TNFα cytokine is one of the most potent mediators of inflammation. It is associated with an increased CVR. It can induce proatherogenic lipid alterations, including increased LDL-cholesterol and HDL-cholesterol [68] and promote hypercoagulability inducing tissue factor (TF) expression in endothelial tissue and suppressing anticoagulant activity through activated thrombomodulin-activated protein C [69]. It also induces endothelial dysfunction through decreasing nitric oxide and regulating adhesion molecules, an early critical step in atherogenesis. Several investigations in animal and human models provide convincing evidence on the action of TNFα as one of the major regulators of vascular homeostasis. Blocking of TNFα results in a significant decrease in Lp (a), homocysteine levels and increases in Apo AI, triglycerides, and Apo B concentration. The prolonged use of TNFα blocking agents interferes with proatherogenic action, reducing the incidence of cardiovascular events. Taken together these studies confirm a critical role of TNFα at the prothrombotic, proinflammatory and metabolic level. An association between TNFα levels with heart failure was observed in chagasic patients. Autopsies specimens confirmed the presence of cardiac inflammatory cell infiltrates showing a Th1 cytokines pattern. Chronic asymptomatic chagasic patients have TNFα plasma concentrations roughly eightfold higher than healthy controls, and TNFα may play a role in progression to heart failure, The increased level of TNFα might also be related to disease severity in chronic Chagas disease as found in patients with DCM. Interestingly TNFα blockage aggravates experimental CCC [70, 73].

8.8. Interleukin-1 (IL-1)

The IL-1 interleukin is a crucial proinflammatory mediator in acute and chronic inflammation, and also a powerful innate immune response inducer. It induces the synthesis and expression of several hundreds of secondary inflammatory mediators in different diseases [74, 75]. The inflammatory response is associated with the expression of numerous cytokines [interferon gamma, interferon alpha, tumor necrosis factor (TNF), and interleukin-3 (IL-3)], which stimulate xanthine oxidoreductase (XOR). The main circulating form of IL-1 is the IL-1β, initially synthesized as the pro IL-1β a precursor which is activated by caspase-1 cleavage in the setting of a macromolecular structure known as the inflammasome [71]. Many potential triggers of the inflammasome have been identified, including microbial agents, ischemia, damaged cells, cholesterol crystals, and TLRs ligands such as danger-associated molecular patterns (DAMPs) or pathogen-associated molecular patterns (PAMPs). The IL-1 molecule has been associated with endothelial dysfunction, hypertension, heart failure, and diabetes [75]. Recent studies indicate that XOR and XO serum levels are considerably increased in both cardiac and asymptomatic patients following *T. cruzi* invasion. Serum levels of IL-1β could be used in predicting the long-term outcome of patients affected by idiopathic DCM [71, 76]. Cardiac fibrosis and heart failure progression in inflammatory dilated DCM might be related to the myeloid differentiation factor-88/IL-1β signaling pathway [72, 77].

8.9. Interleukin-6

IL-6 provides a link between innate and adaptive immunity through the regulation of leukocyte activation, differentiation, and proliferation. During the acute and chronic inflammatory response, macrophages release TNFα in the presence of a variety of stimuli including atherogenic factors. In the macrophages, TNFα triggers the release of TNFα, and of more IL1B, which stimulates endothelial cells to produce IL6 and IL8. To date, both the scientific outcome of experimental studies, and the abundant clinical evidence in atherosclerosis indicate that low-intensity sustained inflammation plays a key role in atherosclerotic plaque formation, progression, and destabilization leading to clinical endpoints like myocardial infarction, sudden death, or stroke. The underlying mechanisms are still unclear, despite the intense research over the past two decades. Both IL6 and its signaling events contribute to atherosclerotic plaque development and destabilization. Increased levels of IL6 [78, 79] and CRP, an accepted CVRF, can also contribute to atherosclerosis and arterial thrombosis by activating tissue factor production, increasing adhesiveness of endothelial cells, fibrinogen and factor VIII and stimulating platelet production, and aggregation [91]. In addition, smooth muscle cells (SMC) also produce abundant IL-6. Other inflammatory factors generated by adipocytes like IL6, CRP, and TNFα are also implicated in the pathophysiology of the metabolic syndrome. The polymorphism of IL6 genes correlates with the severity of coronary artery disease, and with myocardial infarction risk [80, 81], but not with carotid atherosclerosis, which seems to be independent, These findings clearly suggest a strong association between IL6 levels, atherosclerosis, and risk of cardiovascular death. Produced locally IL6 in the endothelial vasculature and by SMC, IL6 induces ROS production, proliferation, and SMC migration. IL6 is an important autocrine and/or paracrine regulator of SMC proliferation and migration, critical steps in atherosclerosis progression. Besides, circulating IL-6 levels (in parallel with an increase in circulating CRP) increase with progression to heart failure in Chagas disease. These observations agree with the polymorphisms analyzed in patients with idiopathic dilated cardiomyopathy (IDCM) that relates to TNF, IL-6, and CRP profile. A recent study shows that a rough increase in serum IL-6 is incidental with chronic IDCM [82].

9. Conclusion

Search results illustrated that immune-activated pathways are the main contributors to systemic inflammation in human CCC due an interplay and active crosstalk between different traditional risk factors, mainly metabolic and inflammatory factors derived from immune-mediated host-parasite interactions, both innate and adaptive.

Tissue damage induces inflammatory reactions leading to dilated cardiomyopathy in genetically predisposed persons. The DCM represents an essential hallmark of CCC. Evidence suggests that the pathway of inflammation in DCM culminates in altered concentrations of various markers in peripheral blood, including oxidative stress molecules and markers of vascular and systemic inflammation. These scenarios necessarily require a means of communicating between different cell populations. Crossroads between "natural and specific immunity effector cells and molecules" and "parasite persistence strategies in blood, adipose tissue and heart and other infected tissue" would appear to contribute to cardiovascular risk. The Suppressor of Cytokine Signaling (SOCS) plays a critical role in the regulation of all crossroads of cytokine inflammatory network that induced pathogenesis of dilated cardiomyopathy and seems to play a critical role as negative regulators of inflammation, hypertrophy, contractile dysfunction and ventricular arrhythmias. However, our understanding of the origins of the individual pathway components and crossroads and their assembly into a functional pathway is limited so far. Unlike classical risk factors, approaches based on inflammatory status needs clinically validated biomarkers and its contribution to the development of cardiomyopathy in chagasic and IDCM needs additional studies, even when there is strong evidence suggesting increased morbidity and mortality associated with the systemic inflammatory burden and inflammatory cardiomyopathy.

Acknowledgements

The authors would like to thank Dr. José Milei for gently providing us with **Figure 1** to illustrate our chapter.

Author details

Rodolfo A Kölliker-Frers[1,2†], Matilde Otero-Losada[3†], Gabriela Razzitte[1], Mariela Calvo[1], Justo Carbajales[4] and Francisco Capani[2*]

*Address all correspondence to: franciscocapani@hotmail.com

1 Parasitology Unit, José María Ramos Mejía Hospital, Buenos Aires, Argentina

2 Laboratory of Cytoarchitecture and Neuronal PlascitICY, Institute of Cardiological Research, "Prof. Dr. Alberto Taquini", ININCA-UBA-CONICET, Buenos Aires, Argentina

3 Laboratory of HPLC, Institute of Cardiological Research, University of Buenos Aires, National Research Council, ININCA-UBA-CONICET, Buenos Aires, Argentina

4 Cardiology Unit, José María Ramos Mejía Hospital, Buenos Aires, Argentina

† RAKF and MOL share authorship of this paper.

References

[1] Rodrigues MM, Oliveira AC, Bellio M. The immune response to *Trypanosoma cruzi:* Role of toll-like receptors and perspectives for vaccine development. Journal of Parasitology Research. 2012;**2012**:507874

[2] Morrot A, Villar SR, González FB, Pérez AR. Evasion and immuno-endocrine regulation in parasite infection: Two sides of the same coin in Chagas disease? Frontiers in Microbiology. 2016;**7**:704

[3] Kolliker Frers RA, Cosentino V, Tau J, Kerzberg EM, Urdapilleta A, Chiocconi M, Kogan N, Otero-Losada M, Capani F. Immune-mediated inflammation promotes subclinical atherosclerosis in recent-onset psoriatic arthritis patients without conventional cardiovascular risk factors. Frontiers in Immunology. 2018;**9**:139. DOI: 10.3389/fimmu.2018.00139

[4] Weintraub RG, Semsarian C, Macdonald P. Dilated cardiomyopathy. Lancet. 2017;**390**: 400-414

[5] Konno T, Chen D, Wang L, Wakimoto H, et al. Heterogeneous myocyte enhancer factor-2 (Mef2) activation in myocytes predicts focal scarring in hypertrophic cardiomyopathy. Proceedings of the National Academy of Sciences of the United States of America. 2010;**107**:18097-18102

[6] Colegrave M, Peckham M. Structural implications of β-cardiac myosin heavy chain mutations in human disease. The Anatomical Record. 2014;**297**:1670-1680

[7] Lynch TL 4th, Ismahil MA, Jegga AG, Zilliox MJ, et al. Cardiac inflammation in genetic dilated cardiomyopathy caused by MYBPC3 mutation. Journal of Molecular and Cellular Cardiology. 2017;**102**:83-93

[8] Ogimoto A, Okayama H, Nagai T, Ohtsuka T, et al. Association of monocyte chemoattractant protein 1 gene polymorphism with susceptibility to nonfamilial idiopathic dilated cardiomyopathy. Journal of Cardiology. 2009;**54**:66-70

[9] Linetzky B, Confine J, Castellani N, De Mayo F, et al. Risk of cardiovascular events associated with positive serology for Chagas: A systematic review. International Journal of Epidemiology. 2012;**41**:1356-1366

[10] Bonney KM, Engman DM. Chagas heart disease pathogenesis: One mechanism or many? Current Molecular Medicine. 2008;**8**:510-518

[11] Añez N, Carrasco H, Parada H, Crisante G, et al. Myocardial parasite persistence in chronic chagasic patients. The American Journal of Tropical Medicine and Hygiene. 1999;**60**:726-732

[12] Jordan KA, Hunter CA. Regulation of CD8+ T cell responses to infection with parasitic protozoa. Experimental Parasitology. 2010;**126**:318-325

[13] Fuenmayor C, Higuchi ML, Carrasco H, Parada H, et al. Acute Chagas disease: Immunohistochemical characteristics of T cell infiltrate and its relationship with *T. cruzi* parasitic antigens. Acta Cardiologica. 2005;**60**:33-37

[14] Nagajyothi F, Machado FS, Burleigh BA, Jelicks LA, et al. Mechanisms of *Trypanosoma cruzi* persistence in Chagas disease. Cellular Microbiology. 2012;**14**:634-643

[15] Giorgi ME, de Lederkremer RM. Trans-sialidase and mucins of *Trypanosoma cruzi*: An important interplay for the parasite. Carbohydrate Research. 2011;**346**:1389-1393

[16] Oliveira AC, Peixoto JR, de Arruda LB, Campos MA, et al. Expression of functional TLR4 confers proinflammatory responsiveness to *Trypanosoma cruzi* glycoinositol-phospholipids and higher resistance to infection with *T. cruzi*. Journal of Immunology. 2004;**173**:5688-5696

[17] Chamond N, Grégoire C, Coatnoan N, Rougeot C, et al. Biochemical characterization of proline racemases from the human protozoan parasite *Trypanosoma cruzi* and definition of putative protein signatures. The Journal of Biological Chemistry. 2003;**278**:15484-15494

[18] Desruisseaux MS, Trujillo ME, Tanowitz HB, et al. Adipocyte, adipose tissue, and infectious disease. Infection and Immunity. 2007;**75**:1066-1078

[19] Halberg N, Wernstedt-Asterholm I, Scherer PE. The adipocyte as an endocrine cell. Endocrinology and Metabolism Clinics of North America. 2008;**37**:753-768. x–xi

[20] Rajala MW, Scherer PE. Minireview: The adipocyte—At the crossroads of energy homeostasis, inflammation, and atherosclerosis. Endocrinology. 2003;**144**:3765-3773

[21] Ferreira AV, Segatto M, Menezes Z, Macedo AM, et al. Evidence for *Trypanosoma cruzi* in adipose tissue in human chronic Chagas disease. Microbes and Infection. 2011;**13**:1002-1005

[22] Pinazo MJ, Espinosa G, Cortes-Lletget C, Posada Ede J, et al. Immunosuppression and Chagas disease: A management challenge. PLoS Neglected Tropical Diseases. 2013;**7**:e1965

[23] Campos MA, Almeida IC, Takeuchi O, Akira S, et al. Activation of toll-like receptor-2 by glycosylphosphatidylinositol anchors from a protozoan parasite. Journal of Immunology. 2001;**167**:416-423

[24] Previato JO, Wait R, Jones C, DosReis GA, et al. Glycoinositolphospholipid from *Trypanosoma cruzi*: Structure, biosynthesis and immunobiology. Advances in Parasitology. 2004;**56**:1-41

[25] Campos MA, Closel M, Valente EP, Cardoso JE, et al. Impaired production of proinflammatory cytokines and host resistance to acute infection with *Trypanosoma cruzi* in mice lacking functional myeloid differentiation factor 88. Journal of Immunology. 2004;**172**:1711-1718

[26] Ha T, Li Y, Hua F, Ma J, et al. Reduced cardiac hypertrophy in toll-like receptor 4-deficient mice following pressure overload. Cardiovascular Research. 2005;**68**:224-234

[27] Mathur S, Walley KR, Wang Y, Indrambarya T, et al. Extracellular heat shock protein 70 induces cardiomyocyte inflammation and contractile dysfunction via TLR2. Circulation Journal. 2011;**75**:2445-2452

[28] Laguens RP, Cabeza Meckert PM, Vigliano CA. Pathogenesis of human chronic chagasic myocarditis. Medicina (Buenos Aires). 1999;**59**(Suppl 2):63-68

[29] Leon JS, Godsel LM, Wang K, Engman DM. Cardiac myosin autoimmunity in acute Chagas heart disease. Infection and Immunity. 2001;**69**:5643-5649

[30] Bryan MA, Guyach SE, Norris KA. Specific humoral immunity versus polyclonal B cell activation in *Trypanosoma cruzi* infection of susceptible and resistant mice. PLoS Neglected Tropical Diseases. 2010;**4**:e733

[31] Calzada JE, Garisto J, Zebedes S, Samudio FE, et al. Prevalence of autoantibodies against autonomic receptors in patients with chronic cardiopathies. Biomédica. 2009;**29**:133-139

[32] Guedes PM, Gutierrez FR, Silva GK, Dellalibera-Joviliano R, et al. Deficient regulatory T cell activity and low frequency of IL-17-producing T cells correlate with the extent of cardiomyopathy in human Chagas disease. PLoS Neglected Tropical Diseases. 2012;**6**:e1630

[33] Liongue C, Taznin T, Ward AC. Signaling via the CytoR/JAK/STAT/SOCS pathway: Emergence during evolution. Molecular Immunology. 2016;**71**:166-175

[34] Kinjyo I, Inoue H, Hamano S, Fukuyama S, et al. Loss of SOCS3 in T helper cells resulted in reduced immune responses and hyperproduction of interleukin 10 and transforming growth factor-beta 1. The Journal of Experimental Medicine. 2006;**203**:1021-1031

[35] Chen Z, Laurence A, Kanno Y, Pacher-Zavisin M, et al. Selective regulatory function of Socs3 in the formation of IL-17-secreting T cells. Proceedings of the National Academy of Sciences of the United States of America. 2006;**103**:8137-8142

[36] Aboulhoda BE. Age-related remodeling of the JAK/STAT/SOCS signaling pathway and associated myocardial changes: From histological to molecular level. Annals of Anatomy. 2017;**214**:21-30

[37] Yajima T, Murofushi Y, Zhou H, Park S, et al. Absence of SOCS3 in the cardiomyocyte increases mortality in a gp130-dependent manner accompanied by contractile dysfunction and ventricular arrhythmias. Circulation. 2011;**24**:2690-2701

[38] de Oliveira FL, Araújo-Jorge TC, de Souza EM, de Oliveira GM, et al. Oral administration of GW788388, an inhibitor of transforming growth factor beta signaling, prevents heart fibrosis in Chagas disease. PLoS Neglected Tropical Diseases. 2012;**6**:e1696

[39] Yang Z, Hulver M, McMillan RP, Cai L, et al. Regulation of insulin and leptin signaling by muscle suppressor of cytokine signaling 3 (SOCS3). PLoS One. 2012;**7**:e47493

[40] Azfar RS, Gelfand JM. Psoriasis and metabolic disease: Epidemiology and pathophysiology. Current Opinion in Rheumatology. 2008;**20**:416-422

[41] Kölliker Frers RA, Bisoendial RJ, Montoya SF, Kerzkerg E, et al. Psoriasis and cardiovascular risk: Immune-mediated crosstalk between metabolic, vascular and autoimmune inflammation. IJC Metabolic and Endocrine. 2015;**6**:43-54

[42] Lanugo M, Prettily LA, da Silva MV, Bazar P, et al. The relationship between heart rate variability and serum cytokines in chronic chagasic patients with persistent parasitemia. Pacing and Clinical Electrophysiology. 2011;**34**:724-735

[43] Bisoendial RJ, Boekholdt SM, Vergeer M, Strokes ES, et al. C-reactive protein is a mediator of cardiovascular disease. European Heart Journal. 2010;**31**:2087-2091

[44] Gonzalez-Juanatey C, Llorca J, Amigo-Diaz E, Dierssen T, et al. High prevalence of subclinical atherosclerosis in psoriatic arthritis patients without clinically evident cardiovascular disease or classic atherosclerosis risk factors. Arthritis and Rheumatism. 2007;**57**:1074-1080

[45] Han C, Robinson DW Jr, Hackett MV, Paramore LC, et al. Cardiovascular disease and risk factors in patients with rheumatoid arthritis, psoriatic arthritis, and ankylosing spondylitis. The Journal of Rheumatology. 2006;**33**:2167-2172

[46] Kimhi O, Caspi D, Bornstein NM, Maharshak N, et al. Prevalence and risk factors of atherosclerosis in patients with psoriatic arthritis. Seminars in Arthritis and Rheumatism. 2007;**36**:203-209

[47] Peters MJ, van der Horst-Bruinsma IE, Dijkmans BA, Nurmohamed MT. Cardiovascular risk profile of patients with spondylarthropathies, particularly ankylosing spondylitis and psoriatic arthritis. Seminars in Arthritis and Rheumatism. 2004;**34**:585-592

[48] Gross MD, Bielinski SJ, Suarez-Lopez JR, Reiner AP, et al. Circulating soluble intercellular adhesion molecule 1 and subclinical atherosclerosis: The coronary artery risk development in young adults study. Clinical Chemistry. 2012;**58**:411-420

[49] Laucella S, De Titto EH, Segura EL, Orn A, et al. Soluble cell adhesion molecules in human Chagas disease: Association with disease severity and stage of infection. The American Journal of Tropical Medicine and Hygiene. 1996;**55**:629-634

[50] Sampietro T, Naglaa D, Bionda A, Dal Pino B, et al. Inflammatory markers and serum lipids in idiopathic dilated cardiomyopathy. The American Journal of Cardiology. 2005;**96**:1718-1720

[51] Noutsias M, Hohmann C, Pauschinger M, Schwimmbeck PL, et al. sICAM-1 correlates with myocardial ICAM-1 expression in dilated cardiomyopathy. International Journal of Cardiology. 2003;**91**:153-161

[52] Paiva CN, Figueiredo RT, Kroll-Palhares K, Silva AA, et al. CCL2/MCP-1 controls parasite burden, cell infiltration, and mononuclear activation during acute *Trypanosoma cruzi* infection. O Biologico. 2009;**86**:1239-1246

[53] Frade AF, Pissetti CW, Ianni BM, Saba B, et al. Genetic susceptibility to Chagas disease cardiomyopathy: Involvement of several genes of the innate immunity and chemokine-dependent migration pathways. BMC Infectious Diseases. 2013;**13**:587

[54] Guo Y, Cen Z, Wei B, Wu W, et al. Increased circulating interleukin 10-secreting B cells in patients with dilated cardiomyopathy. International Journal of Clinical and Experimental Pathology. 2015;**8**:8107-8114

[55] Rubiś P, Wiśniowska-Smiałek S, Wypasek E, Rudnicka-Sosin L, et al. 12-month patterns of serum markers of collagen synthesis, transforming growth factor and connective tissue growth factor are similar in new-onset and chronic dilated cardiomyopathy in patients both with and without cardiac fibrosis. Cytokine. 2017;**96**:217-227

[56] van der Aar AM, Sibiryak DS, Bakdash G, van Capel TM, et al. Vitamin D3 targets epidermal and dermal dendritic cells for induction of distinct regulatory T cells. The Journal of Allergy and Clinical Immunology. 2011;**127**:1532-1540.e7

[57] Wu L, Ong S, Talor MV, Barin JG, et al. Cardiac fibroblasts mediate IL-17A-driven inflammatory dilated cardiomyopathy. The Journal of Experimental Medicine. 2014;**211**:1449-1464

[58] Jialal I, Devaraj S, Venugopal SK. C-reactive protein: Risk marker or mediator in atherothrombosis? Hypertension. 2004;**44**:6-11

[59] Birjmohun RS, Bisoendial RJ, van Leuven SI, Ackermans M, et al. A single bolus infusion of C-reactive protein increases gluconeogenesis and plasma glucose concentration in humans. Metabolism. 2007;**56**:1576

[60] Qamirani E. C-reactive protein inhibits endothelium-dependent NO-mediated dilation in coronary arterioles by activating p38 kinase and NAD(P)H oxidase. Arteriosclerosis, Thrombosis, and Vascular Biology. 2005;**25**:995-1001

[61] Sadahiro T, Kohsaka S, Okuda S, Inohara T, et al. MRI and serum high-sensitivity C reactive protein predict long-term mortality in non-ischaemic cardiomyopathy. Open Heart. 2015;**2**(1):e000298

[62] Fon Tacer K, Kuzman D, Seliskar M, Pompon D, et al. TNF-alpha interferes with lipid homeostasis and activates acute and proatherogenic processes. Physiological Genomics. 2007;**31**:216-227

[63] Valsami S, Ruf W, Leikauf MS, Madon J, et al. Immunomodulatory drugs increase endothelial tissue factor expression in vitro. Thrombosis Research. 2011;**127**:264-271

[64] Rocha Rodrigues DB, dos Reis MA, Romano A, Pereira SA, et al. In situ expression of regulatory cytokines by heart inflammatory cells in Chagas disease patients with heart failure. Clinical & Developmental Immunology. 2012;**2012**:7. Article ID: 361730. http://dx.doi.org/10.1155/2012/361730

[65] Pérez-Fuentes R, López-Colombo A, Ordóñez-Toquero G, Gomez-Albino I, et al. Correlation of the serum concentrations of tumour necrosis factor and nitric oxide with disease severity in chronic Chagas disease (American trypanosomiasis). Annals of Tropical Medicine and Parasitology. 2007;**101**:123-132

[66] D'Angelo-Mendoza E, Rodríguez-Bonfante C, Camacho I. Martínez increased levels of tumor necrosis factor alpha. Investigación Clínica. 2005;**46**:229-240

[67] Bilate AM, Salemi VM, Ramires FJ, de Brito T, et al. TNF blockade aggravates experimental chronic Chagas disease cardiomyopathy. Microbes and Infection. 2007;**9**:1104-1113

[68] Dinarello CA. Interleukin-1 in the pathogenesis and treatment of inflammatory diseases. Blood. 2011;**117**:3720-3732

[69] Dinarello CA, Simon A, van der Meer JW. Treating inflammation by blocking interleukin-1 in a broad spectrum of diseases. Nature Reviews. Drug Discovery. 2012;**11**:633-652

[70] Berry CE, Hare JM. Xanthine oxidoreductase and cardiovascular disease: Molecular mechanisms and pathophysiological implications. The Journal of Physiology. 2004;**555**: 589-606

[71] Stutz A, Golenbock DT, Lat E. Inflammasomes: Too big to miss. The Journal of Clinical Investigation. 2009;**119**:3502-3511

[72] Aleksova A, Beltrami AP, Carriere C, Barbati G, et al. Interleukin-1β levels predict long-term mortality and need for heart transplantation in ambulatory patients affected by idiopathic dilated cardiomyopathy. Oncotarget. 2017;**8**:25131-25140

[73] Blyszczuk P, Kania G, Dieterle T, Marty RR, et al. Myeloid differentiation factor-88/interleukin-1 signaling controls cardiac fibrosis and heart failure progression in inflammatory dilated cardiomyopathy. Circulation Research. 2009;**105**:912-920

[74] Matsuzawa Y. Adipocytokines and metabolic syndrome. Seminars in Vascular Medicine. 2005;**5**:34-39

[75] Yin YW, Hu AM, Sun QQ, Liu HL, et al. Association between interleukin-6 gene-174 G/C polymorphism and the risk of coronary heart disease: A meta-analysis of 20 studies including 9619 cases and 10919 controls. Gene. 2012;**503**:25-30

[76] Rauramaa R, Väisänen SB, Luong LA, Schmidt-Trücksäss A, et al. Stromelysin-1 and interleukin-6 gene promoter polymorphisms are determinants of asymptomatic carotid artery atherosclerosis. Arteriosclerosis, Thrombosis, and Vascular Biology. 2000;**20**:2657-2662

[77] Rundek T, Elkind MS, Pittman J, Boden-Albala B, et al. Carotid intima-media thickness is associated with allelic variants of stromelysin-1, interleukin-6, and hepatic lipase genes: The Northern Manhattan Prospective Cohort Study. Stroke. 2002;**33**:1420-1423

[78] Schuett H. How much is too much? Interleukin-6 and its signaling in atherosclerosis. Thrombosis and Haemostasis. 2009;**102**:215-222

[79] Tedgui A, Mallat Z. Cytokines in atherosclerosis: Pathogenic and regulatory pathways. Physiological Reviews. 2006;**86**:515-581

[80] López L, Arai K, Giménez E, Jiménez M, et al. Proteína C reactiva y la interleucina-6 aumentan los niveles séricos como la enfermedad de Chagas avanza hacia la insuficiencia cardiaca. Revista Española de Cardiología. 2006;**59**:50-56

[81] Liaquat A, Asifa GZ, Zeenat A, Javed Q. Polymorphisms of tumor necrosis factor-alpha and interleukin-6 gene and C-reactive protein profiles in patients with idiopathic dilated cardiomyopathy. Annals of Saudi Medicine. 2014;**34**:407-414

[82] Bironaite D, Daunoravicius D, Bombloads J, Cibiras S, et al. Molecular mechanisms behind progressing chronic inflammatory dilated cardiomyopathy. BMC Cardiovascular Disorders. 2015;**15**:26

5

Efficacy and Safety of Chagas Disease Drug Therapy and Treatment Perspectives

Wilton H. Kawaguchi, Leticia Bonancio Cerqueira, Mariana Millan Fachi, Michel L. Campos, Iara J. Messias Reason and Roberto Pontarolo

Abstract

Chagas disease, also known as American trypanosomiasis, is a neglected disease caused by the protozoan parasite *Trypanosoma cruzi*. The disease affects about 6–7 million people worldwide, mostly in Latin America. Although Chagas disease was discovered more than 100 years ago, and the first treatments over 40, only 2 drugs were used to treat this pathology, it is still considered one of the neglected diseases. In this chapter, the subjects related to conventional etiological therapies, benznidazole and nifurtimox, such as the drug, the mechanism of action, the therapy schedule for treatment, efficacy and safety and their adverse effects will be discussed. Additionally, it will address alternative therapies of comorbidities related to the progression of Chagas' disease in patients with chronic disease, such as heart disease and dysfunction of the digestive system. Finally, novel pharmacological strategies and their related compounds will be reviewed accounting for their progression in pharmacological studies and their success rate.

Keywords: Chagas disease, benznidazole, nifurtimox, symptomatic treatment, new strategies

1. Introduction

Chagas disease or American trypanosomiasis is caused by the protozoan parasite *Trypanosoma cruzi* (*T. cruzi*). Endemic largely in Latin American countries, it is transmitted primarily by vectors, the insect vector triatomine, also known as "kissing bug". It is estimated that 6–7 million people are infected worldwide, and that more than 10,000 people die each year as a result of the disease, with the highest number of cases in Latin American countries [1].

Although Chagas disease has been discovered more than 100 years ago, there are currently only two drugs used to control Chagas disease (CD), benznidazole and nifurtimox [2–4]. Benznidazole has a similar efficacy profile to nifurtimox. They have high cure rates in the acute phase and at the beginning of the chronic phase, being little or ineffective in the late chronic phase [5]. Benznidazole and nifurtimox belong to the nitro heterocycles class of drugs; however, each presents different mechanisms of action that are considered very aggressive and may cause several adverse effects.

In the chronic phase of CD, the treatment at this stage aims to reduce parasitemia and prevent complications that may lead to progression of visceral lesions. However, the administration of benznidazole and nifurtimox remains controversial [5, 6]. To treat the cardiac and gastrointestinal manifestations attributed to this phase of the disease, it requires specific pharmacological approaches, highlighting the combination of diuretics, angiotensin-converting-enzyme inhibitors or angiotensin receptor blockers, and adrenergic beta blockers. The choice of palliative treatment is in relation to the symptoms of the patient.

Currently, the main treatment for CD is benznidazole and nifurtimox and both compounds are effective in the acute phase to reduce parasitemia and the persistence and the clinical severity of the disease [5]. However, in most countries, benznidazole is the primary choice to begin the treatment, since it has shown less adverse events. The predominant reasons to use nifurtimox are the occurrence of benznidazole resistance or its unavailability [6, 7]. Benznidazole can achieve over 70% of cure in cases of congenital and acute phase, while nifurtimox reaches 80% efficacy. However, these compounds have limited efficacy in the chronic phase, with efficacy rates of only 6–10% [8–10]. Treatment complications include, need for increasing doses, duration varying according to the stage of infection, and high occurrence of adverse effects caused by the long-term treatment with high doses. In addition, resistance may occur depending on the *Trypanosoma. cruzi* (*T. cruzi*) strain [10].

Although the aforementioned therapy is over 40 years old, there are limitations in this first line of treatment for CD. Several studies aimed to bring new options to its arsenal, mainly for the chronic phase. Among them, are drugs used to treat other conditions, such as posaconazole, and new compounds, such as E1224. Each of these has been tested in clinical trials. Other strategies have been suggested as groundbreaking approaches to eradicate, or at least control, CD. These include drugs, such as cruzipain and trypanothione reductase which specifically targets the ergosterol biosynthesis pathway.

Considering this the classical treatment of CD, with a focus on the evaluation of efficacy and safety of the current drug therapy, will be properly addressed in this chapter. In addition, a review of new pharmacological therapies will be discussed.

2. Etiological treatment: benznidazole

2.1. Treatment history

Until the publication of the *Manual de Doenças Tropicaes e Infectuosas* in 1935 by Carlos Chagas and Evandro Chagas (Manual of Tropical and Infectious Diseases), there was no pharmacological treatment available for trypanosomiasis. Drugs with trypanocidal activity have been investigated by a number of researchers; however, without success [11]. In 1936, quinolinic compounds were successfully used to treat an acute case of trypanosomiasis [12]. In the following years, nitrofurazone was administered to treat trypanosomiasis in mice and achieve efficacy rates between 20 and 100%, depending on the therapeutic schedule [13]. These results motivated the experimental trials in humans, in which nitrofurazone demonstrated to be effective against trypanosomes in the circulating blood, cerebrospinal fluids [14] as well as other promising clinical results [15, 16].

Novel studies were performed to identify an alternative therapeutic schedule and main side effects [17, 18]. In 1962, Rio de Janeiro was the host city for the "Meeting of Debates on Chagas Disease", where the standardization of the methodology and establishment of criteria for the evaluation of attempted pharmacological treatments was discussed. Nifurtimox and benznidazole remain as the only two drugs available for treatment of CD [19].

2.2. The drug

Benznidazole (BNZ) N-benzyl-2-(2-nitro-imidazol-1-yl)acetamide (**Figure 1**) is a nitro heterocyclic drug. It was nitroimidazolic derivative synthesized in the early 1970s by Wineholt and Liebman and produced by Hoffman-La Roche, Switzerland. In 2003, the rights and manufacturing technology of BNZ was granted to the Laboratório Farmacêutico do Estado de Pernambuco (*LAFEPE*) – Recife/PE – Brazil [5, 9, 10, 20, 21]. According to the Biopharmaceutical Classification System, BNZ is categorized as class 4, thus exhibiting limited and/or variable absorption due to the characteristics such as low solubility and low permeability. Therefore, there are interests in strategies to improve the absorption rate, hence increasing its bioavailability [22, 23].

BNZ is administered orally in a tablet form of 100 mg for adults and 12.5 mg tablets for children [24]. The drug is fully absorbed in the gastrointestinal tract and the plasma peak concentration was achieved within 2–4 hours. The half-life is 12 hours and its metabolites were eliminated in urine and feces [5, 10, 20].

2.3. Mechanism of action

The mechanism of action of BNZ is not fully understood [9, 25]. However, some reports associate its action with the formation of free radicals and/or electrophilic metabolites. In the nitroimidazole derivatives, the reduction of the nitro group (NO_2) in the amino group (NH_2)

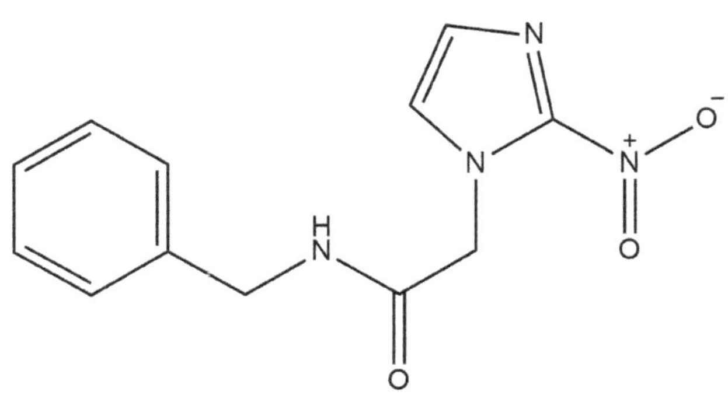

Figure 1. Chemical structure of benznidazole.

occurs by the action of nitroreductase present in protozoan cells or bacteria. This reaction leads to the formation of radical intermediates, as well as electrophilic metabolites. The process is initiated by the action of the enzyme NADPH cytochrome P450 reductase, which acts on the nitro group (R-NO_2) of the molecule nitroimidazole, inducing the production of an intermediate nitro radical (R-NO_2) and the formation of hydroxylamine (R-NHOH). These intermediates act on the covalent modification of macromolecules, such as DNA, causing fragmentation in the chain and destabilization of the helix, inhibiting DNA synthesis leading to cell death of protozoa parasitic and/or bacterial. In addition to this alteration in DNA, it involves the modification of other macromolecules, such as lipids and proteins, affecting *T. cruzi* metabolism. An additional mechanism of action of BNZ is the increase in phagocytosis, leading to lysis and inhibition of *T. cruzi* growth through an interferon-gamma (IFN-γ)-dependent mechanism and through the enzyme NADH-fumarate reductase, respectively [9, 11, 26–28].

Concomitantly, the electrophilic metabolites mentioned above due to their high reactivity and low specificity, may present human host action and cytotoxic effects observed during the treatment of patients [27–29].

2.4. Therapeutic schedule

The dosage of BNZ in the acute phase of the disease should be provided in two or three administrations daily, during the 60-day period. The dose is established according to the patient's age and weight. For adults, it is recommended 5 mg/kg/day, whereas for children weighing less than 40 kg, 5–10 mg/kg/day is recommended. Furthermore for children, the therapeutic regimen should be as small as possible to achieve therapeutic adherence. A recommendation for infants is 10 mg/kg/day. In congenital infections, the treatment is indicated for children born to mothers who were serologically positive for CD with the presence of *T. cruzi* in umbilical cord blood, serum-specific IgM soon after birth, and IgG after 6 months. In the newborn, the recommended etiologic therapy is the administration of BNZ twice a day for 30 days, it is suggested to be provided at 5 mg/kg/day [5, 11, 20, 30–32].

In the chronic phase, the dosage is 5–7 mg/kg/day divided into two administrations with an interval of 12-hour between doses, and for 30–60 consecutive days [5, 20].

2.5. Efficacy and safety

It is considered as the first choice treatment because it exhibits a better safety and efficacy profile when compared to nifurtimox. Moreover, there is evidence of greater efficacy [7, 28]. It has antiprotozoal and antibacterial performance, acting against the trypomastigote and amastigote forms [5].

In the acute phase, if the treatment is initiated immediately following the confirmation of the presence of *T. cruzi* in the direct examination of the peripheral blood, the cure percentages are greater than 70–80%, independent of the transmission route [5, 7, 9, 33]. It should be administered to patients in the early chronic phase, children less than 12 years, laboratory accidents and congenital infection. In newborns treated during the first year of life, the chances of cure are greater than 90%; otherwise, in the late chronic phase the patient has lower chances of cure (~10%) [20, 34–36].

Two placebo-controlled clinical trials were performed in the USA in children between 6 and 12 years old for the evaluation of treatment using BNZ, in which the results were satisfactory. In the first trial, 60% of the children treated had a change from positive to a negative in serology for CD, compared to 14% of them receiving placebo. In the second trial, similar results for children treated with BNZ showed a 55% change from a positive to a negative antibody test, compared to 5% of those receiving placebo [37].

For treatment in cases of organ transplantation, it is essential to know if the donor or recipient presents positive serology and can transmit or reactivate the infection. In cases of absolute requirement for transplantation, the serum-reactive donor in which the recipient is serologically negative for a chagasic infection, the donor should receive BNZ therapy following the traditional dosing regimen, within 60 days prior to transplantation. For the recipient following transplantation, it is recommended to initiate therapy by performing serological tests over time. There is a serum conversion with the treatment for the acute phase. If an acute infection is detected, the treatment need to be started [38–40].

Immunocompromised patients, carriers of hematological malignancies, users of immunosuppressive drugs, or those co-infected with the acquired immunodeficiency virus may reactivate CD. The treatment is the conventional treatment, lasting 60 days, and depending on the clinical conditions of the patient, it may be increased to 90 days [40–42].

When accidental infection occurs, the individual who accidentally had contact with contaminated materials; needle puncture, contact in lesions, wounds or mucous membranes, or any other means that indicates the possibility of having been infected by the parasite, is evaluated by serological tests and treatment begins immediately. During the 10–15 days of the treatment period, the serological tests will be repeated [5, 11].

At the beginning of the chronic phase in children, treatment follows the same reasoning for acute phase cases in children younger than or equal to 12 years with positive serology. For adults, therapy is recommended to prevent or reduce the progression of CD in more severe forms, such as cardiomyopathy, and to prevent congenital transmission in pregnant women [5, 11, 20, 43]. Its use in the chronic phase has generated vast discussions. The BENEFIT project – Benznidazole Evaluation for Interrupting Trypanosomiasis, is an international multicenter, randomized, double-blinded, placebo-controlled trial of BNZ for the treatment of patients with mild to moderate Chagas cardiomyopathy. This study has conducted and produced results that indicated that the use of BNZ in the chronic phase significantly reduced the detection of circulating parasites; however, did not attenuate the cardiac clinical progression [20, 33].

Treatment for patients older than 50 years should take into account the risk of toxicity of the drug against the benefits of the therapy individually [6, 20].

2.6. Adverse effects

Therapy with BNZ contains some challenges, such as the large doses administered, time duration varying according to the stage of infection, and high occurrence of adverse effects. These challenges are less frequent when compared with nifurtimox (**Table 1**). The adverse effects in patients receiving BNZ may be classified into three groups: manifestations of

Adverse effects	Benznidazole	Nifurtimox
Anorexia and weight loss	5–40%	50–75%
Nausea	0–5%	15–50%
Vomiting	0–5%	15–26%
Peripheral neuropathy	0–30%	2–5%
Leukopenia	Rare: <1%	Rare: <1%

Table 1. Frequencies of adverse effects associated with benznidazole and nifurtimox.

hypersensitivity (dermatitis with rashes, generalized or peritoneal edema, fever, lymphadenopathy, muscle and joint pain), bone marrow depression (agranulocytosis, neutropenia, and thrombocytopenic purpura), and peripheral polyneuropathy (paresthesias and polyneuritis) [7, 11].

Adverse effects of dermatological cause appear in approximately 30% of the patients being treated with the drug. Rashes occur due to photosensitization, dermatitis is usually mild to moderate and may be treated with topical systemic corticosteroids. However, treatment should be discontinued immediately in cases of severe or exfoliative dermatitis or associated with fever and adenopathy. Bone marrow suppression is rare, but if occurs the treatment should be discontinued immediately. Additional adverse effects include weight loss, nausea and/or vomiting, anorexia, and insomnia [8, 11, 20, 29, 43].

Treatment is contraindicated in pregnancy and in patients with severe renal or hepatic impairment [11, 20, 44].

According to the World Health Organization (WHO), the ideal requirements for treatment are: parasitological cure in both phases (acute and chronic), effective doses in single or few doses, low cost, no side effects or teratogenic effects, without hospitalization, and induction of resistance. Until now, there is no drug for the treatment of CD that meets each of these WHO requirements.

3. Etiological treatment: nifurtimox

3.1. The drug

Nifurtimox (NFX) (**Figure 2**) belongs to the class of nitrofuran compounds. Her-Linger, Mayer, Petersen and Bock from Bayer™ synthesized it in 1962 in Germany. This was the first drug designed to treat trypanosomiasis, such as sleeping sickness and Chagas diseases [34]. Its production was interrupted in 1980s due to the reduction on world demand [11]. In 2009, the WHO Expert Committee on the Selection and Use of Essential Medicines recommends the inclusion of NFX in the model list of essential medicines (EML) and Bayer resumed the production of NFX [45]. Bayer, through WHO, still provides NFX worldwide in 120 mg and 30 mg tablets under the brand name Lampit [46], in United States and it is redistributed by Center for Disease Control and Prevention (CDC) [47].

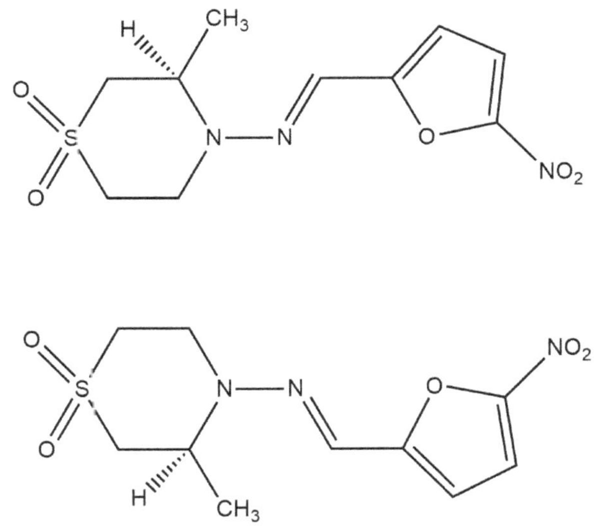

Figure 2. Chemical structure of nifurtimox.

NFX is a 5-nitrofuran (3-methyl-4-(5′-nitrofurfurylideneamine) tetrahydro-4H-1,4-tiazine-1,1-dioxide. NFX possesses an asymmetric center, but it is used as a racemic mixture since pure stereoisomers were not more active or less toxic.

NFX is well absorbed following oral administration. The plasma levels range from 10 to 20 mM and lower concentrations are found in urine and tissues. The therapeutic schedule must vary according to the patient's age and disease phase [9, 11, 48, 49].

3.2. Mechanism of action

The mechanism of action of NFX is based on cellular damage originating from the production of nitro anion radical through two pathways: through a redox cycle with the formation of $O\cdot^{-}$ (superoxide anion) and its reduction to the corresponding amine derivative [50–52].

This mechanism was thoroughly studied by Do Campo and colleagues [51, 53–58]. The reduction of a nitro group by nitroredutase (NTR) is fundamental for NFX mechanism of action. This enzyme catalyzes the reduction of 2-electrons of the compound, producing a nitrous intermediate, followed by a second 2-electron reduction to generate a hydroxylamine. This derivative can directly lead to cell damage, or generate other cytotoxic agents (**Figure 3**) [52, 59]. Since the *T. cruzi* detoxification mechanism is insufficient, it becomes more susceptive to reactive nitro compounds [60–62]. The presence of the nitro reductase type I in the parasite is the main responsibility for NFX selectivity. This enzyme is absent in mammals, reducing the formation of toxic agents in human.

3.3. Therapeutic schedule

Several therapeutic schedules were evaluated in the past years. The doses vary between 5 and 30 mg/kg/day, in extended therapies of 30–120 days [63–67]. Based on these experiments and considering the efficacy/tolerance ratio, the ideal therapeutic schedule of NFX is 8–10 mg/kg/day

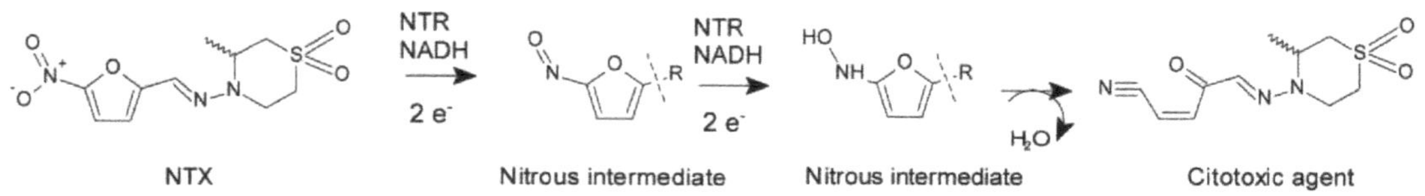

Figure 3. Mechanism of NFX based on nitroreductase type 1 action.

in adults and 15 mg/kg/day in children, for 60, 90 or 120 days, divided into three daily doses, after meals [1, 68]. It must be highlighted that even at these doses, side effects may potentially be present in adults.

3.4. Safety and efficacy

Many studies regarding the efficacy of NFX were performed between the 1960 and 1980s, at the beginning of its development and first years of commercialization [5, 11, 34]. Considering these studies, the activity of the NFX against the *Trypanosoma sp.* is expressive. NFX is capable to achieve efficacy rates of 70–100% in acute parasitemia cases. However, these rates substantially decrease when it comes to adult chronic phase, reaching values of only 7–8% in adults, although in children under 14, it remains around 86% [68, 69].

The primary reason why BNZ is often preferred compared to NFX is due to the presence of adverse effects. NFX frequently produces side effects [5, 11, 34, 70], but the majority are mild and can be managed with dose reduction or temporary suspension of medication [11, 68, 71].

3.5. Adverse effects

The treatment of CD is long and continuous and the presence of adverse effects becomes quite common between 60 and 100% of the patients [68]. The most frequent side effects described in the case of NFX are anorexia, nausea, headache, and amnesia. The possible neurological reactions are restlessness, disorientation, forgetfulness, insomnia, spasms, paresthesias, polyneuritis, and convulsive seizures. Most of the adverse effects (93%) are mild and disappear through dose reduction or after suspending the treatment [68, 70].

4. Symptomatic treatment of chronic phase

CD is classified evolutionary into two phases: an initial acute phase, followed by a chronic phase. Each phase has distinct clinical characteristics, diagnostic parameters, and treatment [72–76]. The acute phase is characterized by intense parasitism related with nonspecific symptoms, including fever, eyelid edema (denominated Chagoma), edema, and myocarditis. In general, the progression of disease can take years to reach the chronic phase, which presents four clinical forms: indeterminate (without clinical manifestations), cardiac, digestive, and mixed (association of cardiac and digestive) [77–81].

4.1. Chronic Chagas cardiomyopathy (CCC)

Chronic Chagas cardiomyopathy (CCC) is associated with high rates of morbidity and mortality, and it is categorized into stages of cardiac impairment (A, B, C, and D) according to the manifestations, electrocardiograph, radiological alterations, and changes in ventricular function [72, 74, 75, 82, 83]. Approximately 20–40% of patients with the indeterminate form will develop CCC. Several mechanisms contribute to this including the persistence of the parasite and autoimmunity. Moreover, factors such as dysautonomia (neurogenic mechanisms) and microvascular dysfunctions may potentiate and amplify this damage [74, 75, 77, 79–81, 84].

The cardiac form of Chagas can occur with or without ventricular failure [25, 82, 84]. Although the most common is the coexistence of arrhythmic manifestations with the congestive form, some patients have only arrhythmias and intraventricular and atrioventricular conductions compromising with normal ventricular function. Management of CCC treatment is based on the following clinical manifestations such as heart failure, cardiac arrhythmia, and thromboembolism [25, 79, 84].

Although, Chagas disease represents an important cause of heart failure (HF), limited studies have established the use of these drugs in Chagas patients. The treatment of CCC aims to reduce symptoms, delay the evolution of ventricular dysfunction, and prolong survival. In the asymptomatic or mild stages of HF, it is intended to delay the evolution of the disease. In the advanced stages, the objective is to improve the quality of life and the survival of patients. The efficacy and tolerability of these drugs in patients with CCC is extrapolated from the results obtained for other etiologies. Therefore, the CCC treatment is suggested to be performed in accordance with the general guidelines for HF treatment and should consist of the combination of three therapeutic classes: angiotensin-converting enzyme inhibitors (ACEI) or angiotensin receptor blockers (ARB), diuretics, and adrenergic beta blockers (BB) [40, 72, 82].

Angiotensin-converting enzyme inhibitors (ACEI) or angiotensin receptor blockers (ARB) have an essential role in adverse cardiac remodeling and ventricular dysfunction progression of HF [40, 72, 82]. In experimental studies reported in the literature, captopril and enalapril demonstrated to diminish myocarditis and fibrosis of CCC [85–88]. These drugs should be administrated initially in low doses. In spite, some physicians report that CCC does not tolerate high doses of ACEI, according to the degree of tolerability; the dose can be progressively increased [25, 78, 81]. ACEI is recommended to patients with a left ventricular ejection fraction (LVEF) <45% [82, 83]. Regarding ARB, spironolactone and eplerenone have been evaluated in studies and data have shown that these drugs are effective in improving the quality of life and reduction of symptoms associated with CCC [89–91] and this class is considered as the treatment of choice for Chagas patients with LVEF <45%, or patients with LVEF<35% and New York Heart Association (NYHA) Class III/IV [82, 83]. In addition, in cases that are contraindicated to ACEI and ARB (hyperkalemia and progressive renal failure), the combination of hydralazine and isosorbide dinitrate should be prescribed [25, 73, 79, 83].

Beta-adrenergic blockers (carvedilol, bisoprolol, or metoprolol) are suggested in association with ACEI and ARB due to autonomous nervous system involvement in CCC and the production of antibodies against β-1 adrenergic and M-2 muscarinic receptors [25, 73, 79, 83]. Limited reports address the efficacy of this therapeutic class to treat Chagas patients with ventricular dysfunction [86, 92–96]. Beta blockers have been avoided because of the presence of frequent bradycardia; therefore these drugs are not indicated for patients with bradycardia ≤50 bpm or AV conduction disorders (PR > 280 ms) [25, 73, 79, 83].

Moreover, digoxin and diuretics are considered a pharmacological option in CCC, justifying the use of digoxin for patients with symptomatic LVEF ≤45%, principally in the presence of atrial fibrillation when the ventricular frequency is increased and diuretics to improve congestive symptoms and signs. For advanced HF stages, the combination of thiazides with loop diuretics has been proven to be more effective [25, 72, 73, 79, 83].

The annual incidence of thromboembolism in Chagas patients is between 1 and 2%, affecting mainly patients with HF. Occasionally, this aggravation is the first manifestation of the CD. Cardiac emboli can reach both the pulmonary and systemic circulation, with the cerebral territory being the most clinically evident [40, 79, 82]. The treatment of thromboembolism is performed based on the established recommendations, alternating according to the extension and compromised organ. For this, a score derived from a prospective cohort study with 1043 patients was recently available to evaluate the risk and to implement preventing thromboembolisms in CCC. Through risk-benefit analysis, warfarin is indicated for patients with 4–5 point. In the case of 3 points, acetylsalicylic acid (AAS) or warfarin could be used. For 2 points, it is suggested to use AAS or no prophylaxis, and 0–1 points do not need prophylaxis [79, 81, 97].

Patients with CCC usually present ventricular arrhythmia. The most frequent ventricular arrhythmias in Chagas patients are ventricular ectopies, isolated or repetitive. The presence of these arrhythmias in asymptomatic patients with preserved ventricular function does not require antiarrhythmic treatment, whereas in symptomatic cases, the antiarrhythmic treatment can be individualized. The goal of pharmacological treatment of arrhythmias is the control of symptoms. Amiodarone is widely used, despite the high incidence of adverse events. At the usual doses of 200–400 mg/day, it can be associated with alternative agents recommended for cardiopathies of other etiologies, such as propafenone, sotalol, and beta blockers, to reduce severe arrhythmic events. However, drugs belonging to class I (sodium-channel blockers) should be avoided, principally in patients with ventricular dysfunction due to proarrhythmic effects, whereas propafenone is contraindicated in patients with left ventricular dysfunction [77, 79, 83, 98]. Bradyarrhythmia is related with sinus node dysfunction or atrioventricular blocks. For the treatment of symptomatic bradyarrhythmias in CCC, a permanent pacemaker implant is usually performed [98].

4.2. Digestive form of CD

The digestive manifestations of the CD correspond to the functional alterations observed in the esophagus and intestine, which result in the formation of mega-esophagus or megacolon, respectively. These deformations are related with the involvement of the enteric nervous system, especially the Auerbachs plexus. Degenerative phenomena in this region are caused by the presence of inflammatory processes associated with autoimmune responses. Therefore, both megacolon and mega-esophagus results in alterations in motility, and consequently, in slow transit and difficulty to empty, followed by increased organ caliber [99–102].

Mega-esophagus is classified into four groups with the objective of situating the different radiological aspects within the evolutionary spectrum of the affection. In addition, the classification of the mega-esophagus is important for the choice of treatment [99–101, 103].

The symptoms commonly reported in mega-esophagus are: dysphagia, regurgitation and esophageal pain. Treatment of mega-esophagus included clinical, pharmacological measures, dilatation and surgical procedure to aid in the transit of foods and liquids. The choice of treatment to be applied depends on the following factors: patient agreement, relevance of symptoms, degree of classification, nutritional status, clinical condition, comorbidities, age and available hospital infrastructure [40, 103, 104].

Clinical and pharmacological treatment is indicated for patients in group I, or patients at high risk of being treated with other forms of treatment, or in cases refusing invasive treatment. Patients must frequently drink water during the meals, eat slowly, and give preference to food in a pasty consistency. Hot and cold foods and drink and eating prior to bedtime are not recommended because food may be retained in the esophagus, causing pain or nocturnal regurgitation during sleep. The pharmacological treatment is based on substances that aim to relax the esophageal sphincter; however, the beneficial effect of these drugs is restricted to the period of action, being only a symptomatic treatment. The nitric derivatives (isosorbitol dinitrate) and the calcium channel blockers (nifedipine) are recommended [40, 101, 104, 105].

Alternative treatment is forced dilation of the distal segment of the esophagus and esophagic junction using a pneumatic or hydrostatic balloon or surgery. Surgery is performed for patients classified in group II (according to the intensity of the symptoms), III, and IV, and for patients without adequate response to clinical treatment. Another alternative is the injection of botulinum toxin, which acts to inhibit acetylcholine release [40, 101, 105].

The most frequent symptoms in megacolon consist of intestinal constipations, abdominal distension discomfort, occlusive phenomena associated with fecaloma, and sigmoid volvulus [106, 107]. Megacolon treatment may be clinical or surgical and varies according to patient agreement, level of complications, nutritional status, clinical condition, presence of comorbidity, and age [40]. If the clinical treatment indicates an alteration in the diet, use of laxatives, such as lubrificant laxatives (mineral oils) and emollient laxatives, and intestinal washes with water and glycerin may be used [105].

5. Therapeutic alternatives for Chagas disease treatment

5.1. Clinical trials

As previously described in this chapter, a randomized controlled clinical trial for investigation of BNZ in the treatment of CD was performed only recently: the BENEFIT clinical trial [95]. Therefore, it is not surprising that there is a lack of clinical studies with novel drug candidates for CD, since even the study to evaluate the first choice treatment is very recent.

Posaconazole (POS) (**Figure 4A**) is a triazole derivative with antifungal activity [108], that has been approved for the treatment of invasive fungal infections in humans [109]. It has shown trypanocidal activity in murine models [110, 111]. In addition, POS treatment led to the cure of the infection in one patient, resulting in parasite levels lower than after treatment with BNZ [112]. Therefore, POS efficacy and safety were compared to BNZ in phase II clinical trial CHAGASAZOL NCT01162967 [4], since it has shown trypanocidal activity in murine models. In this study, 78 patients were randomly selected to receive POS at a dose of 400 mg, POS at a dose of 100 mg, or BNZ at a dose of 150 mg. All drugs were orally administered twice daily for 60 days. During the treatment days, only two individual of POS patients treated with the dose of 100 mg had tested positive for *T. cruzi* DNA using a RT-PCR assay. The study duration was 1 year, thus the patients were retested following the treatment period. The outcomes have shown a significantly (p-value lower than 0.01) higher incidence of positive *T. cruzi* DNA results in both POS-treated groups (81–92%) compared to BNZ-treated group, since the last one led to only 38% of patients testing positive for *T. cruzi* DNA using the RT-PCR assay. While all patients from POS groups completed the study, five patients stopped the BNZ treatment, due to severe skin reactions. The adverse reactions of the current treatment with BNZ are some of the reasons why superior treatments must be pursued. However, BNZ treatment failed in fewer patients than POS [4].

CHAGASAZOL was not the only clinical trial testing the potential application of POS in Chagas Disease treatment. The clinical trial STOP-CHAGAS NCT01377480 [113] investigated if POS or POS plus BNZ were superior to BNZ monotherapy in the reduction of parasites load after 60 days of treatment and 360 days follow up. In this study, 120 subjects were randomly divided into the following groups: POS 400 mg twice a day; BNZ 200 mg and placebo, both twice a day; BNZ 200 mg and POS 400 mg, both twice a day; or placebo 10 mg. Two outcome stages were considered, the persistence of negative RT-PCR in day 180 and the maintenance of this response by the end of the study in day 360. The successful overall outcome was the RT-PCR negative result in both stages. Both groups receiving BNZ achieve 96% subjects with negative RT-PCR at day 360, while placebo group and POS alone group had 16.7% and 23.3% subjects with negative RT-PCR, respectively. Those groups receiving BNZ also had six serious adverse events reported, such as cutaneous reactions, nervous system disorders, and gastrointestinal symptoms. Therefore once again, BNZ monotherapy was superior to POS, and no advantages were observed in the combination therapy.

Ravuconazole (**Figure 4C**) is another triazole compound that has shown potent and specific anti-*T. cruzi* action *in vitro*, but with limited *in vivo* activity, probably as a consequence of its poor pharmacokinetic properties [114]. Therefore, E1224 (**Figure 4D**) was developed as a prodrug of ravuconazole. A phase II Clinical Trial was performed in 2013 to evaluate the prodrug efficacy and safety compared to BNZ, as a randomized double-blinded placebo-controlled proof-of-concept study [115]. The study was performed in 224 patients with chronic indeterminate CD. Two groups received E1224 for 60 days at doses of 200 mg (low dose) and 400 mg (high dose), one group took E1224 for 30 days at a dose of 400 mg (short dose), and one group received BNZ at dose of 5 mg/kg/day. All treatments were able to eliminate blood-circulating parasites during the treatment period. E1224 had a parasite clearance rate of 90, 89, and 76% for the low dose group, short dose group, and high dose group, respectively. However, at the 12-month evaluation clearance of all patients that received E1224 was significantly low, and only the high dose group (29%) led to results significantly better than placebo.

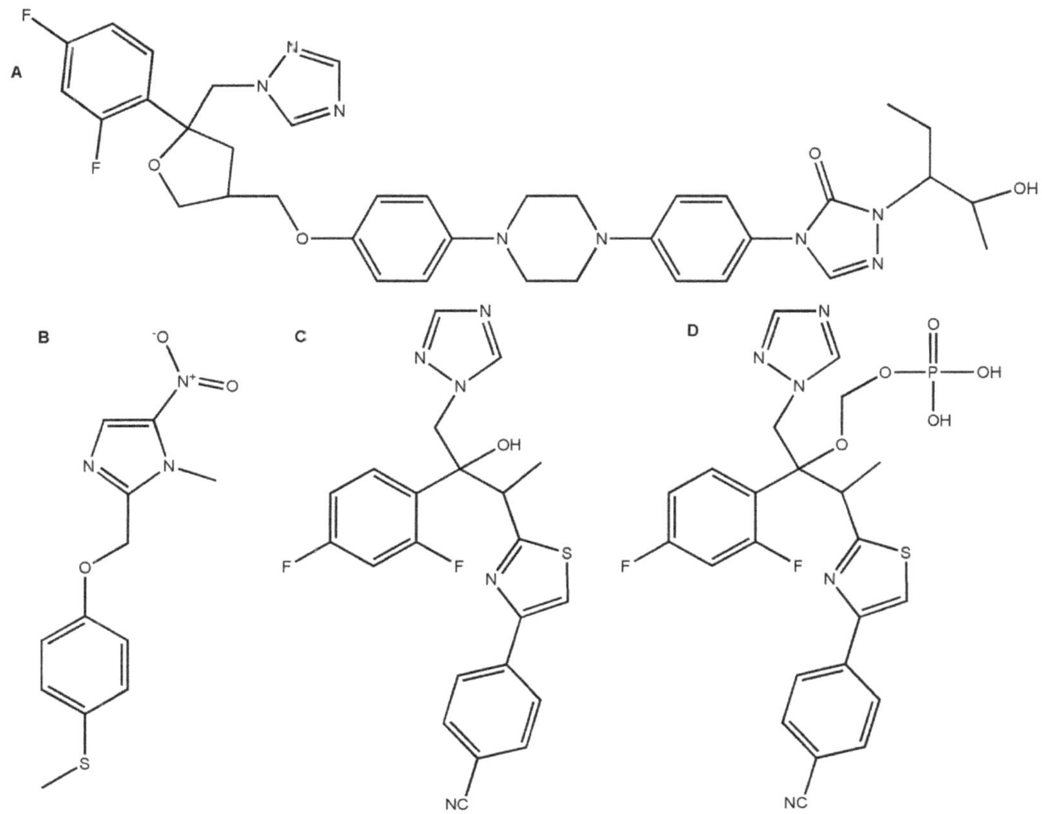

Figure 4. Structures of the compounds posaconazole (A), fexinidazole (B), ravuconazole (C), and E1224/fosravuconazole (D).

Alternatively, the BNZ clearance was 91% at 60 days after treatment and it dropped to 82% at 12 months, also being significant versus placebo. In summary, the drug candidate E1224 was as effective as BNZ at clearing the parasite following the treatment course, but the sustained efficacy 1 year following treatment was very low. Further, BNZ led to significant side effects. Therefore E1224, now called fosravuconazole, will be clinically tested in association to BNZ in order to improve treatment tolerability issues by combining them in the disease therapy.

A search for CD studies of new treatments on the clinical trials website (clinicaltrials.gov) provides one more study, with fexinidazole (**Figure 4B**). This compound is an old nitroimidazole that has shown promising results in preclinical models of CD [116]. According to Drug for Neglected Disease initiative (DNDi), this clinical study NCT02498782 was stopped due to safety and tolerability issues that occurred at the highest tested dose. High efficacy was observed at the lowest dose with acceptable safety and tolerability. Based on this, DNDi claims to be planning a new study in the near future [117].

5.2. Preclinical studies

Considering the lack of new and safer treatment options for CD, it is very encouraging to observe the efforts of many research groups investigating suitable candidates, which may improve the quality of life of many Chagas disease patients. Among the proposed targets for new alternative therapies examples are, ergosterol synthesis, cruzipain, trypanothione reductase, and type I nitroreductase. Studies addressing these targets in several phases of development will be discussed in this text. However, only a few compounds have demonstrated *in vivo* activity and favorable disposition, while none of the published preclinical candidates seems to be in the boundary of the clinical studies.

5.2.1. CYP51

The sterol 14α-demethylase (CYP51) is an important enzyme for *T. cruzi* survival [118], which works as a target of broad-spectrum antifungal agents, such as POS and ravuconazole, or its prodrug fosravuconazole [119]. Since they were clinically tested, as previously mentioned, they are the most close that a new treatment has come to the patients, even though the clinical studies outcomes were not the best [113]. Albaconazole was considered promising after *in vitro* and *in vivo* studies, but its effect was not satisfactory against a resistant strain [120, 121].

Several others inhibitors of sterol biosynthesis have been tested in non-clinical phases. TAK-187 is another antifungal agent [122] tested for CD due to its good drug-like properties and mechanism of action aiming at CYP51. It has shown potent anti-*T. cruzi* activity *in vitro* and *in vivo* [122], while preventing *Trypanosoma cruzi*-induced cardiac damage [123]. Recently, a new formulation of TAK-187 was patented [124], indicating that a clinical study is potentially possible.

Dialkyl imidazoles have shown high potency (EC50 in the 0.4–10 nM range) against *T. cruzi in vitro*, leading two of them to be tested *in vivo* [125]. These derivatives were able to reduce the parasitemia to undetectable levels in a mouse model of acute CD. According to the authors, these compounds are less expensive to be produced than POS. Carrying systematic modifications in the proposed scaffold of the aforementioned candidates led to new candidates with an EC50 better than that of POS (1 nM); however, only *in vitro* studies have been performed [126].

Since tipifarnib has shown potent anti-*T. cruzi* activity, it is being considered as a new lead compound for CD treatment [127]. To evaluate this drug, analogs of the antitumor agent were designed and investigated *in vitro*. They were considered advantageous due to their modest potency for inhibition of human CYP3A4 [128]. One of these analogs, compound 2 was evaluated *in vivo*, but was not better than POS or BNZ [129]. Lack of adequate pharmacokinetic properties, with short half-life and low exposure, may cause the tipifarnib analog to be ineffective.

A very rational study was performed in the development of 4-aminopyridyl-based CYP51 inhibitors [130]. In this study, compounds were developed and tested for their *in vitro* activity. To assess their action *in vivo*, the pharmacokinetic study was previously performed to better understand the compounds disposition and modify the vehicle of administration. Some of the derivatives have demonstrated better *in vivo* activity when compared to the *in vitro* studies. For the authors, the disconnection between *in vitro* and *in vivo* potency raised questions about prioritizing the CYP inhibitors based only on their *in vitro* performance. They achieved lead compounds with good potency and oral bioavailability, while they admit the need for optimization of the elimination half-lives.

A similar study design was followed to evaluate analogs of fenarimol [131], where it was observed that compounds with long half-lives, that is, maintaining plasma concentration above the IC50, were those that led to undetectable parasite levels in bloodstream. The compounds that were less effective to reduce the parasitemia were those with fast elimination and plasma concentrations equals or below the IC50. The two lead compounds were highly bioavailable with a long half-life. The *in vivo* efficacy was superior compared to BNZ and comparable to POS.

Assuming an evolution of the antifungal approach, VNI is an imidazol developed to be specifically active in the inhibition of the CYP51 of *T. cruzi*. It was able to cure the acute and chronic forms of CD in mice, with 100% survival and no observable side effects. Its pharmacokinetics were considered suitable for further development; however, the presented data were not completely explored [132]. The VNI optimization, VFV, overcame the promising results of VNI not only in the animal model of CD cure rate, but also with better pharmacokinetic properties and more information regarding distribution and biotransformation [133]. The reporting of VFV acute toxicity study have shown no observed adverse effect up to 200 mg/kg in mice, but authors did not present data to assure that the absorption was not saturated, that is, the exposure was proportional to the doses used in the acute toxicity study [134]. These imidazole-containing compounds seem to be the most advanced compounds, but the authors highlight the need for further studies.

5.2.2. *Cruzipain*

The cysteine proteinase cruzipain is vital for *T. cruzi* survival, since it is essential for the parasite replication and differentiation. Based on this, cruzipain has been considered as a target for drug discovery, but also for vaccines [135]. Phe-ala-PQ was a prodrug of primaquine, which had the intent to use the proteinase function of cruzipain to release the parent molecule in the parasite [136], but there are others.

Vinyl-sulfone derivatives [137], such as K11777 and WRR-483 have irreversible inhibitory activity in cruzipain, leading them to be effective against *T. cruzi in vitro* and, also *in vivo* [138, 139]. On the other hand, Cz007 and Cz008 are vinyl-sulfones containing nitrile with reversible cysteine proteinase activity that showed *in vivo* anti-*T. cruzi* action following oral administration in a dose lower than that of BNZ [140, 141]. Authors report bioavailability of both new compounds to be approximately 50%, but with short elimination half-life, what led them to administer the compounds for the efficacy study mixed to powdered chow, while BNZ was administered in water.

Additional compounds focusing on cruzipain have their anti-trypanocidal activity published only *in vitro*, such as thiazolyl hydrazones [142], thio semicarbazones [143], acylhydrazones [144], dipeptidyl nitrile derivatives [145], and triazine and purine nitriles [146].

5.2.3. *Trypanothione reductase*

Trypanothione reductase is responsible for the parasite antioxidant protective mechanism, thus inhibitors aiming for this target may disrupt its antioxidant defenses [147]. Some tricyclic compounds already active for other conditions were able to inhibit trypanothione reductase, and clomipramine was the most active with an inhibition constant (Ki) of 6 μM [148]. The testing for new active compounds led to the discovery of inhibitors with a Ki up to 0.33 μM

[149]. Among the phenothiazines, thioridazine is one of the most potent irreversible inhibitors of trypanothione reductase [150], and has shown better *in vivo* activity than the non-treated group [151]. When compared to BNZ, thioridazine animal survival was comparable of BNZ in mice infected with *T. cruzi* [152].

Moreover the trypanothione reductase inhibition, hydroxymethyl nitrofurazone (NFOH) is able to inhibit cruzipain by 60%, showing *in vivo* activity and experimental animal survival comparable to BNZ [153]. The NFOH pharmacokinetics were studied in rats and rabbits [154, 155], and indicated that optimization is needed despite the dual action.

Additional compounds able to inhibit trypanothione reductase *in vitro* include quaternary analogs [156] of chlorpromazine. The dibenzosuberyl-containing analogs of clomipramine were poor inhibitors of trypanothione reductase, while the polyamine derivatives containing dibenzosuberyl were potent inhibitors up to 0.26 μM, even though they were not active *in vivo*, maybe due to poor pharmacokinetic properties, which were not evaluated [157]. Studying the *in vitro* anti-*T. cruzi* activities of ethyl and methyl quinoxaline-7-carboxylate 1,4-di-N-oxide derivatives, three compounds were discovered. However, only one was non-cytotoxic on host macrophage cells [158], and no *in vivo* study was presented.

5.2.4. Type I nitroreductase

Type I nitroreductase is an enzyme responsible for the differentiation of *T. cruzi* and for the activation of nitroheterocycles [159]. Nitroreductases are among the enzymes proposed as responsible for the bioactivation of BNZ [159] and NFX [160]. Based on this hypothesis, the impairment of this enzyme would be responsible for resistance [159].

The type I nitroreductase bioactivation approach supports the *in vitro* action of aziridinyl nitrobenzamide [161] and halogenated nitrobenzylphosphoramide mustards [162] prodrugs; however, the last was assessed in *T. brucei* parasites. Several nitrotriazole-based compounds demonstrated significant *in vitro* antichagasic activity [163, 164]. Further studies identified compounds with promising *in vivo* activity that has shown good *in vitro* ADME properties [165].

Nitrotriazole compounds with dual action aiming type I nitroreductase and inhibition of CYP51 were able to clear the parasites following a 10-day treatment, better than what was observed in the previous mentioned monofunctional 3-nitrotriazole-based derivatives [166]. Prior to the positive results of the dual action compounds, some experiments led to the understanding that nitroheterocylic compounds are better than those able to inhibit ergosterol biosynthesis [167], while it seems that together, they can work better.

Many preclinical candidates have only proven to be effective *in silico* or *in vitro* becoming promising leads or proving the validity of the proposed strategy. Novel drug candidates with *in vivo* activity, in limited cases have published disposition data, such as bioavailability and elimination half-life. The crucial study before clinical studies is the achievement of the NOAEL, since it is necessary to calculate the first in human dose. However, for compounds not showing clear toxicity without the pharmacokinetic assessment, the NOAEL can be overestimated due to saturated absorption, and this can be an challenge for compounds without this data [168].

5.2.5. Combined alternatives in preclinical studies

Based on the safety issues of BNZ and NFX, strategies to reduce their administered amount would prove beneficial as it may decrease the adverse effects. To circumvent the decrease in efficacy due to dose reduction, combined therapies have been proposed.

The combination of the diamidine prodrug DB289 and BNZ orally decreased parasitemia by 99%, while alone they led to 70 and 90% for DB289 and BNZ, respectively. When the combination of BNZ and DB766 was administered, the decrease in the parasitemia was at least 99.5%. Both combined treatments provided 100% protection against mice mortality, while BNZ alone provided only 78% protection [169].

The combination of BNZ and ketoconazole were evaluated in a disease mouse model. This led to better results than single treatments with susceptible and moderately resistant (Y) strains of *T. cruzi*. [170]. The same Y strain of *T. cruzi in vivo* was used to evaluate the combination of BNZ and itraconazole and the results indicated a fourfold improvement in the disease outcome against each single treatment. Additionally, this combination led to a decrease in cardiotoxicity in the experimental CD [171].

The new compound tetrahydro-β-carboline N-butyl-1-(4-dimethylamino)phenyl-1,2,3,4-tetrahydro-β-carboline-3-carboxamide was superior among its peers in reducing the number of infected cells and the number of internalized parasites, with low cytotoxicity [172]. After this observation, the selected compound was evaluated in combination with BNZ *in vitro* and *in vivo*, where a synergic effect was observed, leading to a reduction in parasitemia and mortality rates [173].

An additional compound tested with BNZ was the new drug candidate 2-methyl-1,5-bis(4-nitrophenyl)penta-1,4-dien-3-one, which has shown trypanocidal activity *in vitro*. Next, it was evaluated in combination with BNZ, ketoconazole, and fluconazole. Although the combination with the last one was ineffective, the combination with BNZ and ketoconazole demonstrated strong synergism [174].

These studies indicate that combination of new compounds or compounds used for alternative conditions have the potential to be a successful approach. A similar strategy has been planned for clinical trials to evaluate the combination of benznidazole and fosravuconazole, despite the absence of advantage in the combined therapy using BNZ and POS.

6. Conclusion

Once no new therapeutic alternatives have been included in its treatment portfolio after benznidazole and nifurtimox introduction there is a need for new compounds able to treat patients of CD. Many new drug candidates are evaluated to provide a better treatment for patients in the chronic phase. Benznidazole and nifurtimox are very effective, but their adverse effects cause many patients to discontinue treatment. Symptomatic treatment of the chronic phase of the disease is as important as the treatment directed in the reduction of the parasite. It is necessary to evaluate the patient conditions correctly to improve the quality of life. It is comprehensible that the chase for new options against this disease begins with a search of new molecules, but it is important to keep in mind that this is just a small step. Significance can only be measured if the following steps are performed and the patient treatment is reached. The combined therapy and the repurposing approaches may discover the next treatment option; however, the research must not be completed until the ideal treatment is achieved.

Acknowledgements

The authors wish to acknowledge the CP 01/2016 Programa Pesquisa para o Sistema Único de Saúde: Gestão Compartilhada em Saúde – PPSUS Edição 2015 Fundação Araucária-PR /SESA-PR/CNPq/MS-Decit (CV 45) and CAPES for their valuable contribution.

Author details

Wilton H. Kawaguchi[1], Leticia Bonancio Cerqueira[1], Mariana Millan Fachi[1], Michel L. Campos[1], Iara J. Messias Reason[2] and Roberto Pontarolo[1]*

*Address all correspondence to: pontarolo@ufpr.br

1 Department of Pharmacy, Federal University of Paraná, Curitiba, Paraná, Brazil

2 Clinical Hospital, Federal University of Paraná, Curitiba, Paraná, Brazil

References

[1] WHO. Chagas Disease (American Trypanosomiasis). 2017. Available from: http://www.who.int/chagas/disease/en/ [Accessed: Aug 22, 2017]

[2] Kropf S, Sá M. The discovery of *Trypanosoma cruzi* and Chagas disease (1908–1909): Tropical medicine in Brazil. História, Ciências, Saúde-Manguinhos. 2009;**16**(Suppl 1):13-34

[3] Malafaia G, Rodrigues ASDL. Centenário do descobrimento da doença de Chagas: Desafios e perspectivas [Centenary of the discovery of Chagas disease: Challenges and perspectives]. Revista da Sociedade Brasileira de Medicina Tropical. 2010;**43**(5):483-485

[4] Molina I, Gómez i Prat J, Salvador F, Treviño B, Sulleiro E, Serre N, et al. Randomized trial of posaconazole and benznidazole for chronic Chagas' disease. New England Journal of Medicine. 2014;**370**:1899-1908

[5] do Alexandre JP, Teston APM, Júnior GZ. Tratamento etiológico da doença de Chagas: Um antigo problema de saúde pública [Etiologic treatment of Chagas' disease: An old public health problem]. Revista UNINGÁ Review. 2014;**20**:91-96

[6] Parker ER, Sethi A. Chagas disease: Coming to a place near you. Dermatologic Clinics. 2011;**29**:53-62

[7] Bern C. Chagas' disease. New England Journal of Medicine. 2015;**373**:456-466

[8] Dias J, Coura J. Clínica e terapêutica da Doença de Chagas, uma abordagem prática para o clínico geral [Clinic and therapy of Chagas disease, a practical approach for the general practitioner]. Revista da Sociedade Brasileira de Medicina Tropical. 1997;**30**:263

[9] Oliveira M, Dias A, Pontes V, Souza Júnior A, Coelho H, Coelho I. Tratamento etiológico da doença de Chagas no Brasil [Etiologic treatment of Chagas' disease in Brazil]. Revista de Patologia Tropical. 2008;**37**(3):207-228

[10] Soares Sobrinho JL, de Moraes Medeiros FP, De La Roca MF, Ramos Silva KE, Antunes Lima LN, Rolim Neto PJ. Delineamento de alternativas terapêuticas para o tratamento da doença de Chagas [Design of therapeutic alternatives for the treatment of Chagas' disease]. Revista de Patologia Tropical. 2007;**36**:103-118

[11] Coura J, Castro S. A critical review on Chagas disease chemotherapy. Memorias do Instituto Oswaldo Cruz. 2002;**97**:3-24

[12] Mazza S, Cossio R, Zucardi E. Primer caso agudo de enfermedad de Chagas comprobado en Tucuman y en tratamiento con Bayer 7602 [First acute case of Chagas disease verified in Tucuman and in treatment with Bayer 7602]. Mission de Estudios de Patologia Regional de Argentina. 1937;**32**(3):3-18

[13] Packchanian A. Chemotherapy of African sleeping sickness. I. Chemotherapy of experimental *Trypanosoma gambiense* infection in mice (*Mus musculus*) with nitrofurazone. American Journal of Tropical Medicine and Hygiene. 1955;**4**(4):705-711

[14] Evens F, Niemegeers K, Packchanian A. Nitrofurazone Therapy of *Trypanosoma Gambiense* Sleeping Sickness in Man. The American Society of Tropical Medicine and Hygiene. 1957;**6**(4):665-678

[15] Ferreira HO. Forma aguda da doença de Chagas tratada pela nitrofurazona [Acute form of Chagas' disease treated by nitrofurazone]. Revista do Instituto de Medicina Tropical de Sao Paulo. 1961;**3**:287-289

[16] Ferreira HO. Fase aguda da doença de Chagas [Acute phase of Chagas' disease]. Journal of Hospital. 1962;**61**:307-311

[17] Coura J, Ferreira L, Saad E, Mortel R, Silva J. Tentativa terapêutica com a nitrofurazona (Furacin) na forma crônica da doença de Chagas. Journal of Hospital. 1961;**60**:425-429

[18] Coura J, Ferreira L, Silva J. Experiências com nitrofurazona na fase crônica da doença de Chagas [Experiments with nitrofurazone in the chronic phase of Chagas disease]. Journal of Hospital. 1962;**62**:957-964

[19] Rodriques Coura J, de Castro SL. A critical review on Chagas disease chemotherapy. Memorias do Instituto Oswaldo Cruz. 2002;**97**(1):3-24

[20] Bern C, Montgomery SP, Herwaldt BL, Rassi Jr A, Marin-Neto JA, Dantas RO, et al. Evaluation and treatment of Chagas disease in the United States: A systematic review. Journal of the American Medical Association. 2007;**298**(18):2171-2181

[21] Serafim EOP, Chin CM, Ribeiro ML, Araújo DS. Abordagem da latenciação de fármacos como ferramenta para descoberta de novos antichagásicos [Approach of drug latency as a tool for the discovery of new antichagasics]. Revista Uniara. 2011; **14**:140-157

[22] Palmeiro-Roldán R, Fonseca-Berzal C, Gómez-Barrio A, Arán VJ, Escario JA, Torrado-Durán S, et al. Development of novel benznidazole formulations: Physicochemical characterization and in vivo evaluation on parasitemia reduction in Chagas disease. International Journal of Pharmaceutics. 2014;**472**:110-117

[23] Priotti J, Ferreira MJG, Lamas MC, Leonardi D, Salomon CJ, Nunes TG. First solid-state NMR spectroscopy evaluation of complexes of benznidazole with cyclodextrin derivatives. Carbohydrate Polymers. 2015;**131**:90-97

[24] Romina Manarin MCL, Bottasso E, Serra E, Silvia Revelli CJS. Efficacy of novel benznidazole solutions during the experimental infection with *Trypanosoma cruzi*. Parasitology International. 2013;**62**(1):79-81

[25] Benziger CP, do Carmo GA, Ribeiro AL. Chagas cardiomyopathy: Clinical presentation and Management in the Americas. Cardiology Clinics. 2017;**35**(1):31-47

[26] Buschini A, Ferrarini L, Franzoni S, Galati S, Lazzaretti M, Mussi F, et al. Genotoxicity revaluation of three commercial nitroheterocyclic drugs: Nifurtimox, benznidazole, and metronidazole. Journal of Parasitology Research. 2009;**2009**:1-11

[27] Perdomo VG, Rigalli JP, Villanueva SSM, Ruiz ML, Luquita MG, Echenique CG, et al. Modulation of biotransformation systems and ABC transporters by benznidazole in rats. Antimicrobial Agents and Chemotherapy. 2013;**57**:4894-4902

[28] Trochine A, Creek DJ, Faral-Tello P, Barrett MP, Robello C. Benznidazole biotransformation and multiple targets in *Trypanosoma cruzi* revealed by metabolomics. PLoS Neglected Tropical Diseases. 2014;**8**:e2844

[29] Campos MCO, Leon LL, Taylor MC, Kelly JM. Benznidazole-resistance in *Trypanosoma cruzi*: Evidence that distinct mechanisms can act in concert. Molecular and Biochemical Parasitology. 2014;**193**:17-19

[30] Ministério da Saúde. Guia de Vigilância em saúde [Health Surveillance Guide]. Ministério da Saúde – Guia de Vigilância em saúde. 2016;**1**:607-619

[31] PAHO. Doença de Chagas: Guia para vigilância, prevênção, controle e manejo clínico da doença de chagas aguda transmitida por alimentos [Chagas disease: A guide for surveillance, prevention, control and clinical management of acute foodborne illness]. Journal of Chemical Information and Modeling. 2009;**12**:160

[32] Rocha MO, Teixeira MM, Ribeiro AL. An update on the management of Chagas cardiomyopathy. Expert Review of Anti-infective Therapy. 2007;**5**:727-743

[33] Morillo CA, Marin-Neto JA, Avezum A, Sosa-Estani S, Rassi A, Rosas F, et al. Randomized trial of benznidazole for chronic Chagas' cardiomyopathy. New England Journal of Medicine. 2015;**373**:1295-1306

[34] Boainain E, Rassi A. Atualização Terapêutica – Terapêutica etiologica da doença de Chagas [therapeutic update – Chagas disease etiological therapy]. Arquivos Brasileiros de Cardiologia. 1979;**6**:395-399

[35] Cançado JR. Long term evaluation of etiological treatment of Chagas disease with benznidazole. Revista do Instituto de Medicina Tropical de Sao Paulo. 2002;**44**:29-37

[36] Costa M, Tavares VR, Aquino MVM, Moreira DB. Doença de chagas: uma revisão bibliográfica [Chagas disease: A literature review]. 2013

[37] FDA. FDA Approves First U.S. Treatment for Chagas disease. Accessed: Aug 29, 2017. Available in: https://www.fda.gov/NewsEvents/Newsroom/PressAnnouncements/ucm573942.htm

[38] Altclas J, Sinagra A, Dictar M, Luna C, Verón MT, De Rissio AM, et al. Chagas disease in bone marrow transplantation: An approach to preemptive therapy. Bone Marrow Transplantation. 2005;**36**:123-129

[39] Fiorelli AI, Stolf NAG, Honorato R, Bocchi E, Bacal F, Uip D, et al. Later evolution after cardiac transplantation in Chagas' disease. Transplantation Proceedings. 2005;**37**:2793-2798

[40] Ministerio da Saúde. Consenso brasileiro em doença de Chagas [Brazilian consensus on Chagas' disease]. Revista da Sociedade Brasileira de Medicina Tropical. 2005;**38**(3):7-29

[41] Sartori AMC, Ibrahim KY, Westphalen E, Braz L, Oliveira O, Gakiya E, et al. Manifestations of Chagas disease (American trypanosomiasis) in patients with HIV/AIDS. Annals of Tropical Medicine & Parasitology. 2007;**101**:31-50

[42] Vaidian AK, Weiss LM, Tanowitz HB. Chagas' disease and AIDS. Kinetoplastid Biology and Disease. 2004;**3**:2

[43] Ribeiro CM, Budni P, Pedrosa RC, Farias MS, Parisotto EB, Dalmarco EM, et al. Antioxidant therapy attenuates oxidative insult caused by benzonidazole in chronic Chagas' heart disease. International Journal of Cardiology. 2010;**145**:27-33

[44] Ministerio da Saúde. Guia de Vigilância Epidemiológica [Epidemiological Surveillance Guide]. Série A Normas e Manuais Técnicos. 2009;**7**:819

[45] Schofield CJ, Jannin J, Salvatella R. The future of Chagas disease control. Trends in parasitology. 2006;**22**(12):583-588

[46] Brener Z. Terapêutica experimental na doença de Chagas. [Experimental therapy in Chagas' disease]. In: Andrade ZB, BarraL-Neto Z, editors. *Trypanosoma cruzi* e doença de Chagas. 2nd ed. Rio de Janeiro: Guanabara Koogan; 2000. pp. 379-388

[47] CDC. Infectious Disease Laboratory – Formulary: U.S. Department of Health & Human Services. 2016. Available from: https://www.cdc.gov/laboratory/drugservice/formulary.html [updated Sep 22, 2016; cited Oct 15, 2017]

[48] Castro JA, de Mecca MM, Bartel LC. Toxic side effects of drugs used to treat Chagas' disease (American trypanosomiasis). Human & Experimental Toxicology. 2006;**25**(8): 471-479

[49] Coura J, de Abreu L, Willcox H, Petana W. Comparative controlled study on the use of benznidazole, nifurtimox and placebo, in the chronic form of Chagas' disease, in a field area with interrupted transmission. I. Preliminary evaluation. Revista da Sociedade Brasileira de Medicina Tropical. 1997;**30**(2):139-144

[50] Núñez-Vergara LJ, Squella JA, Aldunate J, Letelier ME, Bollo S, Repetto Y, et al. Nitro radical anion formation from nifurtimox. Part 1: Biological evidences in *Trypanosoma cruzi*. Bioelectrochemistry and Bioenergetics. 1997;**43**(1):151-155

[51] Docampo R, Mason RP, Mottley C, Muniz RP. Generation of free radicals induced by nifurtimox in mammalian tissues. The Journal of biological chemistry. 1981;**256**(21): 10930-10933

[52] Wilkinson SR, Bot C, Kelly JM, Hall BS. Trypanocidal activity of nitroaromatic prodrugs: Current treatments and future perspectives. Current Topics in Medicinal Chemistry. 2011;**11**(16):2072-2084

[53] Docampo R, Dubin M, Martino EE, Moreno SN, Stoppani AO. Influence of nifurtimox on the glutathione content of the liver and bile in rats. Medicina. 1983;**43**(1):33-40

[54] Docampo R, Moreno SN. Free radical metabolism of antiparasitic agents. Federation Proceedings. 1986;**45**(10):2471-2476

[55] Docampo R, Moreno SN. Free radical metabolites in the mode of action of chemotherapeutic agents and phagocytic cells on *Trypanosoma cruzi*. Reviews of Infectious Diseases. 1984;**6**(2):223-238

[56] Docampo R, Moreno SN, Stoppani AO, Leon W, Cruz FS, Villalta F, et al. Mechanism of nifurtimox toxicity in different forms of *Trypanosoma cruzi*. Biochemical Pharmacology. 1981;**30**(14):1947-1951

[57] Docampo R, Stoppani AO. Generation of superoxide anion and hydrogen peroxide induced by nifurtimox in *Trypanosoma cruzi*. Archives of Biochemistry and Biophysics. 1979;**197**(1):317-321

[58] Docampo R, Stoppani AO. Mechanism of the trypanocidal action of nifurtimox and other nitro-derivatives on *Trypanosoma cruzi*. Medicina. 1980;**40**(Suppl 1):10-16

[59] Patterson S, Wyllie S. Nitro drugs for the treatment of trypanosomatid diseases: Past, present, and future prospects. Trends in Parasitology. 2014;**30**(6):289-298

[60] Morello A. The biochemistry of the mode of action of drugs and the detoxication mechanisms in *Trypanosoma cruzi*. Comparative Biochemistry and Physiology C, Comparative Pharmacology and Toxicology. 1988;**90**(1):1-12

[61] Boveris A, Sies H, Martino EE, Docampo R, Turrens JF, Stoppani AO. Deficient metabolic utilization of hydrogen peroxide in *Trypanosoma cruzi*. The Biochemical Journal. 1980;**188**(3):643-648

[62] Docampo R, de Boiso JF, Boveris A, Stoppani AO. Localization of peroxidase activity in *Trypanosoma cruzi* microbodies. Experientia. 1976;**32**(8):972-975

[63] Cançado JR, Salgado AA, Marra UD, Alvares JM, Machado JR. Ensaio terapêutico clínico na doença de Chagas crônica com o nifurtimox era três esquemas de duração prolongada [Clinical therapeutic trial in chronic Chagas' disease with nifurtimox was three schemes of prolonged duration]. Revista do Instituto de Medicina Tropical de São Paulo. 1975;**17**:111

[64] Cerisola JA, Rohwedder R, Segura EL, del Prado CE, Alvares M, de Martini GJW. El xenodiagnóstico [The xenodiagnosis]. Imprenta dei Instituto Nacional de Investigaciones Cardiovasculares. 1974;**1**:127

[65] Rassi A, Ferreira HO. Tentativas de tratamento especifico da fase aguda da doença de chagas com nitrofuranos em esquemas de duração prolongada [Specific treatment attempts of the acute phase of chagas disease with nitrofurans in long duration regimens]. Revista da Sociedade Brasileira de Medicina Tropical. 1971;**5**(2):35

[66] Schenone H, Concha L, Aranda R, Rojas A, Knierim F, Rojo M. Treatment of chronic Chagas' infection with Lampit. Boletin chileno de parasitologia. 1972;**27**(1):11-14

[67] Silva NN, Kuhn G, Santos JFC, Eye GV, Chaher JAB. Eficácia e tolerância do nitrofurfurilidene na fase crônica da moléstia de Chagas [Efficacy and tolerance of nitrofurfurylidene in the chronic phase of Chagas' disease]. Revista da Sociedade Brasileira de Medicina Tropical. 1974;**8**:325

[68] Forsyth CJ, Hernandez S, Olmedo W, Abuhamidah A, Traina MI, Sanchez DR, et al. Safety profile of nifurtimox for treatment of Chagas disease in the United States. Clinical Infectious Diseases: An Official Publication of the Infectious Diseases Society of America. 2016;**63**(8):1056-1062

[69] Sanchez G, Coronado X, Zulantay I, Apt W, Gajardo M, Solari S, et al. Monitoring the efficacy of specific treatment in chronic Chagas disease by polymerase chain reaction and flow cytometry analysis. Parasite. 2005;**12**(4):353-357

[70] Murcia L, Carrilero B, Albajar Vinas P, Segovia M. Nifurtimox chemotherapy: Collateral effects in treated *Trypanosoma cruzi* infected patients. Revista espanola de quimioterapia : publicacion oficial de la Sociedad Espanola de Quimioterapia. 2012;**25**(1):74-75

[71] Streiger ML, del Barco ML, Fabbro DL, Arias ED, Amicone NA. Longitudinal study and specific chemotherapy in children with chronic Chagas' disease, residing in a low endemicity area of Argentina. Revista da Sociedade Brasileira de Medicina Tropical. 2004; **37**(5):365-375

[72] Bestetti RB. Chagas heart failure in patients from Latin America. Journal of Cardiac Failure Reviews. 2016;**2**(2):90-94

[73] Bestetti RB, Theodoropoulos TA, Cardinalli-Neto A, Cury PM. Treatment of chronic systolic heart failure secondary to Chagas heart disease in the current era of heart failure therapy. American Heart Journal. 2008;**156**(3):422-430

[74] Cunha-Neto E, Chevillard C. Chagas disease cardiomyopathy: Immunopathology and genetics. Mediators of Inflammation. 2014;**2014**:683230

[75] Higuchi M d L, Benvenuti LA, Martins Reis M, Metzger M. Pathophysiology of the heart in Chagas' disease: Current status and new developments. Cardiovascular Research. 2003;**60**(1):96-107

[76] Strasen J, Williams T, Ertl G, Zoller T, Stich A, Ritter O. Epidemiology of Chagas disease in Europe: Many calculations, little knowledge. Clinical Research in Cardiology. 2014; **103**(1):1-10

[77] Barbosa MP, Carmo AA, Rocha MO, Ribeiro AL. Ventricular arrhythmias in Chagas disease. Revista da Sociedade Brasileira de Medicina Tropical. 2015;**48**(1):4-10

[78] Botoni FA, Ribeiro AL, Marinho CC, Lima MM, Nunes Mdo C, Rocha MO. Treatment of Chagas cardiomyopathy. BioMed Research International. 2013;**2013**:849504

[79] de Cardiologia SB. I Latin American guideline for the diagnosis and treatment of Chagas' heart disease. Journal of Sociedade Brasileira de Cardiologia. 2011;**97**(2):1-48

[80] Rassi Junior A, Rassi A, Marin-Neto J. Chagas heart disease: Pathophysiologic mechanisms, prognostic factors and risk stratification. Memorias do Instituto Oswaldo Cruz. 2009;**104**(1):152-158

[81] Ribeiro AL, Nunes MP, Teixeira MM, Rocha MO. Diagnosis and management of Chagas disease and cardiomyopathy. Nature Reviews. Cardiology. 2012;**9**(10):576-589

[82] Andrade J, Marin Neto J, de Paola A, Vilas-Boas A, Oliveira G, Bacal F, et al. I Latin American guidelines for the diagnosis and treatment of Chagas' heart disease – Executive summary. Arquivos Brasileiros de Cardiologia. 2011;**96**(6):434-442

[83] Mora G. Chagas cardiomyopathy. Journal of Cardiology Practice. 2016;**14**(31):1-7

[84] Bilate AM, Cunha-Neto E. Chagas disease cardiomyopathy: Current concepts of an old disease. Revista do Instituto de Medicina Tropical de Sao Paulo. 2008;**50**(2):67-74

[85] Batlouni M, Barretto AC, Armaganijan D, Vichi FL, Spritzer N, Simoes R, et al. Treatment of mild and moderate cardiac failure with captopril. A multicenter study. Arquivos Brasileiros de Cardiologia. 1992;**58**(5):417-421

[86] Botoni FA, Poole-Wilson PA, Ribeiro AL, Okonko DO, Oliveira BM, Pinto AS, et al. A randomized trial of carvedilol after renin-angiotensin system inhibition in chronic Chagas cardiomyopathy. American Heart Journal. 2007;**153**(4):544 e1-544e8

[87] Leon JS, Wang K, Engman DM. Captopril ameliorates myocarditis in acute experimental Chagas disease. Circulation. 2003;**107**(17):2264-2269

[88] Roberti RR, Martinez EE, Andrade JL, Araujo VL, Brito FS, Portugal OP, et al. Chagas cardiomyopathy and captopril. European Heart Journal. 1992;**13**(7):966-970

[89] Pitt B, Remme W, Zannad F, Neaton J, Martinez F, Roniker B, et al. Eplerenone, a selective aldosterone blocker, in patients with left ventricular dysfunction after myocardial infarction. The New England Journal of Medicine. 2003;**348**(14):1309-1321

[90] Pitt B, Zannad F, Remme WJ, Cody R, Castaigne A, Perez A, et al. The effect of spironolactone on morbidity and mortality in patients with severe heart failure. Randomized Aldactone evaluation study investigators. The New England Journal of Medicine. 1999;**341**(10):709-717

[91] Ramires FJ, Salemi VM, Ianni BM, Fernandes F, Martins DG, Billate A, et al. Aldosterone antagonism in an inflammatory state: Evidence for myocardial protection. Journal of the Renin-Angiotensin-Aldosterone System. 2006;**7**(3):162-167

[92] Bestetti RB, Otaviano AP, Cardinalli-Neto A, da Rocha BF, Theodoropoulos TA, Cordeiro JA. Effects of B-blockers on outcome of patients with Chagas' cardiomyopathy with chronic heart failure. International Journal of Cardiology. 2011;**151**(2):205-208

[93] Bestetti RB, Theodoropoulos TA, Cardinalli-Neto A. Treating patients with Chagas' cardiomyopathy with chronic heart failure in the contemporary era. American Heart Journal. 2007;**154**(5):e35. Author reply e3

[94] Issa VS, Amaral AF, Cruz FD, Ferreira SM, Guimaraes GV, Chizzola PR, et al. Beta-blocker therapy and mortality of patients with Chagas cardiomyopathy: A subanalysis of the REMADHE prospective trial. Circulation. Heart Failure. 2010;**3**(1):82-88

[95] Marin-Neto JA, Rassi Jr A, Avezum Jr A, Mattos AC, Rassi A. The BENEFIT trial: Testing the hypothesis that trypanocidal therapy is beneficial for patients with chronic Chagas heart disease. Memorias do Instituto Oswaldo Cruz. 2009;**104**:319-324

[96] Quiros FR, Morillo CA, Casas JP, Cubillos LA, Silva FA. CHARITY: Chagas cardiomyopathy bisoprolol intervention study: A randomized double-blind placebo force-titration controlled study with Bisoprolol in patients with chronic heart failure secondary to Chagas cardiomyopathy [NCT00323973]. Trials. 2006;**7**:21

[97] Sousa AS, Xavier SS, Freitas GR, Hasslocher-Moreno A. Prevention strategies of cardioembolic ischemic stroke in Chagas' disease. Arquivos Brasileiros de Cardiologia. 2008;**91**(5):306-310

[98] Bestetti R. Cardiomiopatia chagásica crônica: diagnóstico e tratamento. Revista da Sociedade de Cardiologia do Estado de São Paulo. 2016;**26**(4):246-252

[99] de Oliveira AP, Bernardo CR, Camargo AV, Ronchi LS, Borim AA, de Mattos CC, et al. Genetic susceptibility to cardiac and digestive clinical forms of chronic Chagas disease: Involvement of the CCR5 59029 A/G polymorphism. PLoS One. 2015;**10**(11):e0141847

[100] Prata A. Clinical and epidemiological aspects of Chagas disease. The Lancet Infectious Diseases. 2001;**1**(2):92-100

[101] Rassi Junior A, Rassi A, Marin-Neto J. Chagas disease. The Lancet. 2010;**375**:1388-1402

[102] Gullo C, Estofolete C, Gil C, Christiano A, Gomes NJ. Formas digestivas da doença de Chagas e carcinogênese: um estudo de associação [Digestive forms of Chagas' disease and carcinogenesis: an association study]. Revista do Colégio Brasileiro. 2012;**39**(2): 146-150

[103] Matsuda NM, Miller SM, Evora PR. The chronic gastrointestinal manifestations of Chagas disease. Clinics (São Paulo, Brazil). 2009;**64**(12):1219-1224

[104] Dias JCP, Coura JR. org. Clínica e terapêutica da doença de Chagas: uma abordagem prática para o clínico geral [Clinical and therapeutic of Chagas disease: a practical approach for the general practitioner]. In: Rezende JM, editor. O Aparelho Digestivo na doença de Chagas [The Digestive Tract in Chagas Disease]. Rio de Janeiro: Editora FIOCRUZ. 1997;**1**:486

[105] Menegheli U. Clinical treatment of the digestive form of Chagas disease. Memorias do Instituto Oswaldo Cruz. 1999;**94**(1):341-342

[106] Braga C, Guimarães L, Amaral R, Bonani A, Moreira N, Gomes M, et al. Megacólon de Doença de Chagas: Uma Abordagem Interdisciplinar [Megacolon of Chagas disease: An interdisciplinary approach]. Revista de Saúde e Biologia. 2013;**8**(1):36-43

[107] Posada E, Pell C, Angulo N, Pinazo MJ, Gimeno F, Elizalde I, et al. Bolivian migrants with Chagas disease in Barcelona, Spain: A qualitative study of dietary changes and digestive problems. International Health. 2011;**3**(4):289-294

[108] Patterson TF. Role of newer azoles in surgical patients. Journal of Chemotherapy. 1999; **11**(6):504-512

[109] Kwon DS, Mylonakis E. Posaconazole: A new broad-spectrum antifungal agent. Expert Opinion on Pharmacotherapy. 2007;**8**(8):1167-1178

[110] Molina J, Martins-Filho O, Brener Z, Romanha AJ, Loebenberg D, Urbina JA. Activities of the triazole derivative SCH 56592 (Posaconazole) against drug-resistant strains of the protozoan parasite *Trypanosoma* (*Schizotrypanum*) *cruzi* in immunocompetent and immunosuppressed murine hosts. Antimicrobial Agents and Chemotherapy. 2000;**44**(1):150-155

[111] Urbina JA, Payares G, Contreras LM, Liendo A, Sanoja C, Molina J, et al. Antiproliferative effects and mechanism of action of SCH 56592 against Trypanosoma (Schizotrypanum) cruzi: *In vitro* and *in vivo* studies. Antimicrobial Agents and Chemotherapy. 1998;**42**(7): 1771-1777

[112] Pinazo MJ, Espinosa G, Gallego M, Lopez-Chejade PL, Urbina JA, Gascon J. Successful treatment with posaconazole of a patient with chronic Chagas disease and systemic lupus erythematosus. American Journal of Tropical Medicine and Hygiene. 2010;**82**(4): 583-587

[113] Morillo CA, Waskin H, Sosa-Estani S, del Carmen Bangher M, Cuneo C, Milesi R, et al. Benznidazole and posaconazole in eliminating parasites in asymptomatic *T. cruzi* carriers. Journal of the American College of Cardiology. 2017;**69**(8):939-947

[114] Urbina JA, Payares G, Sanoja C, Lira R, Romanha AJ. *In vitro* and *in vivo* activities of ravuconazole on *Trypanosoma cruzi,* the causative agent of Chagas disease. International Journal of Antimicrobial Agents. 2003;**21**(1):27-38

[115] Torrico F, Gascon J, Ortiz L, Alonso-Vega C, Pinazo MJ, Schijman A, Almeida IC, Alves F, Strub-Wourgaft N, Ribeiro I. Treatment of adult chronic indeterminate Chagas disease with benznidazole and three E1224 dosing regimens: A proof-of-concept, randomised, placebo-controlled trial. The Lancet Infectious Diseases. 2018. DOI:10.1016/S1473-3099 (17)30538-8

[116] Bahia MT, Nascimento AFS, Mazzeti AL, Marques LF, Goncalves KR, Mota LWR, et al. Antitrypanosomal activity of fexinidazole metabolites, potential new drug candidates for Chagas disease. Antimicrobial Agents and Chemotherapy. 2014;**58**(8):4362-4370

[117] DNDi DfNDi. Fexinidazole (Chagas). 2017. Available from: https://www.dndi.org/diseases-projects/portfolio/fexinidazole-chagas/ [updated Aug 2017; cited Aug 23, 2017]

[118] Lepesheva GI, Zaitseva NG, Nes WD, Zhou W, Arase M, Liu J, et al. CYP51 from*Trypanosoma cruzi*. Journal of Biological Chemistry. 2006;**281**(6):3577-3585

[119] Buckner FS, Urbina JA. Recent developments in sterol 14-demethylase inhibitors for Chagas disease. International Journal for Parasitology: Drugs and Drug Resistance. 2012;**2**:236-242

[120] Urbina JA, Lira R, Visbal G, Bartroli J. In vitro antiproliferative effects and mechanism of action of the new triazole derivative UR-9825 against the protozoan parasite *Trypanosoma (Schizotrypanum) cruzi*. Antimicrobial Agents and Chemotherapy. 2000;**44**(9):2498-2502

[121] Guedes PMM, Urbina JA, de Lana M, Afonso LCC, Veloso VM, Tafuri WL, et al. Activity of the new triazole derivative albaconazole against *Trypanosoma* (*Schizotrypanum*) *cruzi* in dog hosts. Antimicrobial Agents and Chemotherapy. 2004;**48**(11):4286-4292

[122] Schell WA, De Almeida GM, Dodge RK, Okonogi K, Perfect JR. *In vitro* and *in vivo* efficacy of the triazole TAK-187 against *Cryptococcus neoformans*. Antimicrobial Agents and Chemotherapy. 1998;**42**(10):2630-2632

[123] Corrales M, Cardozo R, Segura MA, Urbina JA, Basombrio MA. Comparative efficacies of TAK-187, a long-lasting ergosterol biosynthesis inhibitor, and benznidazole in preventing cardiac damage in a murine model of Chagas' disease. Antimicrobial Agents and Chemotherapy. 2005;**49**(4):1556-1560

[124] Ueki Y. WO2013157584 A1. Google Patents; 2013

[125] Suryadevara PK, Olepu S, Lockman JW, Ohkanda J, Karimi M, Verlinde CLMJ, et al. Structurally simple inhibitors of Lanosterol 14α-Demethylase are efficacious in a rodent model of acute Chagas disease. Journal of Medicinal Chemistry. 2009;**52**(12):3703-3715

[126] Suryadevara PK, Racherla KK, Olepu S, Norcross NR, Tatipaka HB, Arif JA, et al. Dialkylimidazole inhibitors of *Trypanosoma cruzi* sterol 14α-demethylase as anti-Chagas disease agents. Bioorganic & Medicinal Chemistry Letters. 2013;**23**(23):6492-6499

[127] Hucke O, Gelb MH, Verlinde CLMJ, Buckner FS. The protein farnesyltransferase inhibitor Tipifarnib as a new lead for the development of drugs against Chagas disease. Journal of Medicinal Chemistry. 2005;**48**(17):5415-5418

[128] Kraus JM, Tatipaka HB, McGuffin SA, Chennamaneni NK, Karimi M, Arif J, et al. Second generation analogues of the cancer drug clinical candidate Tipifarnib for anti-Chagas disease drug discovery. Journal of Medicinal Chemistry. 2010;**53**(10):3887-3898

[129] Buckner FS, Bahia MT, Suryadevara PK, White KL, Shackleford DM, Chennamaneni NK, et al. Pharmacological characterization, structural studies, and in vivo activities of anti-Chagas disease lead compounds derived from Tipifarnib. Antimicrobial Agents and Chemotherapy. 2012;**56**(9):4914-4921

[130] Calvet CM, Vieira DF, Choi JY, Kellar D, Cameron MD, Siqueira-Neto JL, et al. 4-Aminopyridyl-based CYP51 inhibitors as anti-*Trypanosoma cruzi* drug leads with improved pharmacokinetic profile and *in Vivo* potency. Journal of Medicinal Chemistry. 2014;**57**(16):6989-7005

[131] Keenan M, Chaplin JH, Alexander PW, Abbott MJ, Best WM, Khong A, et al. Two analogues of fenarimol show curative activity in an experimental model of Chagas disease. Journal of Medicinal Chemistry. 2013;**56**(24):10158-10170

[132] Villalta F, Dobish MC, Nde PN, Kleshchenko YY, Hargrove TY, Johnson CA, et al. VNI cures acute and chronic experimental Chagas disease. The Journal of infectious diseases. 2013;**208**(3):504-511

[133] Lepesheva GI, Hargrove TY, Rachakonda G, Wawrzak Z, Pomel S, Cojean S, et al. VFV as a new effective CYP51 structure-derived drug candidate for Chagas disease and visceral Leishmaniasis. Journal of Infectious Diseases. 2015;**212**(9):1439-1448

[134] Guedes-da-Silva FH, Batista DGJ, Da Silva CF, De Araújo JS, Pavão BP, Simões-Silva MR, et al. Antitrypanosomal activity of sterol 14α-Demethylase (CYP51) inhibitors VNI and VFV in the Swiss mouse models of Chagas disease induced by the *Trypanosoma cruzi Y* strain. Antimicrobial Agents and Chemotherapy. 2017;**61**(4):e02098-16

[135] Duschak V, Couto A. Cruzipain, the major cysteine protease of *Trypanosoma cruzi*: A sulfated glycoprotein antigen as relevant candidate for vaccine development and drug target. A review. Current Medicinal Chemistry. 2009;**16**(24):3174-3202

[136] Chung MC, Gonçalves MF, Colli W, Ferreira EI, Miranda MTM. Synthesis and in vitro evaluation of potential antichagasic dipeptide prodrugs of primaquine. Journal of Pharmaceutical Sciences. 1997;**86**(10):1127-1131

[137] Kerr ID, Lee JH, Farady CJ, Marion R, Rickert M, Sajid M, et al. Vinyl sulfones as antiparasitic agents and a structural basis for drug design. Journal of Biological Chemistry. 2009;**284**(38):25697-25703

[138] Rodriguez A, Chen YT, Brinen LS, Kerr ID, Hansell E, Doyle PS, et al. *In vitro* and *in vivo* studies of the trypanocidal properties of WRR-483 against *Trypanosoma cruzi*. PLoS Neglected Tropical Diseases. 2010;**4**(9):e825

[139] Doyle PS, Zhou YM, Engel JC, McKerrow JH. A cysteine protease inhibitor cures Chagas' disease in an immunodeficient-mouse model of infection. Antimicrobial Agents and Chemotherapy. 2007;**51**(11):3932-3939

[140] Ndao M, Beaulieu C, Black WC, Isabel E, Vasquez-Camargo F, Nath-Chowdhury M, et al. Reversible cysteine protease inhibitors show promise for a Chagas disease cure. Antimicrobial Agents and Chemotherapy. 2013;**58**(2):1167-1178

[141] Beaulieu C, Isabel E, Fortier A, Massé F, Mellon C, Méthot N, et al. Identification of potent and reversible cruzipain inhibitors for the treatment of Chagas disease. Bioorganic & Medicinal Chemistry Letters. 2010;**20**(24):7444-7449

[142] Leite ACL, Moreira DR de M, Cardoso MV de O, Hernandes MZ, Alves Pereira VR, Silva RO, et al. Synthesis, cruzain docking, and in vitro studies of aryl-4-oxothiazolylhydrazones against *Trypanosoma cruzi*. ChemMedChem 2007;**2**(9):1339-1345

[143] Du X, Guo C, Hansell E, Doyle PS, Caffrey CR, Holler TP, et al. Synthesis and structure-activity relationship study of potent trypanocidal thio semicarbazone inhibitors of the trypanosomal cysteine protease cruzain. Journal of Medicinal Chemistry. 2002;**45**(13):2695-2707

[144] dos Santos Filho JM, Leite AC, de Oliveira BG, Moreira DR, Lima MS, Soares MB, et al. Design, synthesis and cruzain docking of 3-(4-substituted-aryl)-1,2,4-oxadiazole-N-acylhydrazones as anti-*Trypanosoma cruzi* agents. Bioorganic & Medicinal Chemistry. 2009;**17**(18):6682-6691

[145] Pollastri MP, Avelar LAA, Camilo CD, de Albuquerque S, Fernandes WB, Gonçalez C, et al. Molecular design, synthesis and trypanocidal activity of dipeptidyl nitriles as cruzain inhibitors. PLOS Neglected Tropical Diseases. 2015;**9**(7):e0003916

[146] Mott BT, Ferreira RS, Simeonov A, Jadhav A, Ang KK-H, Leister W, et al. Identification and optimization of inhibitors of trypanosomal cysteine proteases: Cruzain, rhodesain, and TbCatB. Journal of Medicinal Chemistry. 2010;**53**(1):52-60

[147] Flohé L. The trypanothione system and its implications in the therapy of trypanosomatid diseases. International Journal of Medical Microbiology. 2012;**302**(4–5):216-220

[148] Benson TJ, McKie JH, Garforth J, Borges A, Fairlamb AH, Douglas KT. Rationally designed selective inhibitors of trypanothione reductase. Phenothiazines and related tricyclics as lead structures. The Biochemical Journal. 1992;**286**(Pt 1):9-11

[149] Richardson JL, Nett IRE, Jones DC, Abdille MH, Gilbert IH, Fairlamb AH. Improved tricyclic inhibitors of trypanothione reductase by screening and chemical synthesis. ChemMedChem. 2009;**4**(8):1333-1340

[150] Gutierrez-Correa J, Fairlamb AH, Stoppani AO. *Trypanosoma cruzi* trypanothione reductase is inactivated by peroxidase-generated phenothiazine cationic radicals. Free Radical Research. 2001;**34**(4):363-378

[151] Lo Presti MS, Rivarola HW, Bustamante JM, Fernández AR, Enders JE, Fretes R, et al. Thioridazine treatment prevents cardiopathy in *Trypanosoma cruzi* infected mice. International Journal of Antimicrobial Agents. 2004;**23**(6):634-636

[152] Bustamante JM, Presti MSL, Rivarola HW, Fernández AR, Enders JE, Fretes RE, et al. Treatment with benznidazole or thioridazine in the chronic phase of experimental Chagas disease improves cardiopathy. International Journal of Antimicrobial Agents. 2007;**29**(6):733-737

[153] Davies C, Cardozo RM, Negrette OS, Mora MC, Chung MC, Basombrio MA. Hydroxymethylnitrofurazone is active in a murine model of Chagas' disease. Antimicrobial Agents and Chemotherapy. 2010;**54**(9):3584-3589

[154] Nogueira Filho MA, Padilha EC, Campos ML, Pontes Machado DV, Davanço MG, Pestana KC, et al. Pharmacokinetics of hydroxymethylnitrofurazone and its parent drug nitrofurazone in rabbits. Drug Metabolism Letters. 2013;**7**(1):58-64

[155] Serafim EOP, ATdAe S, Moreno AH, Vizioli EO, Ferreira EI, Peccinini RG, et al. Pharmacokinetics of hydroxymethylnitrofurazone, a promising new Prodrug for Chagas' disease treatment. Antimicrobial Agents and Chemotherapy. 2013;**57**(12):6106-6109

[156] Parveen S, Khan MOF, Austin SE, Croft SL, Yardley V, Rock P, et al. Antitrypanosomal, antileishmanial, and antimalarial activities of quaternary arylalkylammonium 2-amino-4-chlorophenyl phenyl sulfides, a new class of trypanothione reductase inhibitor, and of N-acyl derivatives of 2-amino-4-chlorophenyl phenyl sulfide. Journal of Medicinal Chemistry. 2005;**48**(25):8087-8097

[157] O'Sullivan MC, Durham TB, Valdes HE, Dauer KL, Karney NJ, Forrestel AC, et al. Dibenzosuberyl substituted polyamines and analogs of clomipramine as effective inhibitors of trypanothione reductase; molecular docking, and assessment of trypanocidal activities. Bioorganic & Medicinal Chemistry. 2015;**23**(5):996-1010

[158] Villalobos-Rocha JC, Sánchez-Torres L, Nogueda-Torres B, Segura-Cabrera A, García-Pérez CA, Bocanegra-García V, et al. Anti-*Trypanosoma cruzi* and anti-leishmanial activity by quinoxaline-7-carboxylate 1,4-di-N-oxide derivatives. Parasitology Research. 2014;**113**(6):2027-2035

[159] Wilkinson SR, Taylor MC, Horn D, Kelly JM, Cheeseman I. A mechanism for cross-resistance to nifurtimox and benznidazole in trypanosomes. Proceedings of the National Academy of Sciences. 2008;**105**(13):5022-5027

[160] Kubata BK, Kabututu Z, Nozaki T, Munday CJ, Fukuzumi S, Ohkubo K, et al. A key role for old yellow enzyme in the metabolism of drugs by *Trypanosoma cruzi*. The Journal of Experimental Medicine. 2002;**196**(9):1241-1251

[161] Bot C, Hall BS, Bashir N, Taylor MC, Helsby NA, Wilkinson SR. Trypanocidal activity of aziridinyl nitrobenzamide prodrugs. Antimicrobial Agents and Chemotherapy. 2010;**54**(10):4246-4252

[162] Hall BS, Wu X, Hu L, Wilkinson SR. Exploiting the drug-activating properties of a novel trypanosomal nitroreductase. Antimicrobial Agents and Chemotherapy. 2009;**54**(3):1193-1199

[163] Papadopoulou MV, Trunz BB, Bloomer WD, McKenzie C, Wilkinson SR, Prasittichai C, et al. Novel 3-nitro-1H-1,2,4-triazole-based aliphatic and aromatic amines as anti-chagasic agents. Journal of Medicinal Chemistry. 2011;**54**(23):8214-8223

[164] Papadopoulou MV, Bloomer WD, Rosenzweig HS, Chatelain E, Kaiser M, Wilkinson SR, et al. Novel 3-nitro-1H-1,2,4-triazole-based amides and Sulfonamides as potential antitrypanosomal agents. Journal of Medicinal Chemistry. 2012;**55**(11):5554-5565

[165] Papadopoulou MV, Bloomer WD, Rosenzweig HS, Ashworth R, Wilkinson SR, Kaiser M, et al. Novel 3-nitro-1H-1,2,4-triazole-based compounds as potential anti-chagasic drugs:In vivostudies. Future Medicinal Chemistry. 2013;**5**(15):1763-1776

[166] Papadopoulou MV, Bloomer WD, Lepesheva GI, Rosenzweig HS, Kaiser M, Aguilera-Venegas B, et al. Novel 3-Nitrotriazole-based amides and carbinols as bifunctional antichagasic agents. Journal of Medicinal Chemistry. 2015;**58**(3):1307-1319

[167] Moraes CB, Giardini MA, Kim H, Franco CH, Araujo-Junior AM, Schenkman S, et al. Nitroheterocyclic compounds are more efficacious than CYP51 inhibitors against *Trypanosoma cruzi*: Implications for Chagas disease drug discovery and development. Scientific Reports. 2014;**4**(1):1-11

[168] Guidance for Industry: Estimating the Maximum Safe Starting Dose in Initial Clinical Trials for Therapeutics in Adult Healthy Volunteers. U.S. Department of Health and Human Services. Food and Drug Administration. Center for Drug Evaluation and Research (CDER); 2005

[169] Moreno SN, Batista DDGJ, Batista MM, Oliveira GMD, Britto CC, Rodrigues ACM, et al. Combined treatment of heterocyclic analogues and benznidazole upon *Trypanosoma cruzi in vivo*. PLoS One. 2011;**6**(7):e22155

[170] Araujo MS, Martins-Filho OA, Pereira ME, Brener ZA. Combination of benznidazole and ketoconazole enhances efficacy of chemotherapy of experimental Chagas' disease. The Journal of Antimicrobial Chemotherapy. 2000;**45**(6):819-824

[171] Costa FTM, Assíria Fontes Martins T, de Figueiredo Diniz L, Mazzeti AL, da Silva do Nascimento ÁF, Caldas S, et al. Benznidazole/Itraconazole combination treatment enhances anti-*Trypanosoma cruzi* Activity in experimental Chagas disease. PLoS One. 2015;**10**(6):e0128707

[172] Valdez RH, Tonin LTD, Ueda-Nakamura T, Filho BPD, Morgado-Diaz JA, Sarragiotto MH, et al. Biological activity of 1,2,3,4-tetrahydro-β-carboline-3-carboxamides against *Trypanosoma cruzi*. Acta Tropica. 2009;**110**(1):7-14

[173] Valdez RH, Tonin LTD, Ueda-Nakamura T, Silva SO, Dias Filho BP, Kaneshima EN, et al. *In vitro* and *in vivo* trypanocidal synergistic activity of N-butyl-1-(4-dimethylamino)phenyl-1,2,3,4-tetrahydro-carboline-3-carboxamide associated with benznidazole. Antimicrobial Agents and Chemotherapy. 2011;**56**(1):507-512

[174] Peron F, Lazarin-Bidóia D, Ud Din Z, Rodrigues-Filho E, Ueda-Nakamura T, SDO S, et al. Effects of (1E,4E)-2-methyl-1,5-bis(4-nitrophenyl)penta-1,4-dien-3-one on *Trypanosoma cruzi* and its combinational effect with benznidazole, ketoconazole, or fluconazole. BioMed Research International. 2017;**2017**:1-11

6

Biochemical, Cellular, and Immunologic Aspects during Early Interaction between *Trypanosoma cruzi* and Host Cell

Rosa Lidia Solís-Oviedo, Víctor Monteon,
Ruth López and Ángel de la Cruz Pech-Canul

Abstract

The close parasite-host relationship involves different aspects such as the biochemical, physiological, morphological, and immunological adaptations. Studies on parasite-host interaction have provided a myriad of information about its biology and have established the building blocks for the development of new drug therapies to control the parasite. Several mechanisms for the parasite invasion have been proposed through *in vivo* or *in vitro* experimental data. Since the first histological studies until the studies on the function/structure of the involved molecules, this complex interaction has been roughly depicted. However, new recent strategies as genetic and proteomic approaches have tuned knowledge on how the host reacts to the parasite and how the parasite avoids these host's reactions in order to survive.

Keywords: *Trypanosoma cruzi*, immune system, parasite interactions, animal model studies, *in vitro* models, phagocytic, non-phagocytic

1. Introduction

The life cycle of *Trypanosoma cruzi* comprises several morphological transformations involving both mammalian and vector hosts, where three different major developmental stages are identified: epimastigotes, trypomastigotes, and amastigotes (**Figure 1**). The developmental stages of *T. cruzi* alternate between non-infective and infective forms. Epimastigote and amastigote are non-infective but replicative stages in the gut of the triatomine vector and inside the

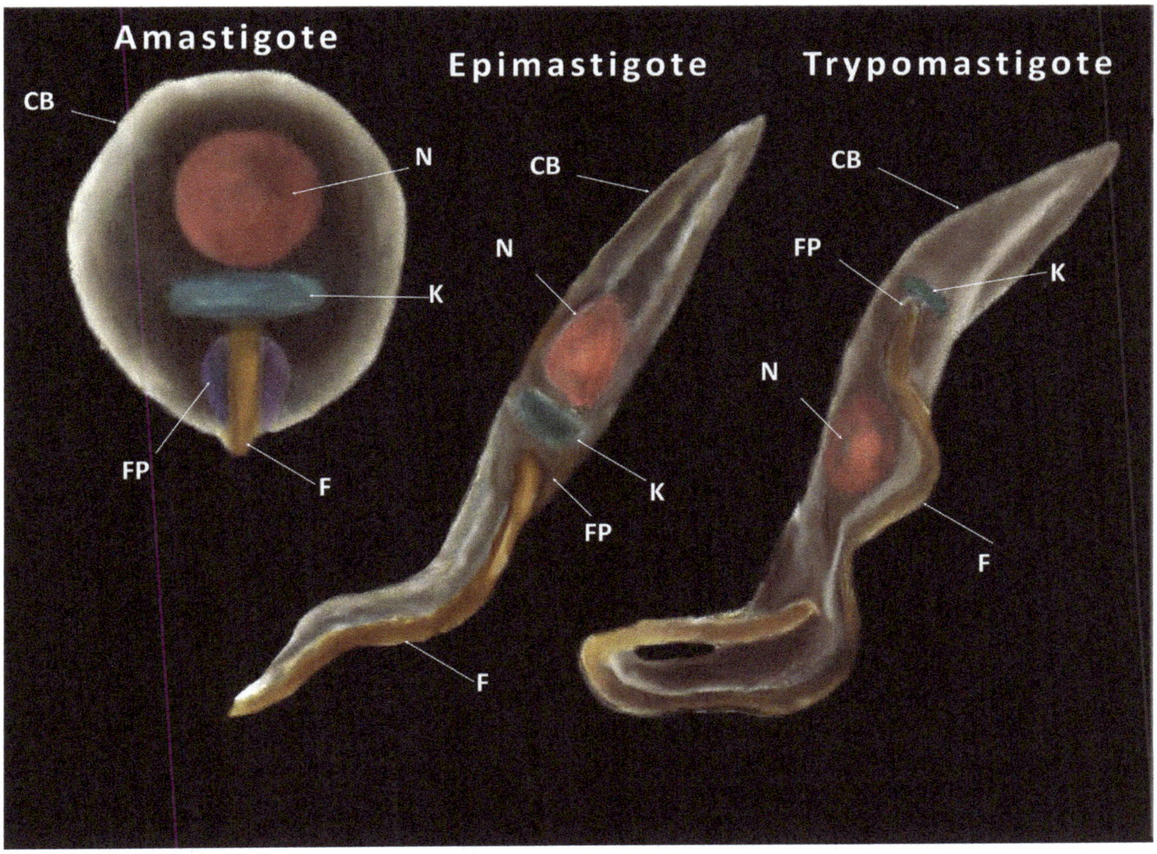

Figure 1. The different stages of *Trypanosoma cruzi*. The image depicted the amastigote, epimastigote, and trypomastigote stages from *T. cruzi* and their membrane domains: Nucleus (N), Kinetoplast (K), Flagellum (F), Flagellar Pocket (FP), and Cell Body (CB). Reprinted with permission from Ángel de la Cruz Pech-Canul et al. [1], Copyright © 2017.

mammalian cell, respectively. Trypomastigote stage is infective but non-replicative and can also be considered as two different developmental stages: the bloodstream trypomastigotes, found in the blood of the mammalian host, and the metacyclic trypomastigotes, found in the rectum of the triatomine vector .

T. cruzi is internalized by phagocytic and non-phagocytic nucleated host cells via multiple pathways. The first general steps through the interaction process of the *T. cruzi* and its mammalian host cell can be divided into three stages: (1) adhesion/recognition, (2) signalling, and (3) invasion [2, 3]. During the adhesion/recognition stage, diverse molecules with cell-adhesion properties are expressed on the membrane surface of the metacyclic trypomastigotes from of the parasite ; these molecules bind to receptors of the target host cells and are able to trigger signals pathway, toward the parasite invasion [4]. That invasive process allows *T. cruzi* internalization and involves the engulfment of the parasite, the formation of a *T. cruzi* parasitophorous vacuole (TcPV) [5], as well as the late disruption and the dispersion of the TcPV, thereby the parasite is released to the host cytoplasm where its replication and differentiation starts until the infective stage [6, 7]. The aim of this chapter is to discuss and to outline the interaction models during the early interaction between *T. cruzi* and its mammalian host cells.

2. An overview of parasite interaction

One of the first barriers faced by *T. cruzi* during host cell invasion is the complexity of the host defence system. The skin and mucous membranes act as physical barriers which prevent penetration by microbes. Undoubtedly, they are the site for multiple and diverse types of chemical, physical, and biological contacts. Lipids and proteins are among the main components of the innate immune system in these tissues. Lipids comprise linoleic acid, oleic acid, squalene, ceramides, and sphingolipids, whereas proteins are more diverse, such as keratin on the surface of the skin or the cationic peptides *alpha*- and *beta*-defensins produced by neutrophils and mucosa tissue, respectively [8]. Furthermore, saliva produced by salivary glands of the vector contains a sort of proline-rich proteins and histidine-rich proteins both with antibiotic properties, lysozyme, peroxidase, lactoferrin, cystatins, and mucins [9]. Due to the rich protein content, both pH and salt concentration play a significant role as inhibitory factors during the parasite/host interaction.

The cellular composition of skin and mucous membranes is a fundamental barrier for permissive or refractory colonization/infection. In the skin, the epidermis is composed by 95% of keratinocytes and other cells present at low concentration, such as melanocytes, Langerhans cells, intra-epithelial lymphocyte, and Merkel cells. Keratinocytes express Toll-like receptors (TLRs) 1–6, 9, and 10 which are able to recognize basically all pathogen-associated molecular patterns (PAMPs) with exception of flagenin; as a consequence, they can secrete an array of mediators such as nitric oxide, leukotrienes, cyclooxygenase, metalloprotease 1 and 9, classical cytokines IL-1, IL-6, IL-8, TNF-alpha, and chemokines CXCL1 and CXCL8. Keratinocytes also express receptors for different cytokines (IL-1, IL-3, TNF-alpha, IL-17, IL-21, IL-22) and chemokines (CXCL9, CXCL10, CXCL11, and CCL20). Other skin cells present at low concentration have also a broad array of receptors that are able to respond to physical and chemical stimulus. In addition, a dense protein layer is found between epidermis and dermis which is composed by collagen type IV, laminin fibronectin, iodogen, and heparan sulfate; together, they structure the basement membrane [10]. The cellular composition of dermis is more complex and diverse. Fibroblast, myofibroblasts, macrophages, adipocytes, dendritic cells, mast cells, and mesenchymal stem cells are found among resident cells in the dermis (**Figure 2**), whereas transitory cells include lymphocytes, polymorphonuclear cells and monocytes. In addition, dermis presents an intricate network of nerves, lymph, and blood system. As skin, mucosal tissue has the property to react with a complex array of mediators required for immune surveillance and inflammatory response to tissue injury and infection. A remarkable differential feature between skin and mucosa tissue is the bias to immune tolerance and anti-inflammatory response in mucosal compartments [11, 12].

In natural conditions, *T. cruzi* infection is established when metacyclic trypomastigotes are deposited on injured skin or mucosa host tissue by blood feeding triatomine. Thus, metacyclic trypomastigotes has to face the above innate immune responses at the portal entry in order to survive (**Figure 2**). Since the pioneer work published by Romaña [13], where a histology description was done, limited information on this area of concern exists. It is very critical to take into account different factors in the relationship between parasite and host. For example, factors

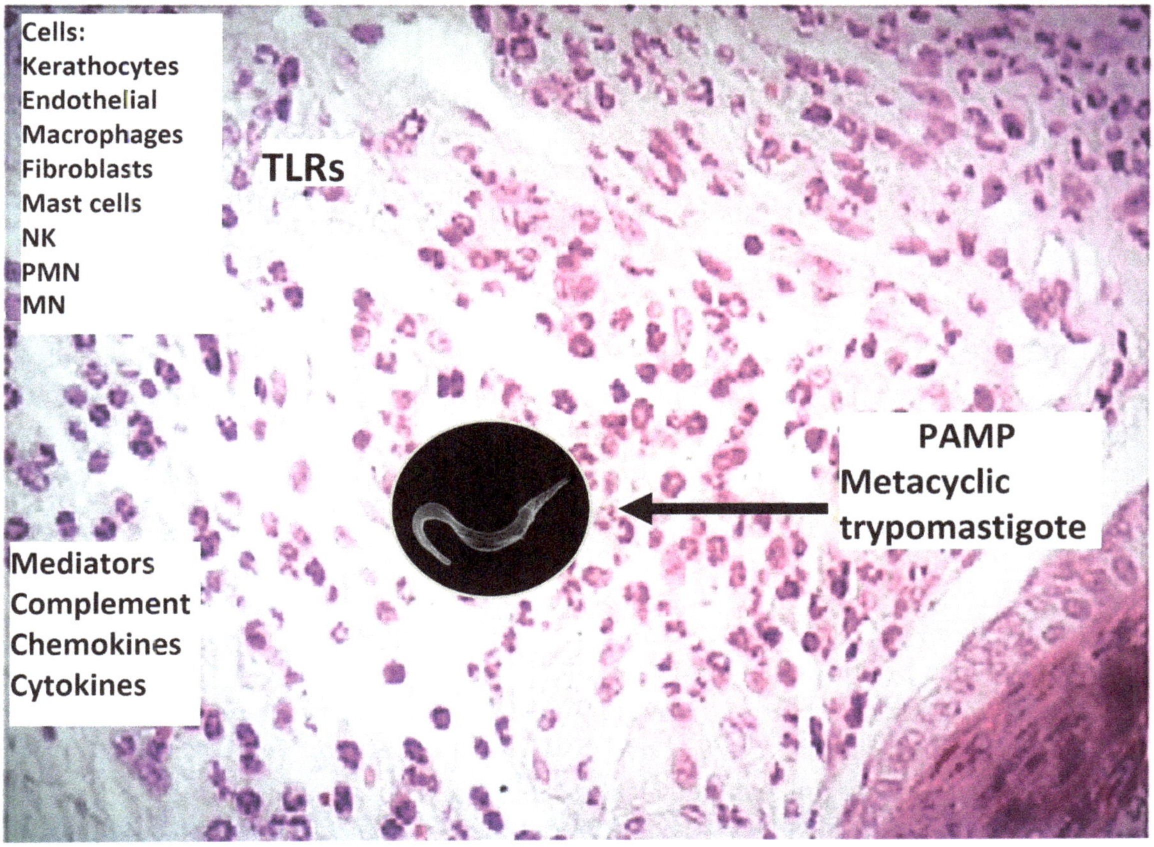

Figure 2. Skin cells of mouse and metacyclic trypomastigote parasite. Host cells were stained with hematoxylin-eosin. A *T. cruzi* trypomastigote is depicted inside the image. Common types of skin cells and some of the mediators for the inflammatory response are listed inside the image: pathogen-associated molecular patterns (PAMPs), natural killer (NK), polymorphonuclear (PMN), mononuclear (MN), and Toll-like receptors (TLRs).

as specie of vector are involved in the transmission, inoculum size, *T. cruzi* phase, portal of entry, *T. cruzi* strain, host immune responses, and microbiota presented in the vector.

3. Specie of vector and *Trypanosoma cruzi*

Firstly, there are many triatomine vector species that transmit the Chagas disease. Some of them have a wide geographical distribution and others are confined to restricted geographical areas. However, all of them can transmit *T. cruzi* infection with different efficacy, a feature that relies on biological behaviour and physiological condition itself. For example, metacyclogenesis involves the process of parasite transformation into the vector; this step is fundamental in order to accomplish the life cycle. The basic transformation that takes place inside the vector is from bloodstream trypomastigote phase to epimastigote and to metacyclic trypomastigotes. This last phase is essential for mammalian infection in as much as epimastigotes are vulnerable to innate immune mechanism. Thus, the metacyclogenesis that takes place into the vector is fundamental in order to switch to mammalian host. Perlowagora-Szumlewicks and Carvalhio-Moreira [14] described triatomine vector species influencing metacyclogenesis with remarkable observation.

They pointed out higher metacyclogenesis rates in *Rhodnius neglectus* and *R. prolixus* (50 and 37%, respectively), whereas in some *Triatoma* species, metacyclogenesis rates were dramatically lower in comparison (5% in *Triatoma sordida*, 7% in *T. brasiliensis*, and 1% in *T. pseudomaculata*). However *T. infestans* can reach up to 42%, in *T. rubrovaria* 27%, in *T. dimidiata* 26%, and *Panstrongylus megistus* metacyclogenesis rates can reach 27%. Other remarkable observation is that metacyclic trypomastigotes rate is not continuous along vector life span. In some cases, it can reach a plateau, but in other cases, it can reach several peaks before metacyclogenesis drops. In natural conditions, *T. barberi* can reach up 76%, in *T. pallidipennis* 15%, whereas in *T. dimidiata* 26% [15].

The metacyclogenesis of *T. dimidiata* in laboratory conditions is similar to natural conditions; in addition, metacyclogenesis is also influenced by the *T. cruzi* strain and the rate of metacyclic parasites change along the age of triatomine vectors [16]. Furthermore, *T. cruzi* strains can moderately influence the rate of metacyclogenesis that take place inside the same triatomine specie but have less impact when compared across triatomine specie [16, 17]. Altogether, the above data highlight the importance of triatomine species and *T. cruzi* strains in the development of metacyclic trypomastigotes: the natural parasite phase that will face mammalian host to complete its life cycle. Due to its importance, this variable should be taken into account for experimental design. Besides, the parasite strains show different virulence relying on virulence factors such as trans-sialidase activity, complement resistance, and cysteine protease cruzipain (TCC) [18]. Trans-sialidase removes and transfers sialic acid from host cells to parasite mucin-like glycoprotein. It is known that trans-sialidase activity is a virulence factor which allows parasite to invade and to escape from parasitophorous vacuole. This enzyme is more expressed in bloodstream and tissue-culture trypomastigotes than in metacyclic trypomastigotes. Trans-sialidase activity also depends on *T. cruzi* lineage and consequently its virulence [19].

Once metacyclic trypomastigotes have overcome the first nonspecific immune mechanical barrier (skin/mucosal tissues), they need to swing into the extracellular matrix proteins in order to find cells to invade for replication and then accomplish their life cycle. GP82, a surface glycoprotein found in both bloodstream and tissue-culture trypomastigotes, has the ability to bind to matrix extracellular proteins such as fibronectin, heparan sulfate, and laminin, serving as bridges for parasite-target cell association and leading to enhanced infection. However, this interaction inhibits cell invasion. The presence of the major cysteine proteinase cruzipain (TCC) helps to degrade these extracellular matrix proteins enabling cell invasion [20]. These surface glycoproteins are very polymorphic among *T. cruzi* strains resulting in different grades of virulence .

The complement system, another unspecific immune mechanism that is essential for inflammation and cellular lysis, can be activated by three pathways. The lectin triggered by mannose-binding lectins (mannose-binding proteins, ficolins, and CL-K1 proteins) that binds to pathogen-associated molecular pattern (PAMPs) rich in *D*-mannose, *L*-fucose, glucose, and *N*-acetyl-glucosamine, *O*-acetylated, and glycan compounds containing sialic acid which activate MASP-1 and MASP-2. The alternative pathway is triggered when the complex C3 (H_2O)-B factor is stabilized on a surface allowing the formation of C3 convertase (C3 (H_2O) Bb). Whereas the classical pathway activation depends on C1 complex interaction with antibodies or LPS and porins present in Gram-negative bacteria, but also with phosphatidylserine on apoptotic cells or via C-reactive proteins synthetized in liver as stress proteins [21].

The four phases of *T. cruzi* (amastigote, epimastigote, metacyclic, and bloodstream trypomastigote) can activate the complement system, but only epimastigotes are susceptible to lysis. However, some strains on metacyclic trypomastigote phase are more vulnerable [22, 23]. Some *T. cruzi* surface molecules enable parasite to evade innate and adaptive immune responses. There are other mechanisms to circumvent the action of complement system such as the presence of calreticulin (TcCRT), the complement regulatory protein (Gp160/TcCRP), the complement C2 receptor inhibitor trispanning (TcCRIT), and the presence of GP58/68 protein and T-DAF. For a comprehensive review, see [21].

Finally, it has been observed that in animal models, metacyclic trypomastigotes induce an inflammatory response at the site of inoculation, as early as 1 h, and it is composed basically of neutrophils while mononuclear infiltrate begins at 24 h with a maximum infiltration at day 15. Nonetheless, poor cytokine expression such as IL-2, Il-4, IL-10, IL-12, and IFN-*gamma* persists over a 2-week post-inoculation, whereas at the regional lymph node to the site of inoculation, it was evident as early as 1 h. The induced pattern of cytokine at the inoculation site is permissive to establishing infection, despite the appropriate immune response in other lymph secondary organs [24–26]. Our group recently reported that pre-exposure to faeces of triatomine decreases parasitemia in mice challenged with metacyclic trypomastigotes. This finding suggests that inflammatory reaction to bacteria faeces in immune individuals helps to control parasite load *in vivo* [27].

4. *In vitro* models

Diverse *in vitro* studies on the *T. cruzi* /host cell interaction process have been described through the years [28]. These studies have included a wide variety of eukaryotic cell lines and parasite strains, as well as the different parasite phases able to infect cells: amastigotes, metacyclic trypomastigotes, or both, bloodstream and tissue-culture trypomastigotes [2, 29]. *T. cruzi* is capable to invade phagocytic or non-phagocytic cells via endocytic mechanisms. Currently, three models for *T. cruzi* invasion have been proposed: lysosomal-dependent, lysosomal-independent, and actin-dependent [3, 6, 30].

Cortez and co-workers [30] recently showed that the participation of lysosomes in the parasite entry site depends on the source of the trypomastigote. They found that the metacyclic trypomastigotes invasion occurs mainly by the lysosome-dependent mechanism, whereas the tissue-culture trypomastigote invasion takes place mostly by the lysosome-independent mechanism. Interestingly, it has been reported that amastigotes are capable of invading host cells by the actin-dependent phagocytic mechanism probably due to their motionless nature [29, 31].

4.1. Lysosomal-dependent

The lysosomal-dependent model is also known as the lysosome exocytosis pathway. Tardieux et al. visualized the recruitment of lysosomes at the parasite entry site during the early event of internalization of tissue-culture trypomastigotes into their mammalian host cells, and they proposed that this process is required for parasite internalization [32]. PGTF is a soluble factor proteolytically generated from trypomastigote which is capable to induce Ca^{2+} signaling in mammalian cells. The addition of PGTF during the host cell invasion of tissue-culture trypomastigotes showed that Ca^{2+} signalling plays a role in the parasite invasion through the reorganization of host cell microfilaments as well as in the migration and fusion of lysosomes [15, 33]. In addition, the increase of Ca^{2+} is required to trigger a form of endocytosis to repair the mechanically injured host cell membrane due to *T. cruzi* invasion [17]. The elevation of intracellular Ca^{2+} concentration triggers the exocytosis of lysosomes. The lysosomal enzyme acid sphingomyelinase (ASM) is released to the host plasma membrane where ASM converts sphingomyelin into ceramide: a lipid capable of forming ceramide-enriched endosomes [34, 35]. Ceramides are also capable to coalesce and to accumulate into the parasitophorous vacuoles, which suggest that this lipid plays an important role in the membrane deformation process required to allow the large trypomastigotes entry into the host cells [32, 36].

4.2. Lysosomal-independent

The lysosomal-independent mechanism depends on phosphatidylinositol-3 (PI 3)-kinase (PI3K) which is activated in the presence of *T. cruzi* bloodstream trypomastigotes. This mechanism is correlated to an efficient parasite invasion of non-phagocytes and phagocytic cells. *In vitro* analysis during *T. cruzi* infection of phagocytic cells has shown the presence of vacuoles enriched with lipids derived from the PI 3-kinase activities: phosphatidylinositol 3-phosphate (PI_3P), phosphatidylinositol 3,4-bisphosphate ($PI(3,4)P_2$), and phosphatidylinositol PI 3,4,5-triphosphate ($PI(3,4,5)P_3$) [37–39].

The inhibition of the class I and III PI 3-kinase activities abolishes the parasite entry into macrophages which suggests a prominent role of the host PI 3-kinase activities during the *T. cruzi* infection process [37]. A class III PI 3-kinase located in *T. cruzi* (TcVps34) is able to produce phosphatidylinositol 3-phosphate, and it has been shown that it plays an important role in vital processes for the parasite survival such as osmoregulation, acidification, and vesicular trafficking [40].

4.3. Actin-dependent

Amastigotes are also capable to penetrate host cell through its plasma membrane via the actin-dependent mechanism. This mechanism contrasts notably from the two models described previously in which trypomastigotes are involved [41, 42]. The invasion capability of amastigotes depends on the *T. cruzi* linage. Amastigotes from the *T. cruzi* I lineage (G strain) have a remarkable ability to invade non-phagocytic cells [29, 43], while the less-infective amastigotes belonging to *T. cruzi* II linage (such as the Y strain) are largely engulfed by phagocytic cells (macrophages) and occasionally by other cell types [43, 44].

Once inside the host cell, amastigotes show the same ability as trypomastigotes to disrupt the parasitophorous vacuole, to replicate in the cytosol, and to differentiate into the infective trypomastigote form. There is also evidence that trypomastigotes are able to differentiate into amastigotes extracellularly while circulating in the bloodstream [45]. This remarkable observation has unravelled an additional mechanism through which the parasite can move among intracellular compartments, elude the host immune system, and sustain the infection.

5. Conclusions

Chagas disease is a potentially life-threatening illness caused by *T. cruzi*. Currently, there are no vaccines which prevent the parasite infection; hence, vector control is still the most useful method to prevent such illness. Although the mammalian host has developed a fine battery of physical and biochemical defences, the parasite has adapted its metabolism to overcome the host defences. *T. cruzi* exhibits multiple strategies to evade the host defenses in order to survive, as summarized here; diverse studies have been conducted trying to unravel the basics of *T. cruzi* infection during the early interaction with its mammalian host. The different *in vivo* and *in vitro* experimental approaches showed a complex interaction depending on both, the parasite and the host characteristics. For example, the amastigote form was relatively recently described as a potentially infective form for host cells. Despite the fact that amastigote form is generally known as a replicative form in the mammalian host, it is capable to infect host cells within the host system in a completely different manner than the one described for the typical infective trypomastigote form. Despite the amount of studies on this topic, the comprehensive understanding of the parasite invasion mechanisms is still incomplete. More efforts should be followed for the elucidation of the early steps of parasite–host interaction as they are crucial for the development of future drugs to prevent the Chagas disease.

Acknowledgements

The authors acknowledge the National Council of Science and Technology from Mexico (CONACyT). Rosa Lidia Solis-Oviedo was supported by CONACyT. Victor Monteon was financial supported by CONACyT (Project CB-2010-2101 153764). Angel de la Cruz Pech-Canul was supported by CONACyT through the "Cátedras CONACyT para Jóvenes Investigadores" Programme.

Conflict of interest

The authors declare that they have no conflicts of interest.

Author details

Rosa Lidia Solís-Oviedo[1], Víctor Monteon[2], Ruth López[2] and Ángel de la Cruz Pech-Canul[3*]

*Address all correspondence to: angelpechcanul@gmail.com

1 Faculty of Chemical Sciences, Autonomous University of Chihuahua, Chihuahua, Mexico

2 Centre for Biomedical Research, Autonomous University of Campeche, Campeche, Mexico

3 CONACyT – Faculty of Chemical Sciences, Autonomous University of Chihuahua, Chihuahua, Mexico

References

[1] de la Cruz Pech-Canul Á, Monteón V, Solís-Oviedo R-L. A brief view of the surface membrane proteins from *Trypanosoma cruzi*. Journal of Parasitology Research. vol. 2017, Article ID 3751403, 13 pages, 2017. DOI: 10.1155/2017/3751403

[2] Barrias ES, de Carvalho TMU, De Souza W. *Trypanosoma cruzi*: Entry into mammalian host cells and Parasitophorous vacuole formation. Frontiers in Immunology. 2013;**4**:186

[3] de Souza W, de Carvalho TMU, Barrias ES. Review on *Trypanosoma cruzi*: Host cell interaction. International Journal of Cell Biology. 2010;**2010**:295394

[4] Maeda F, Cortez C, Yoshida N. Cell signaling during *Trypanosoma cruzi* invasion. Frontiers in Immunology. 2012;**3**(361):1-7

[5] Epting CL, Coates BM, Engman DM. Molecular mechanisms of host cell invasion by *Trypanosoma cruzi*. Experimental Parasitology. 2010;**126**(3):283-291

[6] Romano PS, Cueto JA, Casassa AF, Vanrell MC, Gottlieb RA, Colombo MI. Molecular and cellular mechanisms involved in the *Trypanosoma cruzi*/host cell interplay. IUBMB Life. 2012;**64**(5):387-396

[7] Sibley LD, Andrews NW. Cell invasion by un-palatable parasites. Traffic (Copenhagen, Denmark). 2000;**1**(2):100-106

[8] De Smet K, Contreras R. Human antimicrobial peptides: Defensins, cathelicidins and histatins. Biotechnology Letters. 2005;**27**(18):1337-1347

[9] Fábián TK, Hermann P, Beck A, Fejérdy P, Fábián G. Salivary defense proteins: Their network and role in innate and acquired oral immunity. International Journal of Molecular Sciences. 2012;**13**(4):4295-4320

[10] Nestle FO, Di Meglio P, Qin J-Z, Nickoloff BJ. Skin immune sentinels in health and disease. Nature Reviews Immunology. 2009;**9**(10):679-691

[11] McGettrick HM, Smith E, Filer A, Kissane S, Salmon M, Buckley CD, et al. Fibroblasts from different sites may promote or inhibit recruitment of flowing lymphocytes by endothelial cells. European Journal of Immunology. 2009;**39**(1):113-125

[12] McGettrick HM, Butler LM, Buckley CD, Ed Rainger G, Nash GB. Tissue stroma as a regulator of leukocyte recruitment in inflammation. Journal of Leukocyte Biology. 2012;**91**(3):385-400

[13] Romaña C. Contribuição ao conhecimento da patogenia da Tripanosomose Americana: (período inicial da infecção). Memórias do Instituto Oswaldo Cruz. 1943;**39**:253-264

[14] Perlowagora-Szumlewicz A, Moreira CJ. In vivo differentiation of *Trypanosoma cruzi* – 1. Experimental evidence of the influence of vector species on metacyclogenesis. Memorias do Instituto Oswaldo Cruz. 1994;**89**(4):603-618

[15] Rodriguez A, Rioult MG, Ora A, Andrews NW. A trypanosome-soluble factor induces IP3 formation, intracellular Ca^{2+} mobilization and microfilament rearrangement in host cells. Journal of Cell Biology. 1995;**129**(5):1263-1273

[16] Monteon VGS, Cruz-Zetina G, Balmes J, López R, Hernández O. Caracterización biológica de aislados mexicanos de *Trypanosoma cruzi*: metaciclogénesis, parasitemia y resistencia contra benznidazol. Revista Biomédica. 2009;**20**:206-214

[17] Idone V, Tam C, Goss JW, Toomre D, Pypaert M, Andrews NW. Repair of injured plasma membrane by rapid Ca($^{2+}$)-dependent endocytosis. Journal of Cell Biology. 2008;**180**(5):905-914

[18] San Francisco J, Barria I, Gutierrez B, Neira I, Munoz C, Sagua H, et al. Decreased cruzipain and gp85/trans-sialidase family protein expression contributes to loss of *Trypanosoma cruzi* trypomastigote virulence. Journal of Cell Biology. 2017;**19**(1):55-61

[19] Risso MG, Garbarino GB, Mocetti E, Campetella O, Gonzalez Cappa SM, Buscaglia CA, et al. Differential expression of a virulence factor, the trans-sialidase, by the main *Trypanosoma cruzi* phylogenetic lineages. The Journal of Infectious Diseases. 2004;**189**(12): 2250-2259

[20] Maeda FY, Cortez C, Izidoro MA, Juliano L, Yoshida N. Fibronectin-degrading activity of *Trypanosoma cruzi* cysteine proteinase plays a role in host cell invasion. Infection and Immunity. 2014;**82**(12):5166-5174

[21] Lidani KCF, Bavia L, Ambrosio AR, de Messias-Reason IJ. The complement system: A prey of *Trypanosoma cruzi*. Frontiers in Microbiology. 2017;**8**:607

[22] Cestari I, Ramirez MI. Inefficient complement system clearance of *Trypanosoma cruzi* metacyclic trypomastigotes enables resistant strains to invade eukaryotic cells. PLoS One. 2010;**5**(3):e9721

[23] Leon-Perez F, Gomez-Garcia L, Alejandre-Aguilar R, Lopez R, Monteon VM. Mexican *Trypanosoma cruzi* isolates: In vitro susceptibility of epimastigotes to anti-trypanosoma cruzi drugs and metacyclic forms to complement-mediated lysis. Vector Borne and Zoonotic Diseases. 2007;**7**(3):330-336

[24] Monteon VM, Furuzawa-Carballeda J, Alejandre-Aguilar R, Aranda-Fraustro A, Rosales-Encina JL, Reyes PA. American trypanosomosis: *in situ* and generalized features of parasitism and inflammation kinetics in a murine model. Experimental Parasitology. 1996;**83**(3):267-274

[25] Gomez-Garcia L, Alejandre-Aguilar R, Aranda-Fraustro A, Lopez R, Monteon VM. Description of inflammation and cytokine profile at the inoculation site and in heart tissue of mice re-infected with *Trypanosoma cruzi* vector derived-metacyclic trypomastigotes. Parasitology. 2005;**130**(Pt 5):511-522

[26] Monteon VHO, Lopez R, Reyes PA. Cytokine expression at the inoculation site and nearby tissues in an animal model infected with Metacyclic Trypomastigotes of *Trypanosoma cruzi*. Tropical Medicine and Health. 2009;**37**(4):141-147

[27] Monteon V, Quen-Ramirez E, Macedo-Reyes V, Lopez R, Acosta-Viana K, Pennigton P, et al. Pre-exposure to faeces or saliva of *Triatoma dimidiata* decreases parasitemia in mice

challenged with *Trypanosoma cruzi*: A description of the inflammatory reaction at the inoculation site. Annals of Parasitology. 2016;**62**(3):209-219

[28] Duran-Rehbein GA, Vargas-Zambrano JC, Cuéllar A, Puerta CJ, Gonzalez JM. Mammalian cellular culture models of *Trypanosoma cruzi* infection: A review of the published literature. Parasite. 2014;**21**:38

[29] Mortara RA, Andreoli WK, Fernandes MC, da Silva CV, Fernandes AB, L'Abbate C, et al. Host cell actin remodeling in response to *Trypanosoma cruzi*: Trypomastigote versus amastigote entry. Subcellular Biochemistry. 2008;**47**:101-109

[30] Cortez C, Real FY. N. Lysosome biogenesis/scattering increases host cell susceptibility to invasion by *Trypanosoma cruzi* metacyclic forms and resistance to tissue culture trypomastigotes. Cellular Microbiology. 2016;**18**(5):748-760

[31] Procopio DO, da Silva S, Cunningham CC, Mortara RA. *Trypanosoma cruzi*: Effect of protein kinase inhibitors and cytoskeletal protein organization and expression on host cell invasion by amastigotes and metacyclic trypomastigotes. Experimental Parasitology. 1998;**90**(1):1-13

[32] Tardieux I, Webster P, Ravesloot J, Boron W, Lunn JA, Heuser JE, et al. Lysosome recruitment and fusion are early events required for trypanosome invasion of mammalian cells. Cell. 1992;**71**(7):1117-1130

[33] Burleigh BA. Host cell signaling and *Trypanosoma cruzi* invasion: Do all roads lead to lysosomes? Science's STKE: Signal Transduction Knowledge Environment. 2005; **2005**(293):pe36

[34] Tam C, Idone V, Devlin C, Fernandes MC, Flannery A, He X, et al. Exocytosis of acid sphingomyelinase by wounded cells promotes endocytosis and plasma membrane repair. Journal of Cell Biology. 2010;**189**(6):1027-1038

[35] Trajkovic K, Hsu C, Chiantia S, Rajendran L, Wenzel D, Wieland F, et al. Ceramide triggers budding of exosome vesicles into multivesicular endosomes. Science (New York, N.Y.). 2008;**319**(5867):1244-1247

[36] Fernandes MC, Cortez M, Flannery AR, Tam C, Mortara RA, Andrews NW. *Trypanosoma cruzi* subverts the sphingomyelinase-mediated plasma membrane repair pathway for cell invasion. The Journal of Experimental Medicine. 2011;**208**(5):909-921

[37] Todorov AG, Einicker-Lamas M, de Castro SL, Oliveira MM, Guilherme A. Activation of host cell phosphatidylinositol 3-kinases by *Trypanosoma cruzi* infection. The Journal of Biological Chemistry. 2000;**275**(41):32182-32186

[38] Woolsey AM, Sunwoo L, Petersen CA, Brachmann SM, Cantley LC, Burleigh BA. Novel PI 3-kinase-dependent mechanisms of trypanosome invasion and vacuole maturation. Journal of Cell Science. 2003;**116**(17):3611-3622

[39] Wilkowsky SE, Barbieri MA, Stahl P, Isola ELD. *Trypanosoma cruzi*: Phosphatidylinositol 3-kinase and protein kinase B activation is associated with parasite invasion. Experimental Cell Research. 2001;**264**(2):211-218

[40] Schoijet AC, Miranda K, Girard-Dias W, de Souza W, Flawia MM, Torres HN, et al. A *Trypanosoma cruzi* phosphatidylinositol 3-kinase (TcVps34) is involved in osmoregulation and receptor-mediated endocytosis. Journal of Biological Chemistry. 2008;**283**(46):31541-31550

[41] Fernandes MC, Andrews NW. Host cell invasion by *Trypanosoma cruzi*: A unique strategy that promotes persistence. FEMS Microbiology Reviews. 2012;**36**(3):734-747

[42] Fernandes MC, Flannery AR, Andrews N, Mortara RA. Extracellular amastigotes of *Trypanosoma cruzi* are potent inducers of phagocytosis in mammalian cells. Cellular Microbiology. 2013;**15**(6):977-991

[43] Mortara RA, Andreoli WK, Taniwaki NN, Fernandes AB, Silva CV, Fernandes MC, et al. Mammalian cell invasion and intracellular trafficking by *Trypanosoma cruzi* infective forms. Anais da Academia Brasileira de Ciencias. 2005;**77**(1):77-94

[44] Ley V, Andrews NW, Robbins ES, Nussenzweig V. Amastigotes of *Trypanosoma cruzi* sustain an infective cycle in mammalian cells. The Journal of Experimental Medicine. 1988;**168**(2):649-659

[45] Andrews NW, Hong KS, Robbins ES, Nussenzweig V. Stage-specific surface antigens expressed during the morphogenesis of vertebrate forms of *Trypanosoma cruzi*. Experimental Parasitology. 1987;**64**(3):474-484

7

Slowed Development of Natural Products for Chagas Disease: How to Move Forward?

Javier Varela, Hugo Cerecetto and
Mercedes González

Abstract

Chagas disease, caused by *Trypanosoma cruzi*, is considered an endemic disease that affects millions of people causing generating health, economic and social problems. This study provides a review on research and development of new therapies for Chagas based in natural products of plant origin. We observed that there are more than 400 plant species that have been evaluated against different models of Chagas disease, and in some cases, there are interesting results. Challenge that hinders research work is the purification of the active compound and standardization of the chemical profile of whole extracts. The principal common factor that delays clinical testing is the lack of investment for the development of these products at the clinical phase. In the search of a natural, low cost and available drug for Chagas disease, we propose the use of new methodologies to overcome the existing challenges. The use of plant metabolomic technique is proposed as an option with high potential for the identification of biomarkers that could allow the standardization of chemical profiles. Furthermore, we describe the importance of applying good agricultural and manufacturing practices for reaching a successful development of quality phytotherapeutic products.

Keywords: natural products, metabolomics, *Trypanosoma cruzi*, Chagas disease

1. Introduction

"It does not explode like bombs or sound like shots. As hunger kills silently. As hunger kills the quiet, those who live condemned silence and die doomed to oblivion. The tragedy that does not ring, sick who do not pay, a disease that does not sell. Chagas disease is not a business that appeals to the pharmaceutical industry, nor is it a matter of interest to politicians or journalists. Choose your victims in the pit. He bites them and slowly, little by little, and he ends up with them. Their victims have no rights, no money to buy the rights they do not have. They do not even have the right to know what they die from." *Informe clínico,* by Uruguayan writer Eduardo Galeano, in "*Chagas, una tragedia silenciosa,*" Médicos Sin Fronteras, Editorial Losada, 2005.

Chagas disease is caused by *Trypanosoma cruzi,* transmitted to humans through the bite of *Triatomine* spp. by contaminated defecation rubbed on the mucosa. Transmission can also occur by ingestion of contaminated food, through blood transfusion or vertical transmission from mother to child [1]. It is worth to highlight that this endemic disease causes health, economic, and social problems affecting 6–7 million people in 21 countries from Central and South America. Moreover, 25 million people remain under risk of infection, given the high levels of population mobility from Latin America to the rest of the world or residence in endemic regions [2, 3].

Trypanosoma cruzi (*T. cruzi*) presents a quite complex cycle with different forms throughout its evolutionary cycle. In the insect vector, different stages can be observed. The *spheromastigote,* characterized as the round form of the organism, is predominantly found in the stomach of the organism. The epimastigote stage is found in the gut of the vector, at this stage, the *T. cruzi* is intensively multiplies by binary division. And finally the metacyclic trypomastigote stage, which is the infecting form for the vertebrate host [4, 5]. When the insect feeds on human blood, it defecates on the host's skin, releasing into the feces parasites in the metacyclic trypomastigote form. Upon entry to the organ, trypanosomes are disseminated via the blood or lymphatic, affecting various organs mainly the heart, nervous system, muscle, and digestive system. Once the parasites reach the tissues they reproduce, passing through a non-flagellated stage, called amastigote, which is able to actively multiply themselves forming pseudocysts, where they are to be transformed into trypomastigotes that are later to be released [6]. It is estimated that the incubation period of the disease is between 5 and 12 days relative to each case, as well as the appearance of symptoms and the intensity of them. Often, cases are asymptomatic so timely diagnosis can be very difficult. Undiagnosed individuals may lead to conditions like serious cardiac and digestive conditions begin to arise that may lead to death [7]. It is possible to observe three well-defined stages of the disease. The initial stage is called acute or initial, which lasts approximately 2–4 months after infection. At this stage, many people do not have symptoms. Most patients with symptoms suffer from variable fever, malaise, irritability, headache, enlargement of the liver, spleen, and lymph nodes. When the inoculation is close to the ocular area, the characteristic chagoma is observed as well as a unilateral edema of both eyelids [8]. At this stage, the parasite can be found in the blood. Some acute cases can become deadly and many of these turn out to be young children and patients, who are immunocompromised (e.g. people infected with HIV), who may develop acute myocarditis or meningoencephalitis [9]. Then a second indeterminate or also called latent stage in which the infection becomes undetectable and is usually asymptomatic. It usually occurs between week 8 and 10 of the acute phase and it can last for months or even years. It is estimated that approximately 30% of individuals who reach this stage develop digestive, cardiac, and neurological problems [10]. Finally, the chronic phase which appears in the latter part of the infection, it is characterized by cardiac and intestinal problems. Sudden death can occur without the individual developing heart problems [11].

The diagnosis of this disease is relative to infection of the patient. Direct methods (direct microscopic observation, xenodiagnosis, PCR, etc.) based on the detection of genetic material or parasites or indirect methods (ELISA, IFI, Western blot, etc.) based on the detection of specific antibodies against *T. cruzi*, mainly used in the chronic stage, either symptomatic or asymptomatic. These are usually used mainly in the acute phase, in the case of immunosuppressed persons or under 6 months of age [12].

Unfortunately, an effective chemotherapy for all the clinical forms of the disease has not been reached, although fair enough time has passed by since the discovery of the disease in 1909 by a Brazilian Doctor, Carlos Ribeiro Justiniano Chagas [2]. This intractable situation is the typical case of neglected diseases, where the lack of adequate therapies or effective vaccines provoque health crisis [13]. Despite the revealing evidence of the current situation has not received sufficient attention from the pharmaceutical industry, mainly due to economic considerations. The current pharmacological treatments are based on two nitroheterocycles compounds, which were discovered more than 30 years ago: nifurtimox (Nfx, N-(3-methyl-1,1-dioxo-1,4-thiazinan-4-yl)-1-(5-nitro-2 Methionine, Lampit®, suspended production, and sale by Bayer), and benznidazole (Bnz, N-benzyl-2-(2-nitroimidazol-1-yl) acetamide, Rochagan®, Roche, and currently produced By LAFEPE in Brazil). The problem with these drugs is that the significant side effects including weight loss, nausea and vomiting, rash, tissue abnormalities, leukopenia, neurotoxicity, psychosis, and peripheral neuropathy. On the other hand, Bnz can cause edema, fever, rash, peripheral neuropathy, lymphadenopathy, agranulocytosis, thrombocytopenic purpura, and joint and muscular pain. The use of these drugs during the acute phase of the disease is widely accepted, but its efficacy in the chronic phase is controversial [14].

The medicinal chemistry of Chagas disease has used different approaches in the search for new therapeutic entities. Some are oriented to the chemical development (synthesis) of new agents with interaction with key biomolecules for the parasite, or production of toxic species [15, 16]. Also, the reposition and polypharmacology of drugs have been used [17]. Other strategies have been oriented to the identification and isolation of new agents of natural origin [18]. Despite these efforts, research work in this medical area in order to find new solutions to a problem that seems to have no end is therefore, of utmost importance [14]. This review seeks answers in nature and always remembers the primary motivation: that affected people lacking the necessary resources find in their natural habitat medicinal plants that provide a possible treatment endorsed by science, effective and without side effects.

2. Natural products research

The use of plants for curative purposes dates back to the beginning of human history. The man turned to nature in search of food and health. By means of successes and errors, he learned to know the plants that healed. This knowledge was transmitted from generation to generation and was increased with experimentation. Without the resources offered by nature, humans would not have survived. Gradually humans, by dominating nature, have broken many of the ties that bind him. Today the medicine uses synthetic or semisynthetic drugs to relieve all diseases. Many of these drugs are beneficial, but many also, by misuse or abuse have lost their efficacy and in countless cases cause harmful side effects [19, 20].

In Latin American countries, the use of medicinal plants is the usual practice of indigenous groups and is frequently used by certain sectors of society [21]. This practice is usually an economic alternative to the prices imposed by the pharmaceutical industries and in many cases the only possibility of treatment [21, 22]. Most medicinal plants have multiple physiological effects, due to the presence of more than one active principle. The latter correspond to chemical compounds of the plant, which are subject to variables, such as soil moisture, light conditions, temperature, date of planting and harvesting, drying conditions, and among others [23].

Fortunately, in recent years, there has been an increase in interest in the return to nature, and therefore, it is necessary to build a new relationship with our environment, leading a less artificial life and turning to plants not only to include them in our diet but also to alleviate our conditions [19].

Natural products contribute greatly to the history and landscape of new molecular entities (NMEs). An assessment of all FDA-approved NMEs reveals that natural products and their derivatives represent over one-third of all NMEs. By the end of 2013, the FDA had approved 547 natural products and derivatives. Since the 1970s, the relative and then an absolute number of natural-product-based NMEs began to decline and today stand at fewer than one-quarter (24%) or an average of 7.7 natural product NMEs per year [24]. Plant products represented more than one-fifth (22%) of all NMEs approved before 1950, declining by more than 50–8.7% since that time [24]. Over the past two decades, the pharmaceutical industry has shied away from research into natural products. Attention shifted toward combinatorial chemistry, which seemed to satisfy the need for compound libraries to keep up with high throughput assays based on newly discovered molecular targets. However, this approach did not result in improved productivity, nor did an increase in the number of new drugs. The number of NMEs reached a record low of 24 in 2004 with an average of 40–50 new approved drugs by year in the period of 1981–2014. In the same period of 1981–2014, 16 NMEs were approved as antiparasitic drugs. Newman and Cragg classified these NMEs as unaltered natural products, natural products derivatives, a synthetic drug, synthetic drug (natural product pharmacophore), and mimic of the natural product (**Figure 1**). Among them, 68.7% are related to natural products [25, 26].

Izumi et al. reviewed the prospect of developing new drugs for the Chagas disease, on the screening of almost 400 species belonging to more than 100 plant families for activity against *T. cruzi* [27]. The plant extracts preparation methods have been very variable, from processes involving only one part of the plant to extract with different polarity solvents as well as using all part of the plant in the same solvent. Usually, the plant part in the study is the same that is used traditionally, but this does not assure that the accumulation of the active principles is maximum in the selected part. The plant extracts screened against different intracellular

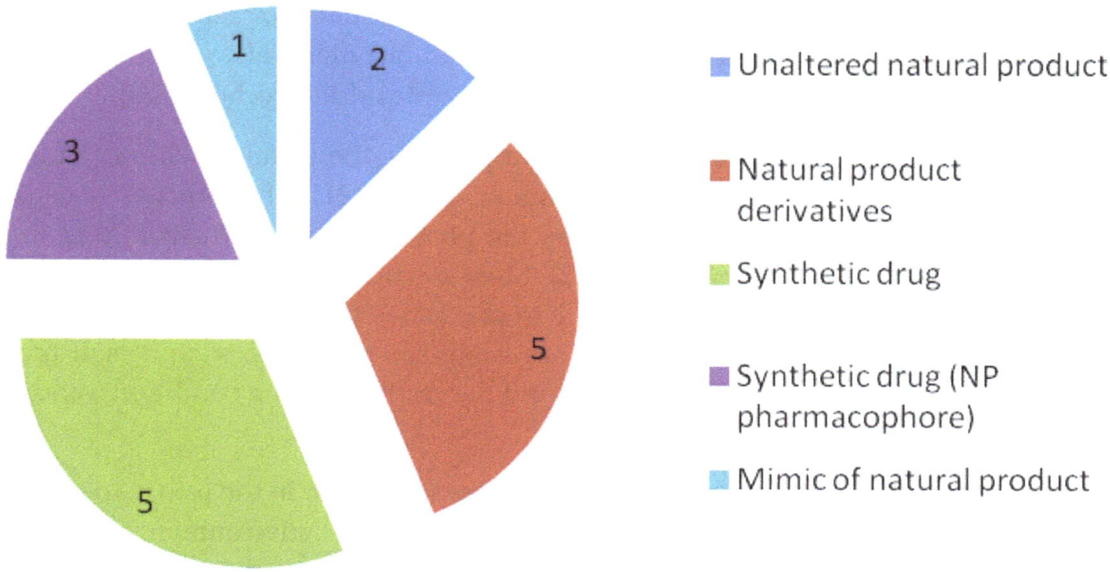

Figure 1. Classification of antiparasitic NMEs approved by FDA in the period 1981–2014.

forms of *T. cruzi* shows promising results. As a result, hexane extracts of *Polygala sabulosa* and aqueous extracts of *Polygala cyparissias* showed 50% inhibition of epimastigote growth after 72 h of treatment at concentrations of 1 and 2 μg/mL, respectively [28]. Ethanol extracts of *Physalis angulata* showed 50% inhibition of epimastigote growth after 120 h of treatment at a concentration of 2.9 μg/mL in Y strain and 7.4 μg/mL in Colombian strain [29]. Ethanol extracts of *Baccharis trimera* and *Baccharis articulata* showed 50% inhibition of epimastigote growth after 120 h of treatment at concentration 13.6 and 16.6 μg/mL in Tulahuen 2 strain, respectively [30]. For trypomastigotes, *Piptadenia africana* methanolic extract caused lysis in 50% of the parasites at 4 μg/mL after 96 h [31], and a methanolic extract from *Gardenia lutea* also promoted the same effect at approximately 22 μg/mL after 72 h [32]. The essential oil from the fruits of *Piper cubeba* showed 50% inhibition of trypomastigote form at a concentration of 45.5 μg/mL [33]. Surprisingly, by applying methanolic extracts of eight different species (*Hypoestes forsskalii, Kleinia odora* and *Psiadia punctulata, Capparis spinosa, Euphorbia schimperiana* and *Ricinus communis, Marrubium vulgare,* and *Solanum villosum*) an inhibition of 50% less than 0.25 μg/mL was found against the amastigote form with a treatment of 7 days [34]. Also for amastigotes, methylene chloride extract from leaves of *Conobea scopari-oides* showed 50% inhibition after 96 h at 1.3 μg/mL [35]. Ethanol extracts of *Baccharis trimera* and *Baccharis articulata* showed 50% inhibition of amastigote growth after 72 h of treatment at concentration 9.9 and 22.3 μg/mL in Dm28c strain, respectively [30]. Given that the financial resources for research on neglected diseases are usually low, most of the laboratories cannot afford the maintenance of infected animal models or cell cultures to perform tests with the infective forms, trypomastigote, and amastigote. This leads to screenings of compounds performed only against non-infective forms, even when promising preliminary results are reached, the isolation of active compounds is not frequent. Despite the screening of hundreds of species, the major, possibly active compound was only isolated, identified, and evaluated for antiparasitic activity in approximately 10% of the cases [27]. *In vivo* studies on the animal model of Chagas disease of plant extracts are less numerous than *in vitro* ones, but there are also reports of promising results. For example, *Serjania yucatanensis* ethanol leaves extract reduced 75% of the parasitemia in infected mice treatment at 100 mg/kg [36] and *Aristeguietia glutinosa* ethanol aerial parts extract reduced 50% of the parasitemia in infected mice at 50 mg/kg [37]. Plants extracts screening performed have been based on isolated efforts directed by research groups worldwide. Moreover, Pereira et al., after conducting an extensive bibliographic review for natural antichagasic products, conclude that there is an important geographic and ethnodirected component in the research initiatives on the relevance of plant derivatives in the treatment of Chagas disease [38]. The main obstacle that stops research work is the gap that needs to be bridged toward clinical phases, given the difficulties in scaling the purification of the active compound, standardization of the chemical profile of whole extracts, and among others. The principal common factor that delays clinical phase is the lack of investment for the development of these products at this stage of investigation [39]. **Figure 2** summarize the progress and current status of research and development of natural products for the Chagas disease.

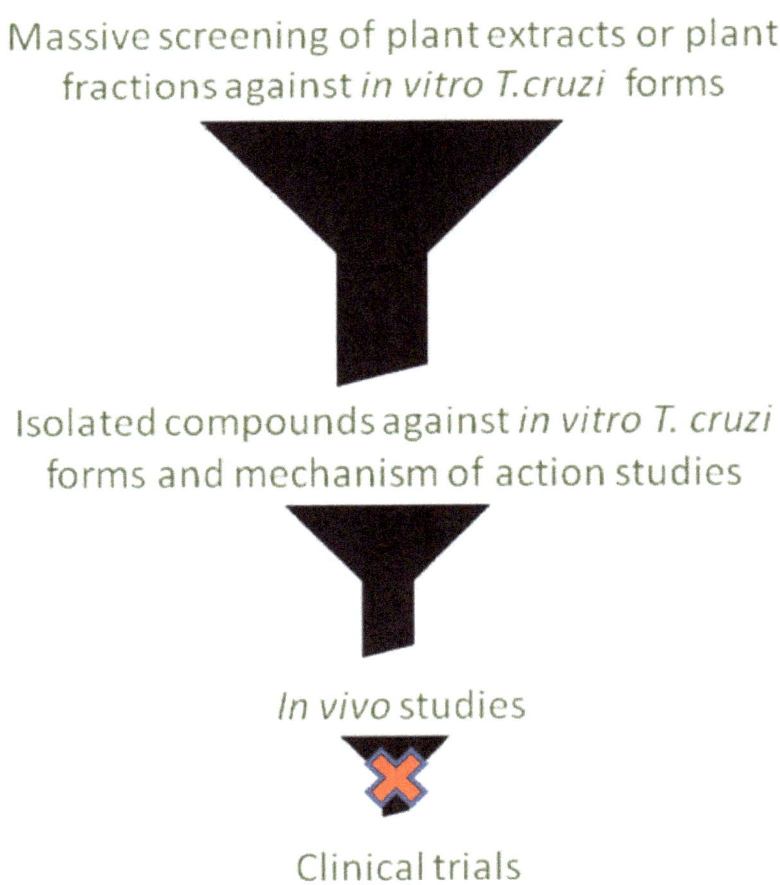

Figure 2. Current status of research and development of natural products for the Chagas disease.

In many cases, the isolation of compounds leads to the loss of biological activity or to the achievement of a really low extraction yield. That is why work with whole extracts should be re-considered as a possible source of new treatment drugs for the Chagas disease. Given the low economic potential of the majority of the affected population, it is clear that the development of new treatment drugs should consider cost-effectiveness. In the search for new therapies for Chagas from plant origin, low cost and easy access for patients, we propose the use of new methodologies to overcome the existing challenges. The use of plant metabolomics technique is proposed as an option with high potential for the identification of biomarkers that could allow the standardization of chemical profiles of whole plant extracts that can be formulated in a simple, quick, and low-cost dosage.

3. Plant metabolomics

Metabolomics can be defined as the detection and quantification of all metabolites of low molecular weight in an organism at a given time and in certain conditions. However, adjusting to our purposes and applications can be better defined as the area of research that seeks to obtain the metabolic fingerprints to detect the differences between them and propose hypotheses that explain the differences.

The field of metabolomics in science marks its beginning when Devaux and Horning publish their research work in the metabolic profile where they apply gas chromatography coupled with mass spectrometry (GC/MS) for the analysis of extracts of human tissues and urine [40]. Immediately, the interest of different groups in using the metabolic profiles for the diagnosis and follow-up of different pathologies [41]. During the 1970s metabolomics studies expanded to a wide range of activities including: novel techniques for detection and elucidation of insect hormones [42], identification of natural products of marine origin [43], and chemotherapeutic agents derived from plant extracts (e.g.: *Hyptis tomentosa*) [44]. At the beginning of the 1980s, the first work on automated metabolic analysis emerged [45] and by the middle of the decade, the first works on metabolic profiling were published using nuclear magnetic resonance (NMR) and high-performance liquid chromatography (HPLC) [46–48]. In order to analyze the mechanism of action of herbicides besides performing GC/MS, a new global approach was developed in 1991 [49]. As a result of scientific cooperation, by the end of twentieth century, it was possible to apply novel technologies to metabolomics and methods of extraction, encouraging the development of metabolite databases [50], which allowed the global development of complete metabolomes [51].

In the last decade, metabolomics has developed as an important field within plant science and natural product chemistry [52–56]. Metabolic fingerprint, also known as a metabolic profile, is an objective analytical approach that seeks to quantify a group or groups of compounds found in an organism or group of organisms. The metabolic profile with gas chromatography and high-performance chromatography coupled to mass spectrometry or proton magnetic resonance (^{1}H NMR) has been successfully used the study plant biochemistry, chemotaxonomy, ecology, pharmacology, and quality control of medicinal plants [57, 58]. The application of NMR has already been demonstrated as a suitable and sufficient method to carry out this type of analysis, since it allows simultaneous detection of various groups of secondary metabolites, in addition to abundant primary metabolites [59]. In addition, ^{1}H NMR spectroscopy has a great advantage over the other techniques, the signal intensity is dependent only on the molar concentration of the metabolites, allowing the direct comparison of these present in the sample [60, 61]. In the last years, several reports on the evaluation of the metabolic differences in *Cannabis sativa*, *Vanilla planifolia*, *Vitis* spp. and *Catharanthus roseus*, among others, and in the classification of *Ilex* species based on their metabolome are published [57, 60, 62, 63]. The major disadvantage in using NMR spectroscopy in the metabolomic analysis is overlapping signals, which however, can be solved by using different 2D-NMR techniques [52, 60, 63].

A typical approach of NMR-based metabolomic application for the identification of new natural products with biological activity that are part of whole extracts (**Figure 3**) was applied for the identification of new natural products with anti-*T. cruzi* activity in Uruguayan plants. Eighty samples of ethanolic extracts from different botanic parts, soils, and seasons, of Uruguayan specimens: *Baccharis trimera*, *Baccharis articulata*, *Baccharis usterii*, *Hydrocotyle bonariensis*,

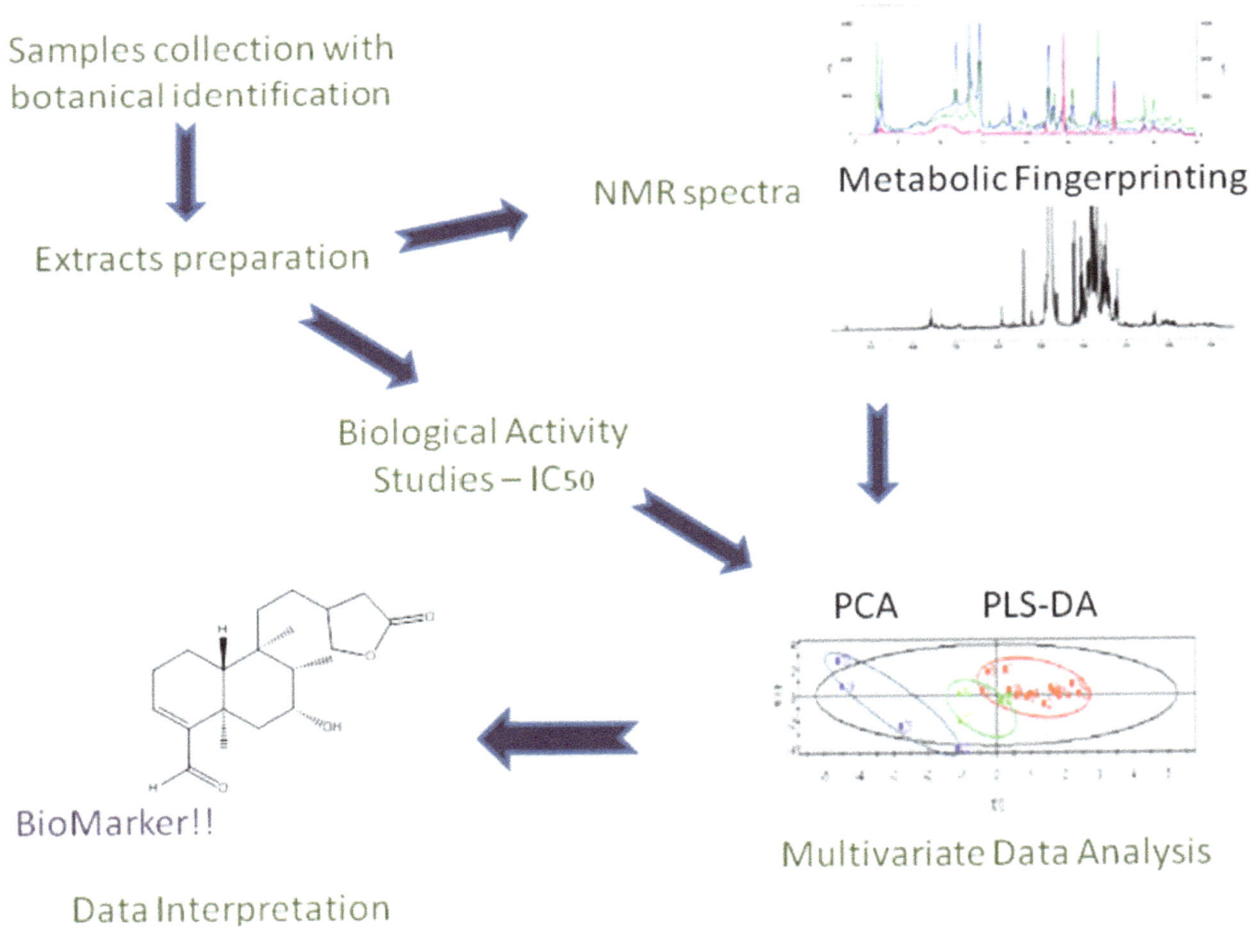

Figure 3. Typical approach of NMR-based metabolomic to identify new active compounds on plant extracts.

Achyrocline satureioides, Taraxacum officinalis, and *Plantago major* were used. As a primary screening the anti-*T. cruzi* activity against the epimastigotes showed that three species of *Baccharis* genus and *Hydrocotyle bonariessis* displayed well to excellent antiproliferative activity. The most active fractions were additionally evaluated for their activity on amastigotes and also for cytotoxicity against mammalian cells. For the identification of the active principles was applied using nuclear magnetic resonance-based metabolomic. Through the metabolomic study of the relationship between the changes in chemical profiles and the biological activities, it was possible to identify the main active principles of the extracts and also the compounds responsible for cytotoxic activity [30]. The technique also allowed us to infer the parts of the plants with greater accumulation of the active compounds as well as the conditions for their maximum expression (soil type, harvest season).

The development of drugs from wild plants with simple growing requirements, allow us to consider the future possibility of creating standardized cultivars, in order to perform *in vivo* assays and clinical trials. We performed the standardization of cultivars of *Baccharis trimera, Baccharis articulata,* and *Baccharis usterii* with relevant results in the expression of their active molecules against *T. cruzi.* The propagation was made by cloning mother plants collected from wild nature and developing their cuttings on an environment controlled greenhouse (**Figure 4**). The plant extracts prepared from the standardized cultivars are being studied *in vivo* in a murine model of the Chagas disease.

When plant cultivars are performed for possible pharmaceutical uses it is important to consider World Health Organization (WHO) guidelines on good agricultural and collection practices (GACP) for medicinal plants [64].

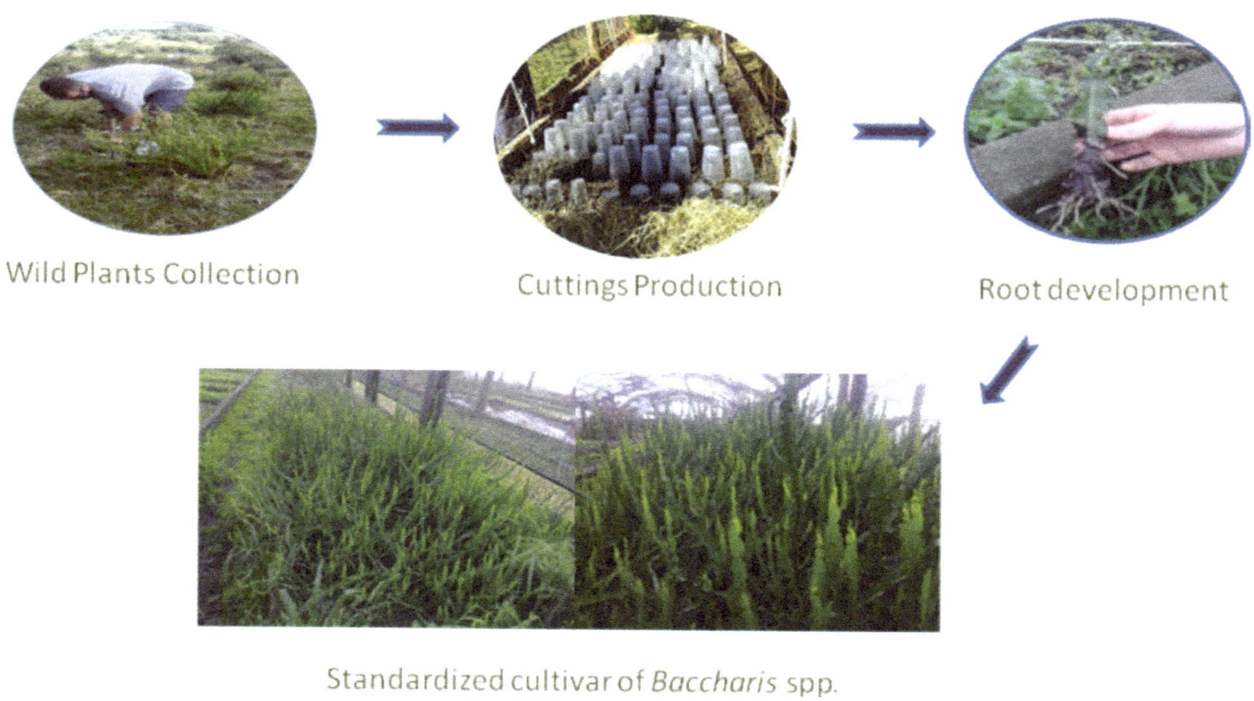
Wild Plants Collection
Cuttings Production
Root development
Standardized cultivar of *Baccharis* spp.

Figure 4. Cultivar propagation of *Baccharis* spp. for standardization of their chemical profile for extracts preparation to be used on *in vivo* test for the Chagas disease.

4. Good agricultural and collection practices (GACP)

Medicinal plant resources are being harvested in increasing volumes, largely from wild populations. Indeed, demand for wild resources has increased by 8–15% per year in Europe, North America, and Asia in recent decades. Various sets of recommendations relating to the conservation of medicinal plants have been developed, such as providing both *in situ* and *ex situ* conservation [65].

The harvest of plants that had a wild growth is considered an efficacious source for medicinal purposes, but domestic cultivation is also a widely used and accepted practice [66–68]. Indeed, domestic cultivation provides advantages for the production of medicinal plants, allowing control for toxic components, avoiding pesticides, increasing the content of active compounds, and having precise information for the identification of botanical origin [69]. In this way, controlling the growing conditions is a relevant tool for production stability and to improve the yields of secondary metabolites, which are frequently the active compounds. Cultivation standards include providing optimal levels of water, nutrients and other environmental factors such as light, humidity, temperature, in order to improved yields of target products [70]. Moreover, controlled cultivation contributes to decrease the harvest of medicinal wild plant resources, also having a positive impact on their prices [71, 72].

This knowledge has been translated into good agricultural and collection practices for medicinal plants that were developed in order to regulate production, assess quality, and lead to the standardization of herbal drugs [73]. The application of these formal practices, summarized in GACP approaches, is important to ensure high quality, safe and pollution free herbal drugs (or crude drugs) [74]. A wide range of problems are controlled by applying GACP including the ecological environment of production, germplasm, cultivation, and collection methods, as well as quality aspects for pesticide detection, authentication in macro and microscopic terms, chemical identification of active compounds, and detection of metal elements [75]. Given the importance of GACP, many countries actively promote their implementation; however, there is still an important gap to bridge concerning knowledge and implementation. This disparity is given by the difficulties encountered for training farmers and other relevant actors for medicinal plant production, such as handlers and processors. While these kind practices are strictly applied at the level of pharmaceutical producers that are used to work in order to meet quality control requirements, it has been more difficult to successfully introduce this practices standard at the level of agricultural producers, handlers, and processors of medicinal plant material. It will be important to focus the efforts on training farmers and other relevant actors to ensure that GACP is adopted and favor the obtainment of high-quality medicinal plant materials [64].

Currently, organic farming is increasingly receiving public attention, given that these practices include a vision of sustainability and economically relevant business without forgetting the well-being of workers and creates integrated production systems for medicinal plants [76, 77]. The main characteristic of organic farming is the avoidance of synthetic fertilizers, pesticides or herbicides, and reaching the standards of organic certification. The defining characteristic of organic farming is the non-use of synthetic fertilizers, pesticides, and herbicides, which are not allowed according to many current organic certification standards in Europe and North America. Instead of applying synthetic fertilizers, organic fertilizers may be continuously supplied to the soil, contributing nutrients, and improving soil stability, while positively impacting the biosynthesis of essential substances. Furthermore, organic farming generates high-quality products and better yields, while taking care of the conservation of those plants. Indeed, when organic fertilizers were applied to the cultivation of *Chrysanthemum balsamita,* the biomass yield was increased and its essential oil content was higher that those free from organic fertilizers [78]. Above all, organic farming is a benign practice for our environment, based upon renewable and sustainable resources that favor the maintenance of a biological equilibrium in the medicinal plants and their ecological systems [74, 76]. For these reasons, the application of organic farming practices is highly relevant for medicinal plant production, encouraging a sustainable, and long-term systemic approach [77].

5. The novel strategy proposed to obtain effective, cheap and standardized phytoterapeutic for treat Chagas disease

Based on the use of metabolomic and the GACP, the following workflow is proposed for obtaining phytoterapeutics for Chagas disease treatment (**Figure 5**).

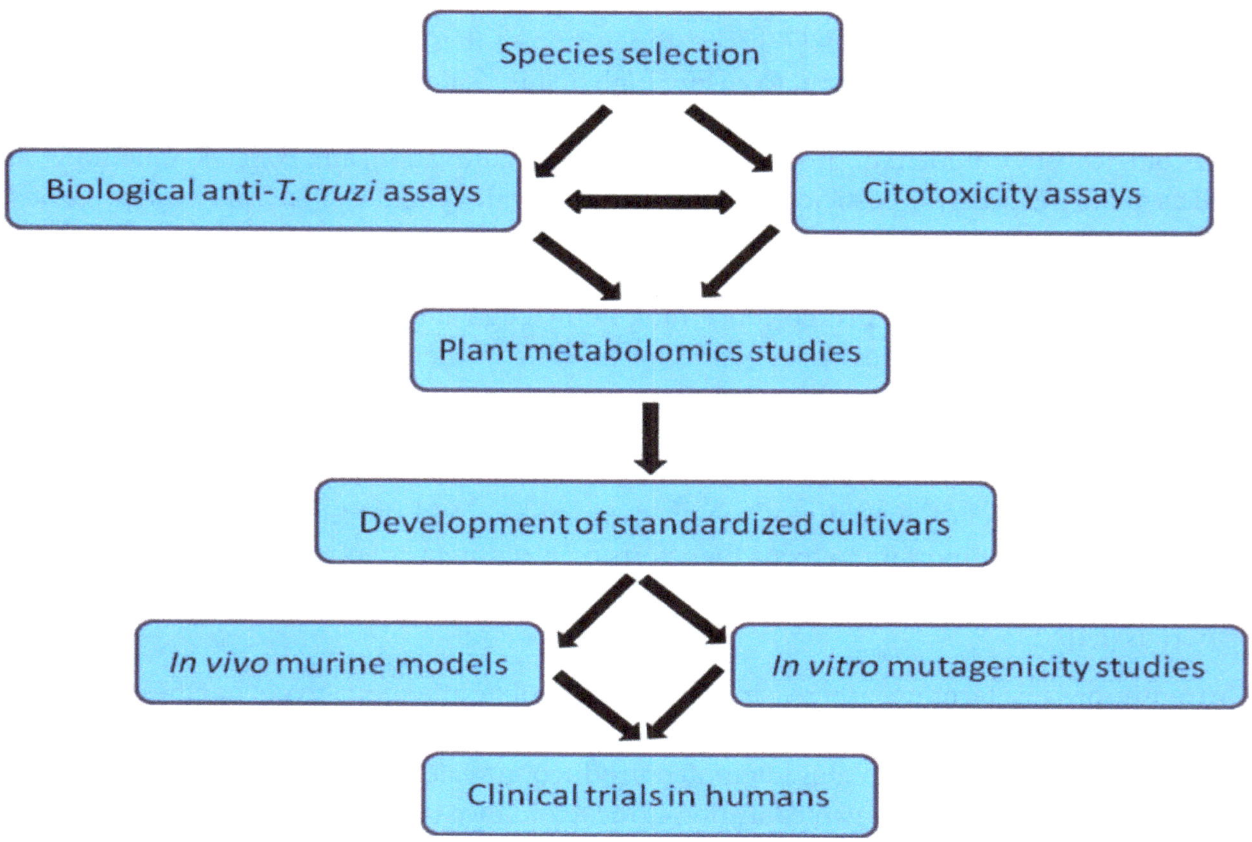

Figure 5. Workflow proposed for research and development of new natural products for Chagas disease treatment.

6. Conclusions

Traditional medicines, particularly herbal medicines have been increasingly used worldwide during the last two decades. On Chagas disease research many plant extracts were evaluated worldwide with relevant results but in most cases, the development is slowed in the scaling of the isolation of the active principle or by the lack of standardization of chemical profiles of the whole extracts. We presented a new novel strategy for the production of effective, cheap and standardized phytotherapeutic products through the use of plant metabolomics technique and the standardization of medicinal plants cultivars applying good agricultural and collection practices.

Author details

Javier Varela[1*], Hugo Cerecetto[1,2] and Mercedes González[1]

*Address all correspondence to: jvarelaubillos@gmail.com

1 Grupo de Química Orgánica Medicinal, Facultad de Ciencias, Universidad de la República, Montevideo, Uruguay

2 Área de Radiofarmacia, Centro de Investigaciones Nucleares, Universidad de la República, Montevideo, Uruguay

References

[1] Maya JD, Orellana M, Ferreira J, Kemmerling U, López-Muñoz R, Morello A. Chagas disease: Present status of pathogenic mechanisms and chemotherapy. Biological Research. 2010;**43**:323-331

[2] Álvarez G, Aguirre-López B, Varela J, Cabrera M, Merlino A, López GV, Lavaggi ML, Porcal W, Di Maio R, González M, Cerecetto H, Cabrera N, Pérez-Montfort R, Gómez-Puyou A. Massive screening yields novel and selective *T. cruzi* triosephosphate isomerase dimer-interface irreversible inhibitors with anti-trypanosomal activity. European Journal of Medicinal Chemistry. 2010;**5**:5767-5772

[3] Chagas disease (American tripanosomiasis). World Health Organization 2016 (Update March 2017). http://www.who.int/mediacentre/factsheets/fs340/en/ [Accessed July 30, 2017]

[4] Storino R, Milei J. Introducción. Enfermedad de Chagas, Vol. 1. Argentina: Mosby-Doyma; 1994. pp. 1-7

[5] Storino R. In: Mautner B y col. Enfermedad de Chagas. En Medicina, Vol. 25. Buenos Aires: Centro Editor Fundación Favaloro; 1998. pp. 774-783

[6] Storino R, Milei, J. Estudio clínico, con métodos complementarios no invasivos y correlación anatomopatologica da la enfermedad de Chagas. Premio Federico Guillermo Scholottman. 1985

[7] Barr SC, Gossett KA, Klei TR. Clinical, clinicopathologic, and parasitologic observations of trypanosomiasis in dogs infected with north American *Trypanosoma cruzi* isolates. American Journal of Veterinary Research. 1991;**52**(6):954-960

[8] Kirchhoff LV. Chagas Disease (American Trypanosomiasis) Clinical Presentation. Departments of Internal Medicine (Infectious Diseases) and Epidemiology, Carver College of Medicine and College of Public Health, University of Iowa, USA; 2011

[9] de Rosa M. Período indeterminado de la enfermedad de Chagas. Revista Argentina de Cardiología. 2002;**70**(1):43-51

[10] Organización Panamericana de la Salud. Zoonosis Y Enfermedades Transmisibles Comunes al Hombre Y a los Animales. Washington, DC: EUA; 2003. pp. 27-39

[11] Schettino S, Paz M, Perera R, Hernandez R. Chagas disease as a cause of symptomatic chronic myocardopathy in Mexican children. The Pediatric Infectious Disease Journal. 2009;**28**:1011-1013

[12] Botero D, Restrepo M. Parasitosis humanas. Colombia: Corporación para las Investigaciones Biológicas; 2003. pp. 220-224

[13] Tekiel V, Alba-Soto CD, González-Cappa SM, Postan M, Sánchez DO. Identification of novel vaccine candidates for Chagas' disease by immunization with sequential fractions of a trypomastigote cDNA expression library. Vaccine. 2009;**27**:1323-1332

[14] Cerecetto H, González M. Synthetic medicinal chemistry in Chagas' disease: Compounds at the final stage of "hit-to-lead" phase. Pharmaceuticals. 2010;**3**:810-838

[15] Merlino A, González M, Cerecetto H. Targets for anti-*T. cruzi* drugs in the post-genomic era. Current Enzyme Inhibition. 2010;**6**(4):195-210

[16] Cerecetto H, González M. Chemotherapy of Chagas' disease: Status and new developments. Current Topics in Medicinal Chemistry. 2002;**2**(11):1187-1213

[17] Bahia MT, Diniz LF, Mosqueira VC. Therapeutical approaches under investigation for treatment of Chagas disease. Expert Opinion on Investigational Drugs. 2014;**23**:1225-1237

[18] Fournet A, Muñoz V. Natural products as trypanocidal, antileishmanial and antimalarial drugs. Current Topics in Medicinal Chemistry. 2002;**2**(11):1215-1237

[19] Hernandez Magaña R, Gally JM. Plantas Medicinales. México: Editorial Árbol; 1981. pp. 7-8

[20] Salas C, Pérez-Vera P, Frías S. Genetic anbormalities in leukemia secondary to treatment in patients with Hodgkin's disease. Revista de Investigación Clínica. 2011;**63**(1):53-63

[21] Bussmann RW, Sharon D. Traditional medicinal plant use in Loja province, Southern Ecuador. Journal of Ethnobiology and Ethnomedicine. 2006;**2**:2-44

[22] Bussmann RW, Sharon D. Traditional plant use in northern Peru: Tracking two thousand years of healing culture. Journal of Ethnobiology and Ethnomedicine. 2006;**2**:47-65

[23] Bravo Díaz L. Farmacognosia. Spain: Elsevier; 2006. pp. 1-9

[24] Patridge E, Gareiss P, Kinch MS, Hoyer D. An analysis of FDA-approved drugs: Natural products and their derivatives. Drug Discovery Today. 2016;**21**(2):204-207

[25] Newman DJ, Cragg GM, Snader KM. Natural products as sources of new drugs over the period 1981-2002. Journal of Natural Products. 2003;**66**:1022-1037

[26] Newman DJ, Cragg GM. Natural products as sources of new drugs from 1981 to 2014. Journal of Natural Products. 2016;**79**:629-661

[27] Izumi E, Ueda-Nakamura T, Prado Dias Filho B, Florencio Veiga Junior V, Vataru Nakamura C. Natural products and Chagas' disease: A review of plant compounds studied for activity against *Trypanosoma cruzi*. Natural Product Reports. 2011;**28**:809-823

[28] Pizzolatti MG, Koga AH, Grisard EC, Steindel M. Trypanocidal activity of extracts from Brazilian Atlantic rain forest plant species. Phytomedicine. 2002;**9**:422-426

[29] Santana Meira C, Teixeira Guimarães E, Andrade Ferreira dos Santos J, Magalhães Moreira D, Campos Nogueira R, Coelho Barbosa Tomassini T, Ribeiro I, Campos de Souza C, Ribeiro dos Santos R, Botelho Pereira Soares M. *In vitro* and *in vivo* antiparasitic activity of *Physalis angulata* L. concentrated ethanolic extract against *Trypanosoma cruzi*. Phytomedicine. 2015;**22**(11):969-974

[30] Varela J, Birriel E, Nargoli J, Faral-Tello P, Robello C, Coqueiro A, Choi YH, Cerecetto H, González M. Identification of new anti-*Trypanosoma cruzi* agents in Uruguayan plants by NMR-based matabolomic profiling. Archives of Natural and Medicinal Chemistry. 2017;**ANMC-105**. DOI: 10.29011/ANMC-105.000005

[31] Mesia GK, Tona GL, Nanga TH, Cimanga RK, Apers S, Cos P, Maes L, Pieters L, Vlietinck AJ. Antiprotozoal and cytotoxic screening of 45 plant extracts from Democratic Republic of Congo. Journal of Ethnopharmacology. 2008;**115**:409-415

[32] Ali H, Konig GM, Khalid SA, Wright AD, Kaminsky J. Evaluation of selected Sudanese medicinal plants for their *in vitro* activity against hemoflagellates, selected bacteria, HIV-RT and tyrosine kinase inhibitory, and for cytotoxicity. Ethnopharmacology. 2002;**83**:219-228

[33] Rodrigues Esperandim V, da Silva FD, Sousa Rezende K, Guidi Magalhães L, Medeiros Souza J, Mendonça Pauletti P, Januário A, da Silva de Laurentz R, Kenupp Bastos J, Venâncio Símaro G, Roberto Cunha W, Andrade M. *In vitro* antiparasitic activity and chemical composition of the essential oil obtained from the fruits of *Piper cubeba*. Planta Medica. 2013;**79**:1653-1655

[34] Abdel-Sattar E, Maes L, Salama MM. *In vitro* activities of plant extracts from Saudi Arabia against malaria, leishmaniasis, sleeping sickness and Chagas disease. Phytotherapy Research. 2010;**24**:1322-1328

[35] Weniger B, Robledo S, Arango G, Deharo E, Aragón R, Muñoz V, Callapa J, Lobstein A, Anton R. Antiprotozoal activities of Colombian plants. Journal of Ethnopharmacology. 2001;**78**:193-200

[36] Polanco-Hernández G, Escalante-Erosa F, García-Sosa K, Acosta-Viana K, Chan-Bacab M, Sagua-Franco H, González J, Osorio-Rodríguez L, Moo-Puc R, Peña-Rodríguez L. *In vitro* and *in vivo* trypanocidal activity of native plants from Yucatan peninsula. Parasitology Research. 2012;**110**:31-35

[37] Varela J, Serna E, Torres S, Yaluff G, Vera de Bilbao N, Miño P, Chiriboga X, Cerecetto H, González M. *In vivo* anti-*Trypanosoma cruzi* activity of hydro-ethanolic extract and isolated active principles from *Aristeguietia glutinosa* and mechanism of action studies. Molecules. 2014;**19**(6):8488-8502

[38] Pereira R, Greco G, Moreira A, Chagas P, Caldas I, Goncalves R, Novaes R. Applicability of plant-based products in the treatment of *Trypanosoma cruzi* and *Trypanosoma brucei* infections: A systematic review of preclinical in vivo evidence. Parasitology. 2017;**144**(10):1275-1287

[39] Rodriguez J, Falcone B, Szajnman S. Detection and treatment of *Trypanosoma cruzi*: A patent review (2011-2015). Expert Opinion on Therapeutic Patents. 2016;**26**(9):993-1015

[40] Devaux P, Horning M, Horning E. Benzyloxime derivatives of steroids. A new metabolic profile procedure for human urinary steroids human urinary steroids. Analytical Letters. 1971;**4**:151-160

[41] Cunnick W, Cromie J, Cortell R, Wright B, Beach E, Seltzer F, Miller S. Value of biochemical profiling in a periodic health examination program: Analysis of 1,000 cases. Bulletin of the New York Academy of Medicine. 1972;**48**:5-22

[42] Judy KJ, Schooley DA, Dunham LL, Hall M, Bergot BJ, Siddall JB. Isolation, structure, and absolute configuration of a new natural insect juvenile hormone from *Manduca sexta*. Proceedings of the National Academy of Sciences of the United States of America. 1973;**70**:1509-1513

[43] Sims JJ, Donnell MS, Leary JV, Lacy GH. Antimicrobial agents from marine algae. Antimicrobial Agents and Chemotherapy. 1975;**7**:320-321

[44] Kingston DG, Rao MM, Zucker WV. Plant anticancer agents. IX. Constituents of *Hyptis tomentosa*. Journal of Natural Products. 1979;**42**:496-499

[45] Vrbanac J, Braselton W, Holland J, Sweeley C. Automated qualitative and quantitative metabolic profiling analysis of urinary steroids by a gas chromatography mass spectrometry-data system. Journal of Chromatography. 1982;**239**:265-276

[46] Nicholson J, O'Flynn MP, Sadler P, Macleod A, Juul S, Sonksen P. Proton nuclear magnetic resonance studies of serum, plasma and urine from fasting normal and diabetic subjects. The Biochemical Journal. 1984;**217**:365-375

[47] Bales JR, Higham DP, Howe I, Nicholson JK, Sadler PJ. Use of high-resolution proton nuclear magnetic resonance spectroscopy for rapid multi-component analysis of urine. Clinical Chemistry. 1984;**30**:426-432

[48] Bales J, Bell J, Nicholson J, Sadler P, Timbrell J, Hughes R, Bennett P, Williams R. Metabolic profiling of body fluids by proton NMR: Self-poisoning episodes with paracetamol (acetaminophen). Magnetic Resonance in Medicine. 1988;**6**:300-306

[49] Sauter H, Lauer M, Fritsch H. Metabolic profiling of plants: a new diagnostic technique. ACS Symposium Series. American Chemical Society. 1991;**443**:288-299

[50] Smith CA, O'Maille G, Want EJ, Qin C, Trauger SA, Brandon TR, Custodio DE, Abagyan R, Siuzdak G. METLIN: A metabolite mass spectral database. Therapeutic Drug Monitoring. 2005;**27**:747-751

[51] Sumner LW, Duran AL, Huhman DV, Smith JT. Chapter three metabolomics: A developing and integral component in functional genomic studies of *Medicago truncatula*. Recent Advances in Phytochemistry. 2002;**36**:31-61

[52] Kim HK, Choi YH, Verpoorte R. NMR-based metabolomics analysis of plants. Nature Protocols. 2010;**5**:536-549

[53] Fiehn O, Kopka J, Dörmann P, Altmann T, Trethewey R, Willmitzer L. Metabolic profiling for plant functional genomics. Biotechnology. 2000;**18**:1157-1161

[54] Rochfort S. Metabolomics revisited: A new "omics" platform technology for systems biology and implications for natural products research. Journal of Natural Products. 2005;**68**:1813-1820

[55] Hall RD. Plant metabolomics: From holistic hope, to hype, to hot topic. The New Phytologist. 2006;**169**:453-468

[56] Verpoorte R, Alfermann AW, Johnson TS. Applications of plant metabolic engineering. Phytochemistry Reviews. 2007;**6**:3-14

[57] Fischedick JT, Hazekamp A, Erkelens T, Choi YH, Verpoorte R. Metabolic fingerprinting of *Cannabis sativa* L., cannabinoids and terpenoids for chemotaxonomic and drug standardization purposes. Phytochemistry. 2010;**71**:2058-2073

[58] Van der Kooy F. Quality control of herbal material and phytopharmaceuticals with MS and NMR based metabolic fingerprinting. Planta Medica. 2009;**75**:763-775

[59] Georgiev MI. Metabolic differentiations and classification of *Verbascum* species by NMR-based metabolomics. Phytochemistry. 2011;**72**:2045-2051

[60] Kim H, Khan S, Wilson EG, Prat Kricun SD, Meissner A, Göraler S, Deelder A, Choi YH, Verpoorte R. Metabolic classification of south American *Ilex* species by NMR-based metabolomics. Phytochemistry. 2010;**71**:773-784

[61] Verpoorte R, Choi YH, Mustafa NR, Kim HK. Metabolomics: Back to basics. Phytochemistry. 2008;**7**:525-537

[62] Choi YH, Tapias EC, Kim HK, Lefeber AW, Erkelens C, Verhoeven JT, Brzin J, Zel J, Verpoorte R. Metabolic discrimination of *Catharanthus roseus* leaves infected by phytoplasma using ^{1}H-NMR spectroscopy and multivariate data analysis. Plant Physiology. 2004;**135**:2398-2410

[63] Ali K, Maltese F, Fortes AM. Monitoring biochemical changes during grape berry development in Portuguese cultivars by NMR spectroscopy. Food Chemistry. 2010;**124**: 1760-1769

[64] WHO Guidelines on Good Agricultural and Collection Practices (GACP) for Medicinal Plants. Geneva: World Health Organization; 2003

[65] Chen S, Yu H, Luo H, Wu Q, Li C, Steinmetz A. Conservation and sustainable use of medicinal plants: Problems, progress and prospescts. Chinese Medicine. 2016;**11**:37-47

[66] Gepts P. Plant genetic resources conservation and utilization: the accomplishments and future of a societal insurance policy. Crop Science. 2006;**46**:2278-2292

[67] Joshi B, Joshi R. The role of medicinal plants in livelihood improvement in Uttarakhand. International Journal of Herbal Medicine. 2014;**1**:55-58

[68] Leung K, Wong A. Pharmacology of ginsenosides: A literature review. Chinese Medicine. 2010;**5**:20-28

[69] Raina R, Chand R, Sharma Y. Conservation strategies of some important medicinal plants. International Journal of Medicinal and Aromatic Plants. 2011;**1**:342-347

[70] Wong K, Wong R, Zhang L, Liu W, Ng T, Shaw P, Kwok P, Lai Y, Zhang Z, Zhang Y, Tong Y, Cheung H, Lu J, Wing S. Bioactive proteins and peptides isolated from Chinese medicines with pharmaceutical potential. Chinese Medicine. 2014;**9**:19-25

[71] Hamilton A. Medicinal plants, conservation and livelihoods. Biodiversity and Conservation. 2004;**13**:1477-1517

[72] Larsen H, Olsen C. Unsustainable collection and unfair trade? Uncovering and assessing assumptions regarding central Himalayan medicinal plant conservation. Biodiversity and Conservation. 2007;**16**:1679-1697

[73] Chan K, Shaw D, Simmonds M, Leon C, Xu Q, Lu A, Sutherland I, Ignatova S, Zhu Y, Verpoorte R, Williamson E, Duezk P. Good practice in reviewing and publishing studies on herbal medicine, with special emphasis on traditional Chinese medicine and Chinese materia medica. Journal of Ethnopharmacology. 2012;**140**:469-475

[74] Muchugi A, Muluvi G, Kindt R, Kadu C, Simons A, Jamnadass R. Genetic structuring of important medicinal species of genus *Warburgia* as revealed by AFLP analysis. Tree Genetics & Genome. 2008;**4**:787-795

[75] Makunga N, Philander L, Smith M. Current perspectives on an emerging formal natural products sector in South Africa. Journal of Ethnopharmacology. 2008;**119**:365-375

[76] Rigby D, Cáceres D. Organic farming and the sustainability of agricultural systems. Agricultural Systems. 2001;**68**:21-40

[77] Macilwain C. Organic: Is it the future of farming? Nature. 2004;**428**:792-793

[78] Suresh B. Organic farming: Status, issues and prospects—A review. Agricultural Economics Research Review. 2010;**23**:343-358

8

Transmitter Insect of Chagas Disease in Northwest Mexico: A Comparative Study of the Cuticular Hydrocarbons Profile of Three Populations of *Triatoma rubida*: Peridomestic, Domestic and Sylvatic

Edgar Alfonso Paredes González,
Gerardo Álvarez Hernandez and
Jesús Ortega-García

Abstract

In México, biogeography data are available for species of triatomas called *Trypanosoma cruzi* transmitters; for example, the phyllosoma complex is distributed in several states of the south-central southeast of the country. In contrast, Northwestern Mexico species such as *Triatoma rubida* are considered sylvatic and in the process of domestication. The lack of research of these northern species of the country has generated an ignorance that contrasts with a growing number of alleged new cases of Chagas disease registered in health institutions in states such as Sonora. From the six species of triatomas that are potential transmitters of the *trypanosoma* in the state of Sonora, *Triatoma rubida* is the only one that has recent studies of distribution and transmission capacity. It is important then to know the degree of domesticity of the native species with the capacity of transmission of *Trypanosoma cruzi* and to define areas of risk. The process of adaptation of the sylvatic triatomines to the peridomestic and the domestic habitat has been understood in terms of environmental and biological variables. In this research, the profile of cuticular hydrocarbons of a peridomestic, domestic and sylvatic population of *Triatoma rubida* was analyzed and compared.

Keywords: *Triatoma rubida*, triatomines, cuticular hydrocarbons

1. Introduction

Chagas disease (CD) is caused in humans and animals by the parasite *Trypanosoma cruzi* (*T. cruzi*) and it is a major cause of mortality in the Americas. It is estimated that about 100 million people are at risk of infection from 6 million people who are infected, generating 56,000 new cases per year for all forms of transmission and 12,000 deaths annually [1–3]. In Mexico, the actual prevalence of CD is unknown and several epidemiological studies have demonstrated the presence of the disease in large urban and rural regions of the country [4]. Even so, it is estimated that there were approximately 1,100,000 infected individuals and 29,500,000 at risk of infection [5, 6]. The most important factors for this to happen are: (1) adaptability of triatomines to human dwellings and the circulation of *T. cruzi* among them and sylvatic and domestic animals; (2) the poverty situation in communities with poor housing and (3) the migration of people between communities and even distant countries where it did not exist [2, 7–10].

In Mexico 32 species are reported; 19 belong to the gender *Triatoma*, 6 to the gender Meccus, 2 to the gender *Panstrongylus* and 1 species of the genders *Belminus, Dipetalogaster, Eratyrus, Paratriatoma and Rhodnius. Triatoma barberi (Usinger), T. dimidiata (Latreille), T. pallidipennis, T. longipennis and T. mazzotti (Usinger)* are the main species found in our country, considered good transmitters of *Trypanosoma cruzi, T. barberi* (usinger), *T. dimidiata* (castreille), *T. pallidipennis, T. longipennis, T. mazzotii* (usinger), *P. picturata, T. mexicana (Herrich-Schaeffer) and T. gerstaeckeri (Stal) Rhodnius prolixus, Dipetalogaster maxima* and *Panstrongylus* spp. [11, 12]. Many of them are described and studied in the central and southern part of the country. However, to date, the factors that predispose the northern part of the country to CD are unknown despite the presence of transmitters in this part of Mexico [13]. The northern arid zones of Baja California Norte (BCN), Baja California Sur (BCS), Chihuahua, Sonora, Durango and Coahuila report a limited presence of domestic triatomines [6, 7]. In the state of Sonora, six species of triatomines have been described: *Triatoma rubida*, they belong to the subgroup *Rubrofasciata*, with five subspecies (*cochimiensis, jaegeri, rubida, sonoriana and uhleri), Triatoma protracta, Triatoma recurva, Paratriatoma hirsuta papagoensis, Triatoma sinaloenses* and *Triatoma incrassata* [14]. All these species are considered sylvatic with little epidemiological value. However, *T. rubida* and *T. recurve* have been associated with human dwellings and with high infection rates (90%) [15–17].

2. Bibliographic revision

2.1. *Triatoma rubida*

This insect has a wide geographic distribution in the Northwest of Mexico, Nayarit, Sinaloa and Sonora, and has been found in the Southwest of the United States in the states of Arizona, California, New Mexico and Texas. It is an established species throughout its range, and there is no information available on its dispersion [18, 19]. The populations of *T. rubida* have been divided into several subspecies based mainly on differences in the pattern and color of transverse spots on the connective border surrounding the abdomen (**Table 1**) [14]. Under laboratory conditions, *T. rubida* completes its life cycle in 130 days, developing 2 generations with very low mortality during their shedding, so that more than 98% of their eggs hatch and 94% complete their development until adulthood. *T. rubida* is distinguished because the female manages to eat in less than 10 min and her time of defecation can be immediate or between 5 and 20 s after her blood intake. The insect behaves very persistently during feeding and has the ability to hang firmly onto the host until it completes its feeding. This is consistent with the information collected during the fieldwork, where people report having seen their pet such as dogs carrying the bugs attached to the body [20, 21]. According to Tropical Disease Research (TDR) and the World Health Organization (WHO), studies on the mobility of sylvatic and domesticated populations in endemic areas of types can potentially be adaptable to the human habitat [22, 23]. The process of adaptation is considered a dynamic and continuous phenomenon that varies from one species to another according to its degree of ecological adaptation to eco-modified man-made ecosystems. It should also be considered that transmission (which becomes important in some areas) can occur without necessarily occurring true habitat events but only cases of invasion in human environments by adult triatomines or human-vector contact in the sylvatic environment [24–26]. The destruction of the ecotopes can cause changes, and eventually the disappearance of sylvatic animals as natural blood resources for triatomines, resulting in the invasion of houses by the vector in the search for human blood and exposure of the population to the risk of contracting Chagas disease [27–29].

Currently in the anti-vectorial fight of CD, in endemic countries like Brazil, Argentina, Bolivia and Peru, morphometric, biochemical, molecular and genetic studies of vector species are being developed, that contribute in the decision-making for the eradication in their houses. One of these lines of work is the analysis of the cuticular hydrocarbons (CH) of the triatomines [30].

2.2. Cuticle of insects

The cuticle of the insect is secreted by a double layer of epidermal and hypodermic cells. The hypodermis is described as a functional syncytium and is formed as a base membrane particularly during deposition and expansion of the old cuticle. The cuticle is formed by an inner procuticle composed of chitin (*N*-acetylglucosamine) and protein and a thinner chitinous outer layer the epicuticle. The pro-cuticle in turn is divided into an inner layer and an outer layer called exocuticle (pre-mutated cuticle) which is formed by sclerosed protein. The inner endocutaneous layer (cuticle after shedding) has remnants of the same sclerosed protein [31, 32].

Subspecies	Geographical Distribution
Triatoma rubida (Uhler)	Baja California Sur, Sonora
Triatoma rubida cochomiensis Ryckman	Baja California
Triatoma rubida jaegeri Ryckman	Isla Estanque BC., Sonora
Triatoma rubida sonoriana Usinger	Sonora, Sinaloa y Nayarit
Triatoma rubida uhleri Usinger	Suroeste de USA, Sonora y Veracruz

*Lent et al., 1979 [14].

Table 1. Geographic distribution of sub-species of ***Triatoma rubida****.

2.3. Insects' cuticular hydrocarbons

The insect's cuticular lipids consist of aliphatic material, which forms a thin layer in its integument. These lipids or surface waxes are presented as highly stable complex mixtures with unique structural characteristics. Among its main compounds hydrocarbons (HCs), fatty alcohols and waxes of high molecular weight predominate. The main function of these lipids in the insect is to restrict water loss and avoid lethal drying. It has been shown that they also participate in the absorption of chemical substances that can affect the activity of microorganisms and intervene in various chemical communication processes [33–35].

Cuticular hydrocarbons (CH) are continuously synthesized in the insect's intrategumenal tissue, through the enzymatic action of fatty acid synthetase (FAS), an acetyl CoA for elongation, a reductase and a decarboxylase that produces hydrocarbons and CO_2. The epidermal cells responsible for its production are the oenocytes that lie beneath the hypodermis. Oenocytes transport hydrocarbons through tissues through a hemolytic lipoprotein called liporin. This lipid synthesis is considered dynamic and changes as the insect passes through its nymphal stages, stopping at the adult stage. De Renobales et al. [36], proposed that the hydrocarbons synthesized by the insect are stored inside their tissues until the next shedding. The insect needs a new layer of lipids as regulators of its permeability [35, 37].

Based on studies conducted in particular on nine species of triatomines of the genus *Triatoma, Pastrongylus* and *Rhodnius*, it has been found that such HCs are alkanes of 27–33 carbon atoms and chains of branched alkanes with 1–3 methyl groups inserted along a carbon skeleton from 29 to 41 carbon atoms [35]. The predominant linear components are nC27, nC29, nC31 and nC33, while in the branched fraction predominate isomers of dimethyl- C37, trimethyl-C37, trimethyl-C35 and trimethyl-C39 as reported by Juárez et al. [38] (**Figure 1**). Williams and Jackson [45] suggested that hydrocarbon differentiation may be an early evolution of specialization; in addition, geographic differentiation also led these authors to suggest that the phenotype may be differentiated prior to species divergence. Similarly, Juárez and Brenner [39, 40], considered that the composition of triatomine HC can be used as a taxonomic criterion to separate individual populations and

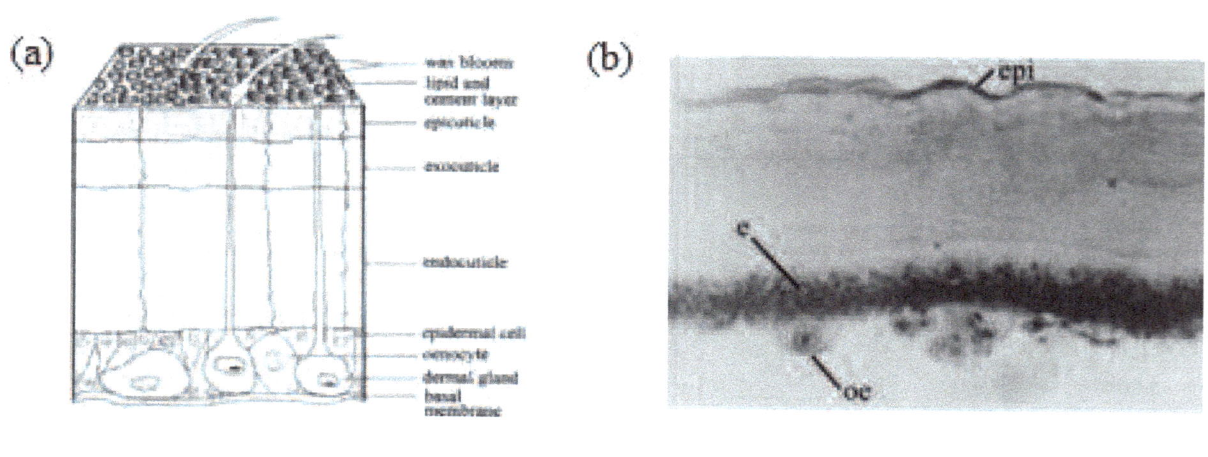

Figure 1. (a) Diagram of a cross-sectional area of the insect integument, illustrating the major layers of the cuticle and (b) cross-sectional view of *T. infestans* integument. Epi, epicuticle; e, epidermal cell layer; oe, oenocytes. Source: Juarez, M.P. 2007.

specimens, based on the graphical comparison of their corresponding profiles (fingerprints) or through the quantitative calculation of numerical indicators such as the determination of HC [41].

Finally, understanding how insect HCs, together with other surface lipids, are involved in the absorption of chemicals is essential for the timely and adequate vector control measures to be applied in the future [42, 43].

This research analyzes and compares the profile of cuticular hydrocarbons of a peridomestic, domestic and a sylvatic population of *Triatoma rubida*; this is an insect that transmits the Chagas disease in the state of Sonora. The rationale for this proposal was to define the hydrocarbon profiles of *T. rubida* peridomestic, domestic and sylvatic, in order to obtain differences between each of the swarms and to be able to differentiate the three populations of insects by their HC profile. Having the knowledge that *T. rubida* participates in the vectorial transmission of *T. cruzi*, the study is very helpful and of high epidemiological value, to take measures to eradicate and/or control it in human dwellings.

3. Materials and methods

3.1. Sampling area

The city of Guaymas Sonora was chosen because it is considered, in this study, to be an endemic area of the CD. The port is situated at 110°53′34″ North latitude and 27°55′30″ West Greenwich, at a height of 15 m. It has a desert or hot climate, with a maximum monthly temperature of 30–35°C in the months from July to August and a minimum average monthly temperature of 18°C. Its average annual temperature is 28°C. Its vegetation is xerophytic type, where mesquite (*Prosopis velutina*), pitahaya (*Stenocereus thurberi*), palo fierro (*Olneya tesota*), palo verde (*Parkinsonia aculeata*), jito (*Forchammeria* watsonii) and scrub subinerme abound [44].

3.2. Sampling and capture of insects

Three districts of the City of Guaymas were monitored to collect the batch of peridomestic and domestic insects, where the epidemic was known: El Rastro, Cerro Gandareño and Yucatán. In these areas, the existence of triatomines was known, particularly *Triatoma rubida sonoriana*, which was the subspecies chosen for this research and had entomological indices indicating infestation in 63%, colonization of 68.4% and density of 8.5% [15].

The sylvatic insects were collected from the surrounding hills, a hill in the northern part was chosen 1400 m away from the city where domestic and peridomestic insects were collected. *Neotoma* spp. were observed in this area and confirmed during visits. Four nests of *Neotoma* were distributed in a radius of 60 m all placed at the base of pitahayas (*Stenocereus thurberi*).

Once collected, the two pairs of main and secondary wings were extracted from the adult insects which were wrapped in foil and transported to the laboratory of parasitology at the University of Sonora, North Caborca Unit. For the identification of the morphological characteristics that define *rubida*, the keys described by Lent and Wygodzinsky [14] were used.

3.3. Analysis and extraction of hydrocarbons

Cuticular hydrocarbons (CHs) were extracted following the methods of Juárez and Blomquist [45], and Juárez et al. [46]. Each pair of specimen wings were given a washing treatment with 2 mL of distilled water twice to remove any contaminants such as feces or soil particles. They were then transferred to a 4 mL glass vial with a screw cap, Teflon septum and properly labeled. A 1 mL of high-performance liquid chromatography (HPLC) grade hexane was added with 99% purity (Sigma-Aldrich, México). With this solvent they were kept for 1 day, at a temperature of 28°C for the extraction of the cuticular lipids.

3.4. Isolation of hydrocarbons

The next step consisted of separating the hydrocarbons from the other cuticular components (lipids, waxes, etc.) present in the extract. For this purpose, the lipid mixture was reconstituted from each vial with hot hexane and then applied to a mini glass column (10 × 5 mm ID) with 1.74 g of silica gel, 60% pore and 70-230 (Sigma-Aldrich, México; cat. 288,624). Previously equilibrated with hexane, the elution was carried out with 4 mL of hexane for each sample (4 mL/mg). The silica from the column was renewed every three samples (**Figure 2**).

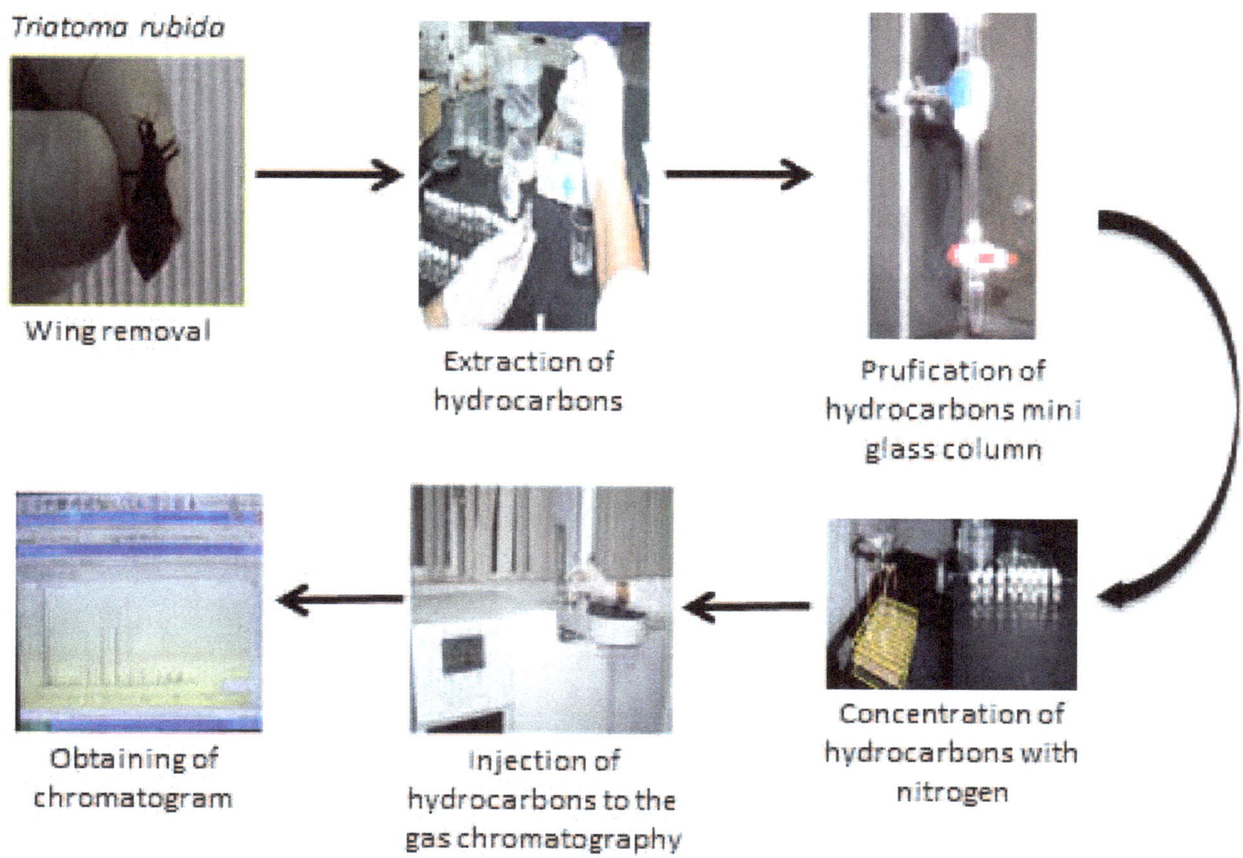

Figure 2. Diagram for the extraction of cuticular hydrocarbons.

3.5. Obtaining the chromatographic profiles of each population

Once the methodology was adjusted, 3 μl of each of the hydrocarbon samples extracted from *Triatoma rubida* was injected into the chromatograph. To do this, 7 μL of hot hexane was taken and poured into the vial containing the hydrocarbons of each specimen, until the largest amount possible from the sample was mixed by circular movements in the bottom of the container, where the required amount was injected in the GC.

3.6. Identification of HC by GC-MS

For the identification of the linear hydrocarbons, an HP 6890 chromatograph coupled to an Agilent 5975C VL mass spectrometer was used. GC conditions were HP-5MS nonpolar column of 30 × 0.25 mm ID × 0.25 μm film; helium carrier gas at 1.5 mL/min constant flow; oven temperature programmed 50°C (1 min) to 200–50°C /min, then to 320–3°C/min (25 min) and the injector was operated in split-less mode at 320°C. The conditions of the MS detector were ionization energy of 70 eV; transfer line at 320°C; the ionization chamber at 230°C and the quadrupole at 150°C. For the analysis of the collected data, an MSD ChemStation Agilent Technologies Inc. was used.

4. Statistical analysis

We estimated central tendency measures and compared the relative means of abundance of hydrocarbons between genera; the significance was tested by a nonpaired t (Excel 2006 package), after normalization of the data with arcosene. Relative means (Tukey's post hoc test) were compared between the three populations through a one-way analysis of variance (ANOVA). The data were presented in tables and graphs. All tests were estimated at one tail and values of $p < 0.05$ were considered as statistically significant. For these analyses the statistical package BioStat 2007 was used.

5. Results

5.1. Collection of insects

A total of 120 peridomestic, 50 domestic and 50 sylvatic specimens were collected. Of the 220 insects, there were nymphs of second stage (NII; 1.4%), nymphs of the third stage (NIII; 11.4%), nymphs of the fourth instar (NIV; 17.3%), 53.6% were nymphs of the fifth instar (NV; 53.6%), 6.8% were adult females (AF) and 9.5% were adult males (AM). No specimens of the first nymphal period were found in all three populations.

5.2. Analysis of the hydrocarbons: Retention times obtained

The gas chromatographic standardization process allowed to obtain the retention times of 14 commercial hydrocarbons standards, AccuStandard Brand, Inc. USA (purity 99%), which were used to estimate Kovats indexes for each sample analyzed (**Table 2**).

Standard	Name	Retention Time (Minutes)
C19	Nonadecane	6.31
C20	Eicosane	7.18
C21	Heneicosane	8.23
C22	Docosane	9.51
C23	Tricosane	10.99
C24	Tetracosane	12.67
C25	Pentacosane	14.49
C26	Hexacosane	16.44
C28	Octacosane	20.45
C30	Triacontane	24.46
C32	Dotriacontane	26.36
C36	Hexatriacontane	35.71
C38	Octatriacontane	38.78
C40	Tetracontane	41.25

Table 2. Retention time of injected standards.

5.3. Identification of the cuticular hydrocarbons profile of *Triatoma rubida*

The 35 components of *T. rubida* were detected (**Figure 3**); however, for this study, only 14 major peaks were considered (**Figure 4**). Five linear hydrocarbons were identified in the three populations of *T. rubida* in both females and males, corresponding to the first five selected peaks of the chromatogram: pentacosano, heptacosano, nonacosano, hentriacontano and tri-triacontano. It is important to note that these five hydrocarbons are present in all three populations (**Figure 5**).

The chromatographic profile was similar for the three populations, and the hydrocarbons corresponded to n-alkanes with a continuous series of C25, C27, C29, C31, C33 and C35. In addition, the Kovats indices identified C35.52, C36.00, C37.74, C37.75, C38.00, C39.41, C39.60 and C39.83, which are likely representations of branched isomers of alkanes. The location of the methyl branches of these hydrocarbons, by the proposal of Katritzky et al. [47], was estimated. The Kovats indexes: IK3552, IK3600, IK3774, IK3775, IK3800, IK3941, IK3960 and IK3983 therefore correspond to the hydrocarbons described in **Table 3**.

5.4. Quantification in percent of area of hydrocarbons analyzed

The relative amounts in the percent of area of each linear and branched hydrocarbon analyzed for each population were obtained. In **Table 4**, the data for the peridomestic, domestic and sylvatic *Triatoma rubida* population are presented.

In **Table 5**, the total amounts for linear and branched hydrocarbons are presented for each of the three populations of *rubida;* also the relative percentage of the majority hydrocarbon is

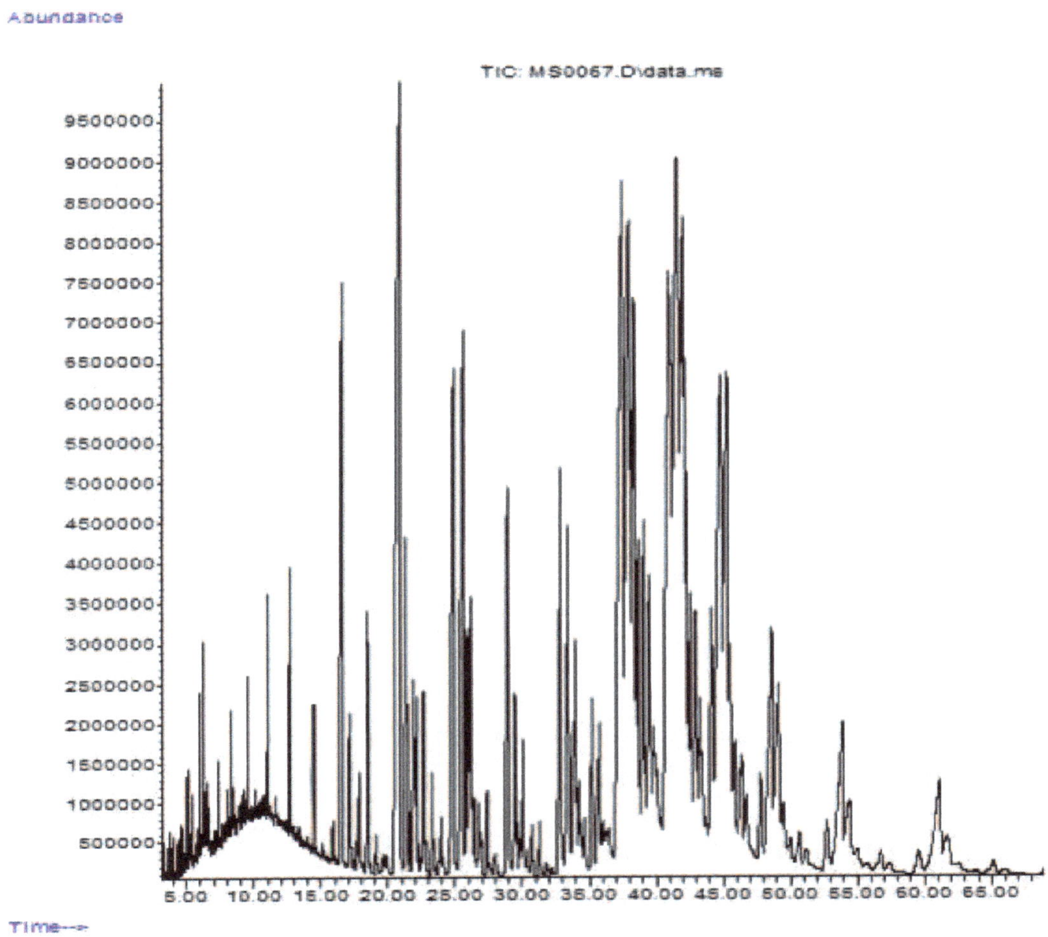

Figure 3. Ion chromatogram total of *Triatoma rubida.*

presented. Using statistical analysis and using the unpaired "t" test, when comparing females and males for each population, a significant difference was found between males and domestic females for the IK2700 peak. When comparing peridomestic males and females, significant differences were found for the IK3100 peak. Regarding the comparison of sylvatic males and females, significant differences were observed for the IK3100 and IK3300 peaks, in addition to the peaks IK2500 and IK2700 (**Figure 6**).

5.5. Comparison of the three populations of *Triatoma rubida*

To analyze the differences between *rubida* species, the one-way parametric analysis of variance (ANOVA) was used. When comparing the three populations of females, significance was found for the relative average abundance of the C27 hydrocarbon. Tukey's post hoc test estimated the differences among the three female populations, finding a significant difference between domestic and sylvatic ones ($p = 0.00001$).

In the comparison of groups of males, significant differences were also found between domestic males and peridomestic males in HC27 ($p = 0.01$) and HC29 ($p = 0.03$), whereas when comparing domestic with sylvatic males, there were significant differences in HC33 ($p = 0.002$). On the other hand, when comparing the populations of females with males, significant differences were observed in the population of domestic females compared to that of peridomestic and sylvatic

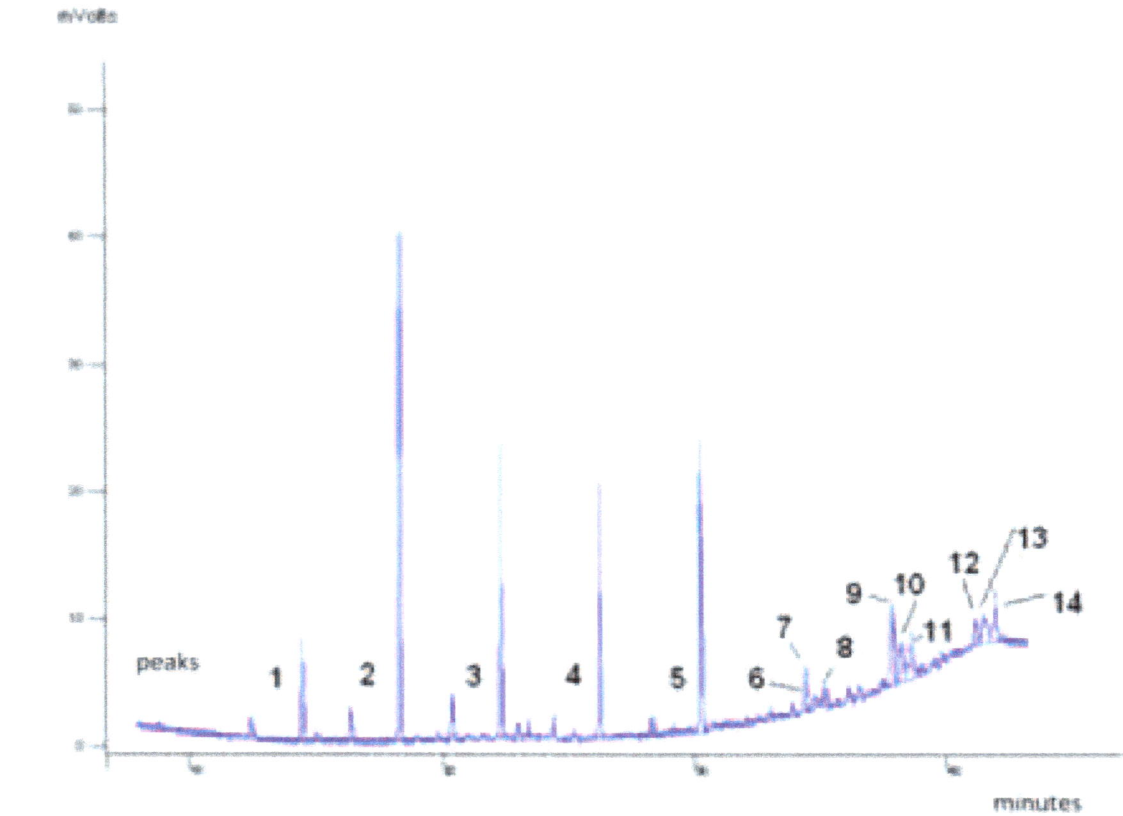

Figure 4. Selection of 14 hydrocarbon peaks, majority in *Triatoma rubida*.

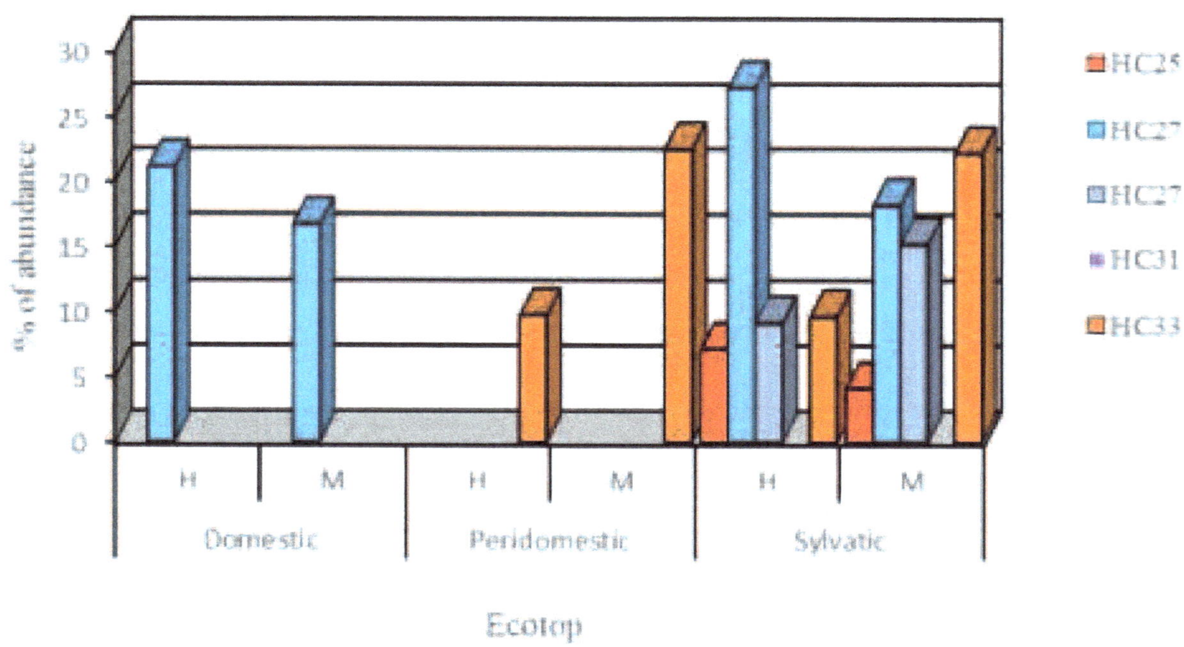

Figure 5. Quantitative variation of cuticular hydrocarbons of *T. rubida* considering its generous.

males in the HC 29 (p = 0.01), 31 (p = 0.03) and 33 (p = 0.001). Meanwhile, the population of peri-domestic females, when compared to domestic males and sylvatic males, had significant differences in HC27 (p = 0.007), HC29 (p = 0.01) and HC33 (p = 0.0009). Finally, in the comparison

Retention rate	Type of hydrocarbon
3574	03 Methyl Pentacontane
3600	3x Dimethyl Pentacontane
3752	13, 23 Dimethyl Heptatriacontane
3775	15,19,23 Dimethyl Heptatriacontane
3800	3x Dimethyl Octariacontane
3941	x Trimethyl Nonatriacontane
3960	xx Dimethyl Nonatriacontane
3983	15.19, 23 Trimethyl Nonatriacontane

*Katritzky et al., 2000 [47].

Table 3. Qualitatively identified branched hydrocarbons.

Peak	Hydrocarbon*	Kovats Index	Domestic[1]		Peridomestic[2]		Sylvatic[3]	
			Male	Female	Male	Female	Male	Female
1	n-25	2500	6.59 ± 2.3	5.50 ± 2.3	4.50[a] ± 0.09	7.56[b] ± 0.9	5.54 ± 1.3	6.18 ± 1.0
2	n-27	2700	16.50[a] ± 1.3	20.90[b] ± 2.0	19.00 [a] ± 3.2	27.88[b] ± 0.8	23.00 ± 1.5	26.64 ± 2.6
3	n-29	2900	9.33 ± 1.2	10.80 ± 2.0	12.82 ± 1.6	13.83 ± 0.8	15.29 ± 0.9	16.10 ± 1.9
4	n-31	3100	11.86 ± 1.8	10.00 ± 1.4	15.69[a] ± 1.2	9.41[b] ± 0.9	14.08 ± 0.7	12.17 ± 2.3
5	n-33	3300	14.06 ± 2.7	12.00 ± 1.8	22.29[a] ± 1.7	9.61[b] ± 0.6	15.72[a] ± 1.3	12.29[b] ± 1.7
6	n-35	3500	5.19 ± 1.7	5.20 ± 0.4	2.98 ± 0.3	3.82 ± 0.5	2.59 ± 1.3	3.03 ± 0.5
7	03 Methyl Pentacontane	3574	2.74 ± 0.3	2.90 ± 0.2	1.55 ± 0.3	1.81 ± 0.3	1.84 ± 1.0	2.00 ± 0.3
8	3x Dimethyl Pentacontane	3600	2.76 ± 0.6	2.00 ± 0.4	1.53 ± 0.1	1.47 ± 0.3	1.70 ± 0.5	1.40 ± 0.3
9	13, 23 Dimethyl Heptatriacontane	3572	6.55 ± 0.2	7.40 ± 1.0	5.61 ± 0.9	7.73 ± 1.2	5.77 ± 0.3	6.00 ± 0.3
10	15,19,23 Dimethyl Heptatriacontane	3775	7.07 ± 0.8	6.80 ± 1.3	4.84 ± 2.7	4.73 ± 1.2	4.13 ± 1.0	4.04 ± 1.4
11	3x Dimethyl Octariacontane	3800	5.63 ± 1.1	4.90 ± 0.5	3.02 ± 1.3	4.00 ± 0.2	3.38 ± 0.6	3.00 ± 1.6
12	x Trimethyl Nonatriacontane	3941	2.14 ± 0.3	1.90 ± 0.3	1.96 ± 0.3	2.22 ± 0.6	1.90 ± 0.2	1.70 ± 1.2
13	xx Dimethyl Nonatriacontane	3960	4.79 ± 0.8	4.50 ± 0.9	3.16 ± 0.9	3.57 ± 0.8	3.18 ± 0.6	3.00 ± 1.1
14	15.19, 23 Trimethyl Nonatriacontane	3983	4.79 ± 1.9	5.20 ± 0.9	2.56 ± 2.2	3.50 ± 0.9	3.07 ± 0.7	3.00 ± 2.2

*The hydrocarbons and peak number are the same as reported in **Figures 6-7**. The means were compared with the unpaired *t* test. [a, b] The differences between males and females were significant among the hydrocarbons in each row. Population analyzed: [1,2] n = 12 females and n = 9 males; [3] n = 9 females and n = 12 males.

Table 4. Relative percent of majority hydrocarbons of ***Triatoma rubida*** peridomestic, domestic and sulvatic (%).

Population /Hydrocarbon	*Triatoma rubida*					
	Domestic		Peridomestics		Sylvatic	
	Female	Male	Female	Male	Female	Male
Linear	56.76	51.75	76.41	76.22	72.11	77.28
Branched	43.24	48.25	23.59	23.78	27.89	22.72
2700*	37.40		49.64		46.88	

*Major component of hydrocarbon detected.

Table 5. Content of cuticle hydrocarbons in ***Triatoma rubida*** (%).

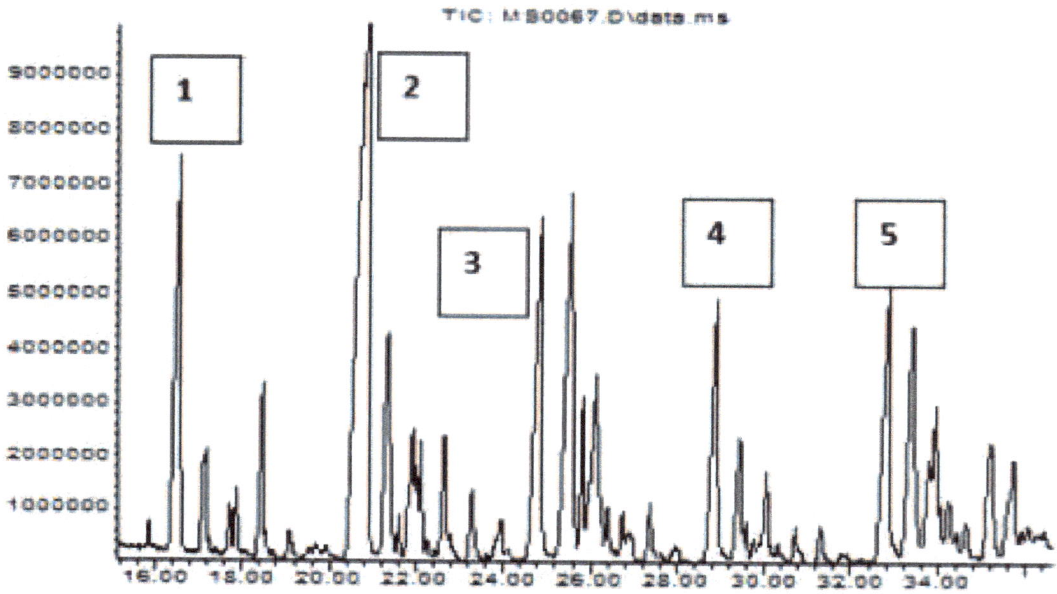

Figure 6. Confirmed linear hydrocarbon mass spectra.

of populations of sylvatic versus domestic males and peridomestic males, significant differences were observed for HC27 (p = 0.0001) and HC29 (p = 0.002).

6. Discussion

6.1. Domestic population

The *GC–MS* analysis showed that in the population of *Triatoma rubida*, domestic, odd chains of HC prevailed, and C27, C29, C31 and C33 predominated, which together represented 56.8% of HC in females and 51.8% for the males. The branched hydrocarbons represented 32.4% in males and 36.5% in females, of total hydrocarbons. The relative amount of pentacosane hydrocarbon was 37.40%. The characteristics of the typical chromatogram of females and males showed that the chromatographic profiles of the cuticular hydrocarbons in domesticated *Triatoma rubida* were qualitatively very similar for both genera. However, their relative amounts were different, as demonstrated in the pentacosane hydrocarbon, where the female had 20.9% and the male had 16.50%.

Based on the graphical representation of the chromatographic profiles, the identification of five of their linear hydrocarbons by mass spectrometry and the statistical analysis when comparing the relative means between genders, we suggest how the typical profile of domestic Triatoma rubida is described in **Figure 7**.

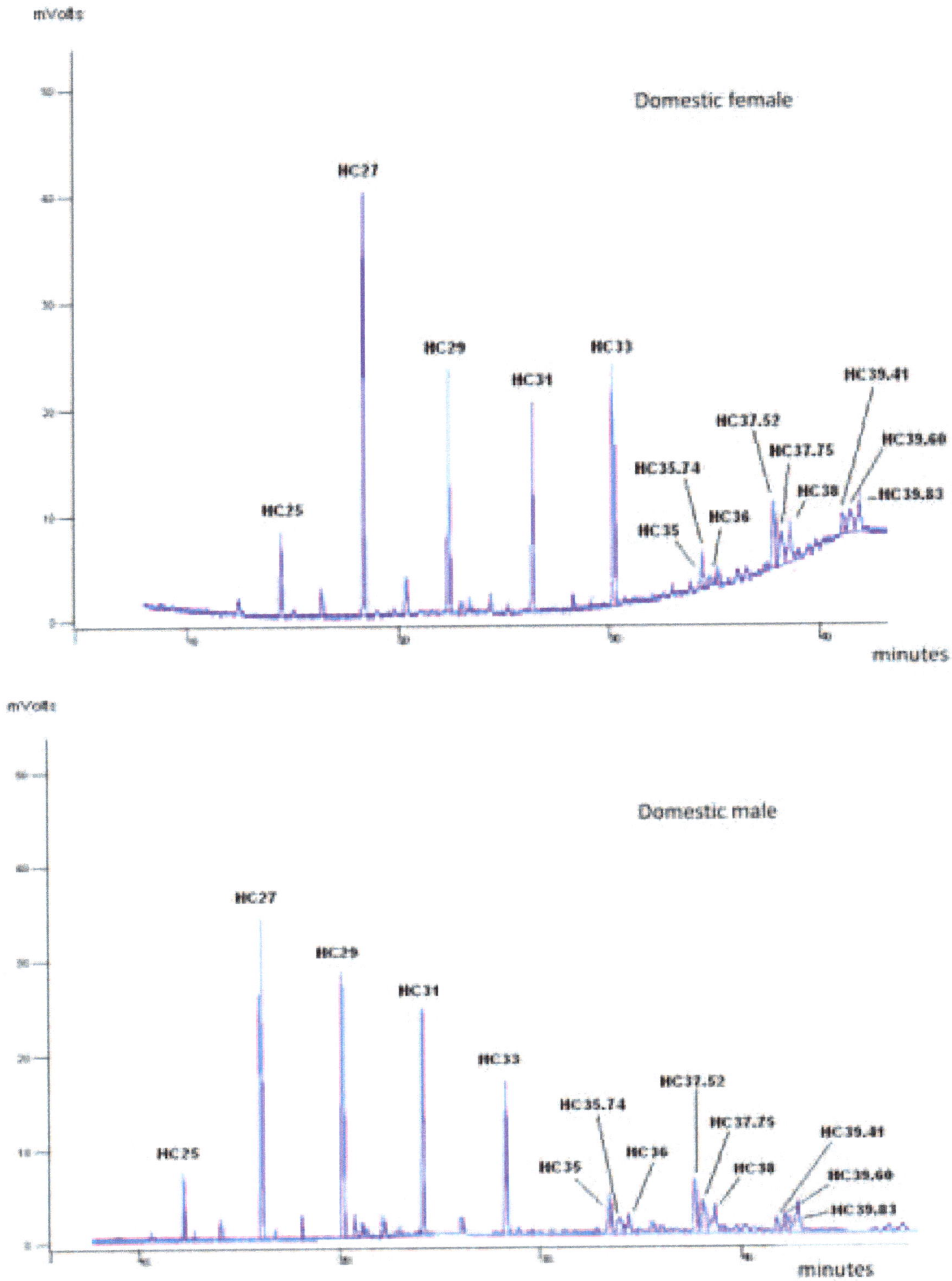

Figure 7. Typical chromatogram of female and domestic male of *Triatoma rubida*.

When comparing this profile of hydrocarbons obtained with studies of other triatomines, a clear differentiation of species can be seen. For example, the literature reports that *T. barberi*, one of the habitat triatomines, is considered to be a transmitter of CD in Mexico, has major alkanes such as C29, C31 along with C33 and C27, respectively and most of its branched components correspond to mono-, di- and trimethyls of C33, C35 and C37 [43]. On the other hand, *T. dimidiata*, considered one of the most important domestic triatomines in Mexico, presents a profile of cuticular hydrocarbons, formed by saturated hydrocarbon chains ranging from C22 to C35. Of these, the odd one strands like C31 followed by C29, C27 and C33 and small amounts of the C22 and C30 hydrocarbons prevail. It also has branched alkanes, most of them mixtures of different isomers: mono-, di- and trimethyl in their internal chains [43]. *Triatoma longipennis* insect belonging to the phyllosoma complex, widely distributed particularly in Central and Southern Mexico, is considered to be a *Triatoma* with a high degree of habitation [48] and has a saturated hydrocarbon profile ranging from C23, C25, C27, C29, C31 to C33, with the majority being C29 (16%) [49].

6.2. Peridomestic population

The GC–MS analysis showed that the chromatographic profiles of the HC in *Triatoma rubida* peridomestic are qualitatively very similar for both genders. As in the domestic population, they corresponded to n-alkanes with a continuous series of C25, C27, C29, C31, C33 C35. In addition, C35.52, C36.00, C37.74, C37.75, C38.00, C39.41, C39.60 and C39.83 were identified, were likely to be representative of branched isomers of alkanes. The location of the methyl branches of these HCs, by the proposal of Katritzky et al. [47], was estimated. The proposal made it possible to estimate that the hydrocarbons IK3552, IK3600, IK3774, IK3775, IK3800, IK3941, IK3960 and IK3983 correspond to the same hydrocarbons identified in the domestic population.

For this population, odd strands prevailed predominantly, C27, C29, C31 and C33, which together represented 76.41% in females and 76.22% in males. The total relative amount of branched hydrocarbons in males and females was 23.59% and 23.78%, respectively. The relative amount of the pentacosane hydrocarbon was 49.64%. Based on the graphical representation of the peridomestic rubida species chromatographic profiles, in their identification by mass spectrophotometry and in the statistical analysis when comparing the relative means between genders. We can suggest as typical profile of Triatoma rubida peridomestic described in **Figure 8**.

6.3. Sylvatic population

The analysis of *GC–MS* showed that sylvatic-type *Triatoma rubida* HC is qualitatively very similar for both sexes. These HCs corresponded to n-alkanes with a continuous series of C25, C27, C29, C31, C33 and C35. In addition, C35.52, C36.00, C37.74, C37.75, C38.00, C39.41, C39.60 and C39.83 were identified, which are likely representations of branched isomers of alkanes. Through the proposal of Katritzky et al. [47], the location of the methyl branches for the identified hydrocarbons was estimated, resulting as qualitatively equal to the two previous populations. Odd numbers, predominantly C27, C29, C31 and C33, chains prevailed in this population, which together represented 72.1% of the relative percentage in females and 72.3% for males. The total relative amount of branched hydrocarbons in males and females

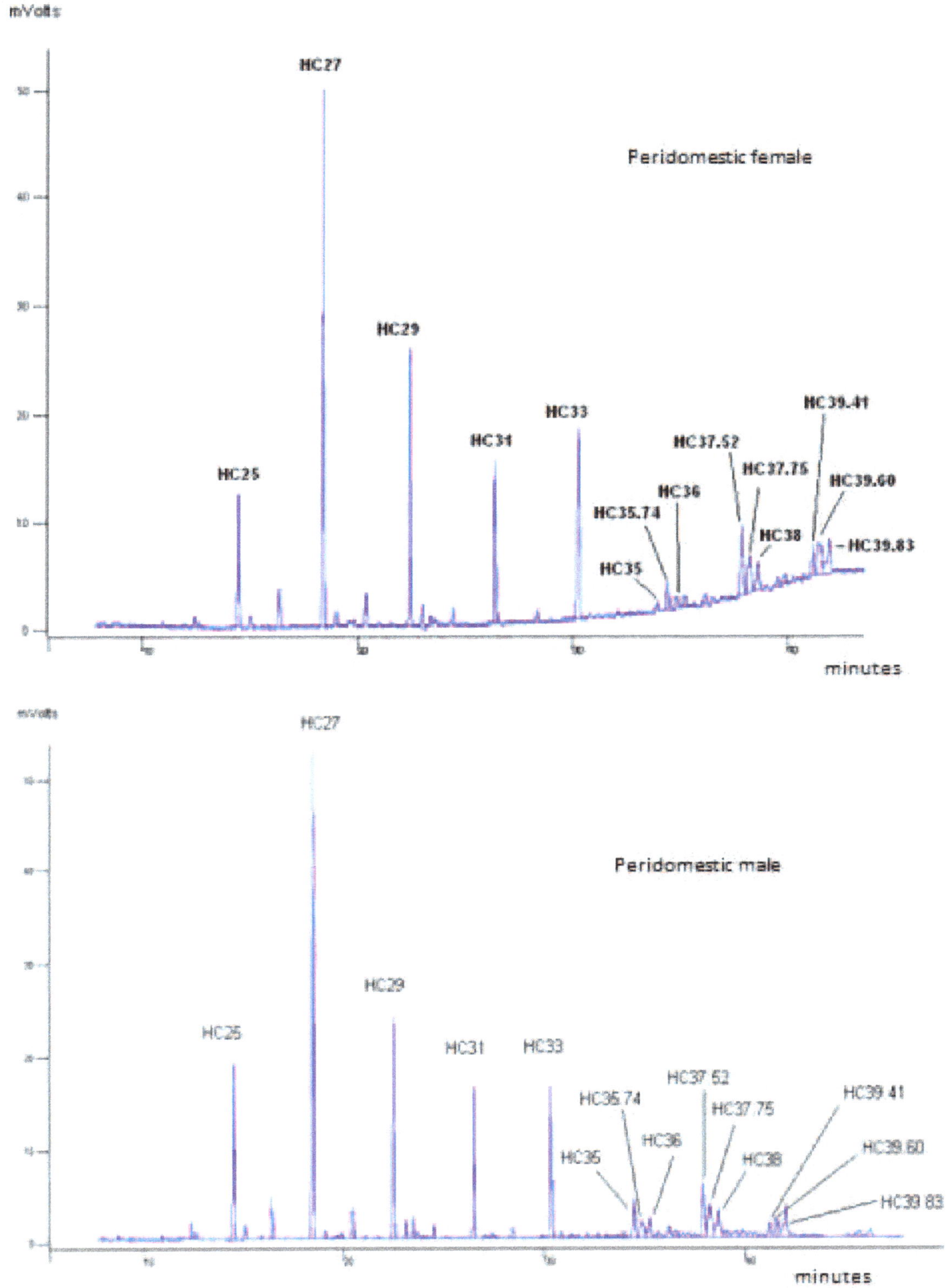

Figure 8. Typical chromatogram of female and peridomestic male of *Triatoma rubida*.

was 27.9 and 22.7%, respectively. The relative amount of the pentacosane hydrocarbon was 46.88%. The pentacosane hydrocarbon of females was present in 27.88% while in the males they presented 19%, similarly the hentriacontano hydrocarbon was 15.59% in males with respect to 9.41% of the females. Likewise, there were differences in the tritriacontano hydrocarbon of females, 9.61% with respect to 22.29% in males.

Based on the graphical representation of the chromatograms of sylvatic *rubida* species, their identification by mass spectrophotometry and statistical analysis when comparing the relative means between sexes, the typical profile of sylvatic Triatoma rubida can be suggested as described in **Figure 9**.

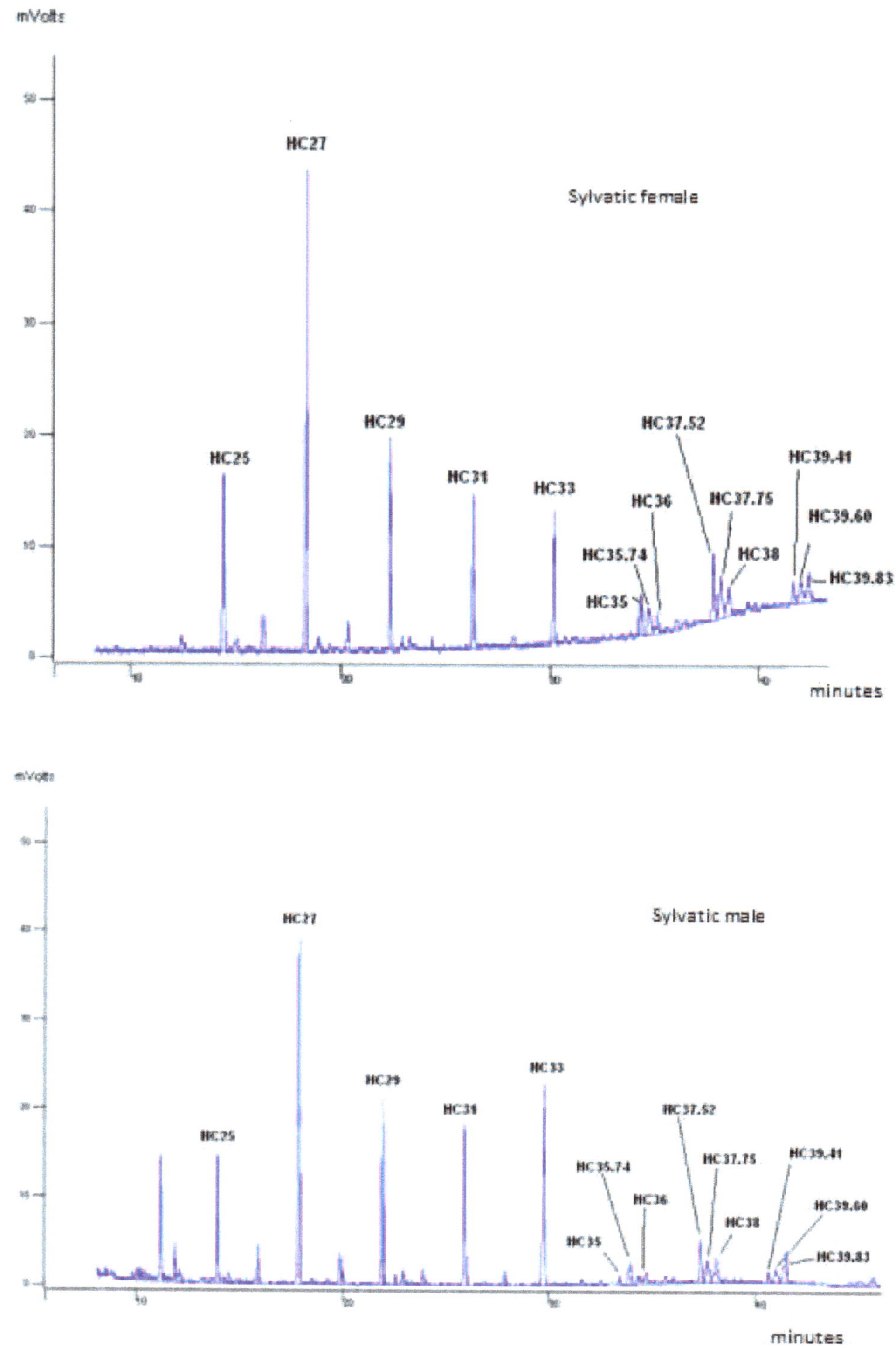

Figure 9. Typical chromatogram of female and sylvatic male of *Triatoma rubida*.

Juárez et al. [38], suggested that quantitative rather than qualitative differences support the idea that cuticular hydrocarbons represent primitive characteristics for *Triatomas*. For example, the study of the tribes *Rhodnius* and *Triatomini* found few common traits among them, however, they converge in their hematophagous habits, even though they come from very different habitats. This led them to suggest that the HC profile obeys an ancestral base set by the selection, favoring the presence of certain hydrocarbons associated with conditions of dry habitats and humid ecotypes such as that of the City of Guaymas.

Therefore, species of triatomines of dry regions present their cuticular profiles as more abundant and complex than their congeners of humid regions. Among Triatoma, *T. brasilinesis* and *T. pseudomaculata* from arid regions of Northeastern Brazil present a more complex profile than *T. infestans* from less dry regions of Central Brazil and Argentina, and in turn the three species mentioned present larger complexity when compared to *T. bimaculata* and *T. vitticeps* from coastal regions [50].

In Mexico, *T. barberi* that lives in dry regions presents a more complex HC model. The population area of *Dipetalogaster maximus* that has been collected from Baja California Sur presents abundant and longer saturated chains and constitutes 60–67.8% of the total hydrocarbon mixture for females and males, respectively. Thus, the relative abundance of n-alkanes may be related to the exposure of adverse conditions [51].

7. Conclusions

This research provides basic knowledge on the cuticular lipids of Triatoma rubida. A unique and very different profile of cuticula hydrocarbons was obtained from *Triatoma barberi, Triatoma dimidiata* and *Dipetalogaster maximus*, species are considered as transmitters of *Trypanosoma cruzi* in Mexico. No characteristic profile in the cuticular hydrocarbons was found in the collected population of females and males of *Triatoma rubida*. However, the cuticular hydrocarbons profile of the peridomestic, domestic and sylvatic populations of the insect is qualitatively similar, but were identified by significant quantitative differences, so it is possible to state that distinctions can be made between populations. The profile of cuticular hydrocarbons, identified in this study, can be used as a reliable chemotaxonomic tool to identify the populations of *T. rubida*, considering the expression of hydrocarbons as the chemical phenotype of the vector that responds to environmental and biological factors of the insect.

Author details

Edgar Alfonso Paredes González[1], Gerardo Álvarez Hernandez[2] and Jesús Ortega-García[1]*

*Address all correspondence to: jortega@guayacan.uson.mx

1 Universidad de Sonora, Unidad regional Norte Caborca México, Mexico

2 Universidad de Sonora, Departamento de Ciencias Químicas, Unidad Centro Hermosillo Sonora, Mexico

References

[1] Pineda-Rodríguez S, Sandra A, Cuevas-Nava JJ, Sánchez-Arriaga J, Rodríguez-Bataz E. Distribución geográfica de vectores de *Trypanosoma Cruzi* y riesgo de infección poblacional en Tecalpulco municipio de Taxco, Guerrero-México. Foro de Estudios sobre Guerrero. 2014;**1**(2):617-621

[2] Molina I, Fernando S, Sánchez-Montalvá A. Actualización en enfermedad de Chagas. Enfermedades Infecciosas y Microbiología Clínica. 2016;**34**(2):132-138

[3] WHO. Research Priorities for Chagas Disease, Human African Trypanosomiasis and Leishmaniasis. Technical Report of the TDR Disease Reference Group on Chagas Disease, Human African Trypanosomiasis and Leishmaniasis. Italia. WHO Library Cataloguing-in-Publication Data; 2012

[4] Portugal-García C, García-Vázquez Z, Monteón-Padilla V, Chávez-López V, Olamendi-Portugal M, Ramos C. Anticuerpos contra *Trypanosoma cruzi* en humanos y perros y presencia del parásito en *Meccus pallidipennis* en la localidad de Puente Pantitlán, Morelos, México. Revista Biomedica. 2011;**22**(3):67-75

[5] Anis R Jr, Rassi A, Marin-Neto JA. Chagas disease. Lancet. 2010;**375**(9723):1388-1402

[6] Salazar Schettino MP, Rojas-Wastavino E, Cabrera-Brabo M, Bucio-Torres MI, Martínez Ibarra JA, Monroy-Escobar MC, Rodas Retana A, Guevara Gómez Y, Bences Blanco MO, Ruiz Hernández AL, Torres Gutiérrez E. Revisión de 13 especies de la familia Triatominae (*Hemiptera*: *Reduviidae*) vectores de la enfermedad de Chagas en México. Journal of the Selva Andina Research Society. 2010;**1**(1):57-80

[7] Ramsey JM, Alvear AL, Ordoñez R, Muñoz G, García R, Leyva R. Risk factors associated with house infestation by the Chagas disease vector *Triatoma pallidipennis* in Cuernavaca metropolitan area, México. Medical and Veterinary Entomology. 2005;**19**(2):219-228

[8] Schmunis AG, Zaida EY. Chagas disease: A Latin American health problem becoming a world health problem. Acta Tropica. 2010;**115**(1-2):14-21

[9] Rodrigues CJ, Borges-Pereira J. Chagas disease: 100 years after its discovery. A systemic review. Acta Tropica. 2010;**115**(1-2):5-13

[10] Steverding D. The history of Chagas disease. Steverding Parasites & Vectors. 2014;**7**(317): 1-8

[11] Lozano-Kasten F, Magallón-Gastélum E, Soto-Gutiérrez M, Kasten-Monges M, Bosseno M, Frédérique S. Conocimiento epidemiológico y situación actual de la enfermedad de Chagas en el estado de Jalisco, México. Salud Pública Méx. 2008;**50**(6):508-514

[12] Velasco-Castrejón Ó, Rivas-Sánchez B. Apuntes para la historia de la enfermedad de Chagas en México. Boletín Médico del Hospital Infantil de México. 2008;**65**(1):57-79

[13] Fernández S. Biología de los triatomitios vectores de Trypanosoma cruzi en el norte de Nuevo León México. Universidad Autónoma de Nuevo León. Facultad de Ciencias Biológicas. División de Estudios de Postgrado; 1987

[14] Lent H, Wygodzinsky PW. Revision of the *Triatominae* (*Hemiptera, Reduvidae*), and their significance as vectors of Chagas disease. American Museum of Natural History. 1979;**163**(3):309-313

[15] Paredes E, Valdéz J, Nogueda B, Alejandre-Aguilar R, Canett R. Vectorial importance of *Triatominae Bugs* (*Hemiptera*: *Reduviidae*) in Guaymas, México. Revista Latinoamericana de Microbiología. 2001;**43**(3):119-122

[16] Espinoza B, Martınez-Ibarra JA, Villalobos G, De La Torre P, Laclette JP, Martınez-Hernandez P. Genetic variation of north American Triatomines (Insecta: *Hemiptera*: *Reduviidae*): Initial divergence between species and populations of Chagas disease vector. The American Journal of Tropical Medicine and Hygiene. 2013;**88**(2):275-284

[17] Paredes-González E, Villa R, Sotelo MI, Ortega-García J. Detección de Triatominos (hemiptera: *Reduviidae*) Domésticos, Peridomésticos y Silvestres en Guaymas, Sonora, México. BIOTECNIA. 2015;**XVII**(2):3-7

[18] Reisenman CE, Lawrence G, Guerenstein PG, Gregory T, Dotson E, Hildebrand JG. Infection of kissing bugs with *Trypanosoma cruzi*, Tucson, Arizona, USA. Emerging Infectious Diseases. 2010;**16**(3):400-405

[19] Caryn B, Kjos S, Yabsley MJ, Montgomery SP. *Trypanosoma cruzi* and Chagas' disease in the United States. Clinical Microbiology Reviews. 2011;**24**(4):655-681

[20] Martínez A, Nogueda-Torres B, Paredes González E, Alejandre-Aguilar R, Solorio-Cibrián M, Barreto SP, Gómez-Estrada HI, Trujillo-García JC. Development of *Triatoma rubida sonoriana*, *Triatoma Barberi* and *Meccus Mazzotti* (*Heteroptera, reduvidae*) under laboratory conditions. Journal of the American Mosquito Control Association. 2005;**21**(3):310-315

[21] Martinez-Ibarra A, Paredes-González E, Licón-Trillo A, Montañez-Valdez OD, Rocha-Chávez G, Nogueda-Torres B. The biology of three Mexican-American species of Triatominae (*Hemiptera*: *Reduviidae*): *Triatoma recurva*, *Triatoma protracta* and *Triatoma rubida*. Memórias do Instituto Oswaldo Cruz, Rio de Janeiro. 2012;**107**(5):659-663

[22] TDR/SWG/VEC. Report of the scientific working group on insect vectors and human health. Ginebra. 2002:23-25

[23] Sommerfeld J, Kroeger A. Innovative community-based vector control interventions for improved dengue and Chagas disease prevention in Latin America: Introduction to the special issue. Transactions of the Royal Society of Tropical Medicine and Hygiene. 2015;**109**(2):85-88

[24] Barrera MA. Dinámica Poblacional de Triatoma dimidiata Vector de la Enfermedad de Chagas, en la Península de Yucatán, México. Tesis. Universidad de Colima. 2003. pp. 11-13

[25] Guhl F. Enfermedad de Chagas: Realidad y perspectivas. Revista Biomedica. 2009;**20**(3): 228-234

[26] González-Brítez N. Dinámica poblacional de triatominos (*Hemiptera-Reduviidae*) relacionados con la transmisión de *Trypanosoma cruzi* en Paraguay, con énfasis en Triato*ma sórdida*. Memorias del Instituto de Investigaciones en Ciencias de la Salud. 2013;**11**(2):105-111

[27] Dias-Lima A, Sherlock AI. Wild vector invading houses and the risk of Emergente of cases of Chagas disease in Salvador, state of Bahia, Norheast Brazil. Memórias do Instituto Oswaldo Cruz, Rio de Janeiro. 2000;**95**(5):611-613

[28] Dos Santos, CB, Luiz, A, Rocha, G, Melim, GE, Fuzari, AA, Falqueto, A. Peridomiciliary colonies of *Triatoma vitticeps* (Stal, 1859) (*Hemiptera, Reduviidae, Triatominae*) infected with *Trypanosoma cruzi* in rural areas of the state of Spírito Santo, Brazil. Memórias do Instituto Oswaldo Cruz, Rio de Janeiro 2005;**100**(5):471-473

[29] Sánchez Z, Russomando G, Chena L, Nara E, Cardozo E, Paredes B, Ferreira E. *Triatoma sordida*: indicadores de adaptación y transmisión de *Trypanosoma cruzi* en intradomicilio del Chaco Paraguayo. Memorias del Instituto de Investigaciones en Ciencias de la Salud. 2016;**14**(3):96-101

[30] Calderón G. Hidrocarburos Cuticulares de Tiatominos: su Aplicación como Marcadores Taxonómicos. Tesis PhD. Universidad Nacional de la Plata Argentina; 2008. pp. 25-28

[31] Kenneth HL. Lipids of the insect cuticle: Origin, composition and function. Journal of Physiology and Biochemistry. 1988;**89B**(4):595-645

[32] Juárez P. Cuticular hydrocarbons of triatomines. Comparative Biochemistry and Physiology, Part A. 2007;**147**(3):711-730

[33] Juárez P. Hydrocarbon biosynthesis in *Triatoma infestans* eggs. Archives of Insect Biochemistry and Physiology. 1994;**25**(3):193-206

[34] Cocchiararo-Bastias LM, Mijailovsky SJ, Calderon-Fernández GM, Nieves A, Figueiras L, Juárez MP. Epicuticle Lipids Mediate Mate Recognition in *Triatoma infestans*. Journal of Chemical Ecology. 2011;**37**(3):246-252

[35] Calderón-Fernández MPJ. The cuticular hydrocarbons of the *Triatoma sordida* species subcomplex (*Hemiptera*: *Reduviidae*). Memórias do Instituto Oswaldo Cruz, Rio de Janeiro. 2013;**108**(6):778-784

[36] De Renobales M. Inhibition of hydrocarbon biosynthesis in the housefly by 2-Octadecynoate. Archives of Insect Biochemistry and Physiology. 1986;**3**(1):75-86

[37] INIBIOLP. Laboratorio de Farmacognosia y Productos Naturales. La Plata, Argentina: Departamento de Química Orgánica; 2002. pp. 1-5

[38] Juárez MP, Fernández R, Schofield CJ, Dujardin JP. Intergeneric comparison of epicuticular hydrocarbons in Triatominae. Research and Reviews in Parasitology. 2000;**60**(3-4): 121-127

[39] William JE, Larry IJ. Epicuticular hydrocarbon variation in drosophila Mojavensis cluster species. Journal of Chemical Ecology. 2001;**10**:2125-2149

[40] Juárez MP, Brenner L. The Epicuticular lipids of *Triatoma infestans* glycerides. Comparative Biochemistry and Physiology. 1984;**78B**(2):427-431

[41] Braga MV, Teixeira Z, Carvalho M, Matsumoto N, Blomquist GJ. Cuticular hydrocarbons as a tool for the identification of insect species: Puparial cases from Sarcophagidae. Acta Tropica. 2014;**128**(3):1-13

[42] Juárez MP, Blomquist GJ. Cuticular hidrocarbons of *Triatoma infestans* and *T. mazzotti*. Com. Biochemistry & Physiology. 1993;**106B**(3):667-674

[43] Juárez MP, Carlson DA, Salazar PM, Mijailovsky S, Rojas G. Cuticular hidrocarbons of Chagas disease vectors in Mexico. Memórias do Instituto Oswaldo Cruz. 2002;**97**(6): 819-827

[44] CONAGUA. Comisión Nacional del Agua. Registro Anual de Temperaturas Período 1980-2004. [Internet]. [Consultado el 03 de abril de 2018]. Disponible en: http://smn.cna.gob.mx/es/

[45] Juárez MP, Blomquist GJ. Cuticular hidrocarbons of *Triatoma infestans* and *T. mazzotti*. Com. Biochemistry & Physiology. 1993;**106B**(3):667-674

[46] Juárez MP, Blomquist GJ, Schofield CJ. Hydrocarbons of *Rhodnius prolixus*, a Chagas disease vector. Comparative Biochemistry and Physiology. 2001;**129B**(4):733-746

[47] Katritzky A, Pozharskii C, Ramsden A, Zhdankin J. Manual de Química Heterocíclica. 2da ed. USA: Elsevier; 2000

[48] Magallón E, Magdaleno-Peñaloza N, Katthain-Duchateau G, Trujillo-Contreras F, Lozano-Kasten FJ, Hernández-Gutiérrez RJ. Distribución de los Vectores de la Enfermedad de Chagas (*Hemiptera, Reduvidae, Triatominae*), en el Estado de Jalisco México. Revista Biomedica. 1998;**9**(3):151-157

[49] Paredes E, Márquez G, Juárez M, Nogueda B, Lugo R, De la Rosa R, Noriega J. Quimiotaxonomía de *Triatoma longipennis* por Análisis de Hidrocarburos Cuticulares. INVURNUS. 2008;**3**(2):3-10

[50] Rodríguez J. Las Enfermedades Transmitidas por Vectores en México. Revista de la Facultad de Medicina de la UNAM. 2002;**45**(3):137-140

[51] Juárez MP, Brenner RR. The epicuticular lipids of Triatoma infestans-II. Hydrocarbon dynamics. Comparative Biochemistry and Physiology Part B: Comparative Biochemistry. 1985;**82**(4):793-803

9

Antiparasitic Mechanisms of the Human Placenta

Castillo Christian, Ana Liempi, Lisvaneth Medina,
Ileana Carrillo and Ulrike Kemmerling

Abstract

Trypanosoma cruzi, during vertical transmission, crosses the placental barrier. The trophoblast, a continuous renewing epithelium, is the first tissue of this anatomical barrier to have contact with the parasite. The epithelial turnover, including the trophoblast, is part of the innate immune response due to the fact that pathogens attach to the surface of cells prior invasion. Cellular processes such as proliferation, differentiation, and apoptotic cell death are part of the trophoblast turnover. Interestingly, *T. cruzi* induces all of them. In addition, the placenta expresses TLRs, whose activation leads to the secretion of pro-inflammatory and immunomodulating cytokines. *T. cruzi* is recognized by TLR-2, TLR-4, TLR-7, and TLR-9. In the present review, we analyze the current evidence about the trophoblast epithelial turnover, the induction of a specific cytokine profile as a local placental innate immune response, as well as other possible defense mechanisms against the parasite.

Keywords: *Trypanosoma cruzi*, placenta, epithelial turnover, TLRs, cytokine profile

1. Introduction

Congenital Chagas disease, caused by *Trypanosoma cruzi* (*T. cruzi*), is associated with premature labor, low birth weight, and stillbirths [1, 2]. The congenital transmission of pathogens is the consequence of complex interactions among the parasite, maternal and fetal/newborn immune responses, and placental factors. The placenta is the least-studied component of this "trilogy" [3, 4] but is essential in determining the probability of transmission since it forms the primary barrier between the maternal and fetal compartments throughout pregnancy [5].

Mother and developing fetus are protected against environmental challenges by the immune system; the placenta is able to modulate fetal as well as maternal immune responses. Maternal immune system presents an enhanced capacity of cellular and molecular recognition and communication between each other. Therefore, during normal pregnancy, the maternal immune defenses assure the health of the mother and developing child. Moreover, the fetus during its development also acquires immune defenses that are able to modulate the maternal immune system. Considering this facts, the immune system responses are unique and particularly effective [6].

The maternal and the fetal developing innate and adaptative immune systems determine the probability of fetal/neonatal infection. Fetal infection is related to diverse pregnancy disorders such as abortion, preterm labor, intrauterine growth retardation, and preeclampsia [7]. Particularly, congenital *T. cruzi* infection can cause abortion, stillbirth, and intrauterine growth restriction [1, 2, 8].

The innate immune system presents a main role in protecting the developing child against *T. cruzi* infection. Thus, increase of pro-inflammatory cytokines is present in the sera of uninfected babies born to infected mothers [9]. However, in newborns who suffer from congenital infection, the levels of inflammation markers as well as active NK cells are low [10]. Therefore, the innate immune response is effective in uninfected newborn from chagasic mothers. The adaptive immune system is also relevant; for instance, maternal anti-*T. cruzi* antibodies are transferred through the placenta to the fetus and where they reduce the parasitemia [9].

Importantly, congenital transmission rates for *Trypanosoma cruzi* (*T. cruzi*) are relatively low (3.9–5.6%) [11, 12]. Moreover, the typical amastigote nests (intracellular parasites) cannot be observed in placentas from mothers with chronic Chagas disease [13] nor in human placental chorionic villi explants (HPCVE) infected in vitro with the parasite [14]. In the latter, only a few parasite antigens and DNA can be identified [14, 15]. In addition, other infections of the placenta are not commonly observed [11]. All these evidences suggest the presence of systemic and local defense mechanisms against pathogen and that the placenta is a key factor against *T. cruzi* infection.

2. Antiparasitic mechanisms of the placenta

Importantly, during congenital transmission, the parasites must cross the placental barrier [8, 16].

2.1. Placenta

The placenta is a temporary organ that provides nutrition and gas exchange for the developing fetus, ensuring normal embryo-fetal growth and development and supporting pregnancy-related changes in maternal physiological systems [17]. The human placenta is classified as discoidal, villous, and hemochorial and consists of a fetal portion, which originates from the *Chorion frondosum*, and a maternal portion, or basal decidua, which originates from the endometrium. The functional units are the floating chorionic villi, formed by the trophoblast, and the villous stroma. The trophoblast comes into contact with maternal blood in the intervillous space (IVS) and is delimited by a basal lamina from the villous stroma, which is the fetal connective tissue containing the fetal capillaries. The placental barrier is formed by the trophoblast, basal laminae, villous stroma, and fetal capillary endothelium (**Figure 1**) [4, 8].

The placenta may contain as much as 500 mL of maternal blood, in the IVS, exposing the trophoblast to pathogens that might be present in it [5]. Therefore, the trophoblast is a key factor against congenital infection since it is the first fetal tissue that comes into contact with pathogens circulating in the maternal blood [11]. On the other hand, the placenta, as an immune regulatory organ, acts as a modulator of fetal as well as maternal immune responses [6]. The placenta, in particular the trophoblast, is also part of a local innate immune response. Three types of defense mechanisms in innate immunity have been described: (i) anatomical barriers, such as the placental barrier (**Figure 1**), (ii) cellular innate immune responses, and (iii) humoral innate immune responses. During tissue invasion, pathogen breaks the anatomical barriers, and innate immune cells are activated and secrete cytokines and chemokines to control pathogen replication [18, 19].

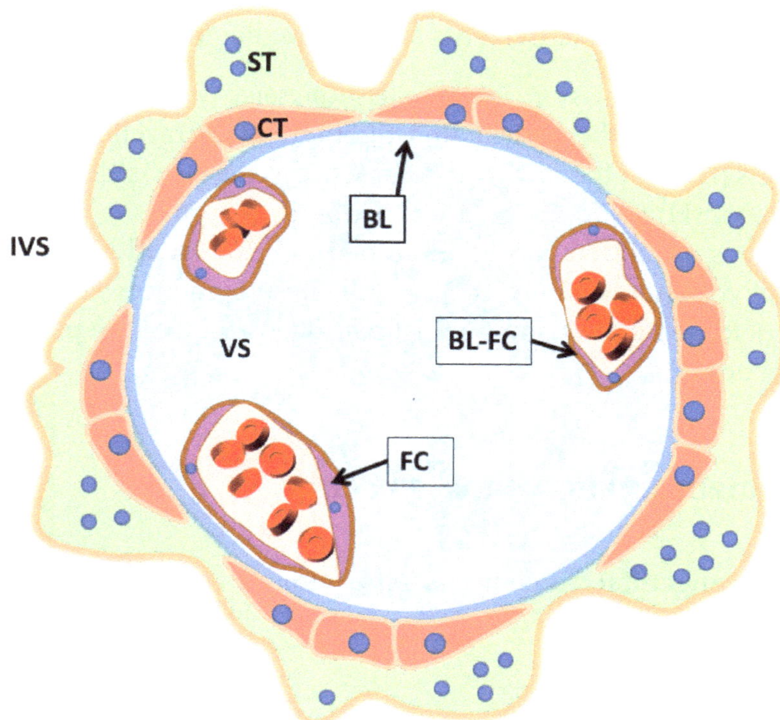

Figure 1. The placental barrier: the placental barrier is formed by the trophoblast composed by the superficial syncytiotrophoblast (ST) that contacts the maternal blood in the intervillous space (IVS) and the cytotrophoblast (CT) which corresponds to the germinative layer of the epithelium. The trophoblast is supported by the fetal connective tissue of the villous stroma (VS) that contains the fetal capillaries (FC). The placental barrier presents also two basal membranes (BM): (1) between villous stroma and trophoblast and (2) around fetal endothelium. The cells of the CT proliferate and afterward differentiate into the ST. The continuous incorporation of CT cells into the ST is counterbalanced by the formation of apoptotic ST knots, which are released into the IVS.

2.2. The trophoblast

The trophoblast is a bistratified epithelium composed of the superficial syncytiotrophoblast (ST) and the basal cytotrophoblast (CT). There is strong evidence that the ST layer is resistant to numerous pathogens, including *T. cruzi* [20, 21]. However, damage of the syncytium might allow the parasite access to the villous core, increasing parasite infection [5, 22].

2.3. The trophoblast epithelial turnover

The basal CT cells are the only ones of the trophoblast with proliferative capacity. The superficial multinucleated ST layer is highly differentiated and is unable to proliferate. Importantly, the ST contacts directly with the maternal blood [23–25], where in case of *T. cruzi* infection, the parasite circulates [11, 26]. The ST is a typical syncytium that is continuous and normally uninterrupted and covers all villous trees of the human placenta. The ST is formed and maintained by the continuous incorporation of CT cells through syncytial fusion, meaning that the CT cells suffer cellular differentiation. The continuous incorporation of CT cells into the ST is counterbalanced by the formation of apoptotic knots that are released into the maternal blood present in the IVS [24, 25]. The normal epithelial turnover assures the integrity of diverse anatomical barriers, including the placental one. The maintenance of the integrity of anatomical barriers is part of the innate immune system due to the fact that pathogens, prior to cell invasion, must attach to the surface of cells. As these cells are continuously eliminated, the attached pathogens are removed with them [3]. Thus, the trophoblast turnover should be considered as a defense mechanism against pathogens, including *T. cruzi*.

2.3.1. Cell proliferation

We have previously shown that the parasite induces, in the trophoblast, cellular proliferation. These experiments were performed in HPCVE and in the trophoblastic cell line BeWo; both models are commonly used in trophoblast studies [27]. In HPCVE *T. cruzi* increases DNA synthesis as well as the PCNA proliferation marker [11]. On the other hand, in BeWo cells the parasite also induces significant DNA synthesis (as determined by BrdU incorporation), increase of the percentage of cells in the ST and G_2/M cell cycle phases, and the expression of the widely used proliferation markers AgNORs, PCNA, and Ki67 [28]. Importantly, it should be taken into account that PCNA acts also as a molecular coordinator in multiple other cellular functions such as DNA damage repair, cell cycle control, cell survival, and gene expression [29]. Therefore, the increase of PCNA expression could also be a response to *T. cruzi*-induced cell and tissue damage. We have previously demonstrated that *T. cruzi* induces during ex vivo infection tissue disorganization of HPCVE [14] as well as apoptosis [30]. However, Ki67, a more specific proliferation marker that can be observed only during the active phases of the cycle [24], was significantly increased together with the other proliferation markers.

2.3.2. Cell differentiation

As described above, CT cells differentiate continuously and fuse with the ST [24, 25]. *T. cruzi* induces cell differentiation in the trophoblast in HPCVE and BeWo cells. Thus, the parasite increases the protein expression of the major biochemical markers of trophoblast differentiation [31]: β-human chorionic gonadotropin (β-hCG) and syncytin [3]. Moreover, *T. cruzi* induces cell fusion in BeWo cells as demonstrated by a two-color fusion assay and by the analysis of the redistribution of the intercellular adhesion protein desmoplakin [3]. Previously, we have shown that *T. cruzi* activates the ERK1/ERK2 MAPK pathway [32]. Interestingly, the induction of trophoblast differentiation is mediated by the activation of the ERK1/ERK2 MAPK and other MAPK signal transduction pathways [33].

2.3.3. Apoptotic cell death

T. cruzi also induces apoptotic cell death in the trophoblast. The ST releases continuously apoptotic knots into the IVS [24]. In HPCVE, the induction of apoptosis has been demonstrated by the determination of the presence of pyknotic nuclei, induction of DNA fragmentation, caspase-3 like activity, and presence of caspase-3 and cleaved cytokeratin 18 [30]. Cellular processes related to apoptosis are also regulating cell differentiation (fusion) in the trophoblast. For instance, CT cell differentiation is regulated by caspases [34, 35]. Particularly, caspase-8, an apoptosis initiator caspase, regulates trophoblast differentiation and fusion. Caspase-8 is activated in highly differentiated CT cells just prior to fusion and escorts the fusing cell content including the nucleus into the ST, and it has not been found in proliferating CT cells [23, 36]. Moreover, the fusion of the trophoblast has been visualized by localizing caspase-8 [34]. *T. cruzi* induces in BeWo cells as well as HPCVE the expression and activation of caspase-8 [11, 37]. Moreover, the inhibition of caspase-8 increases the amount of parasite DNA and the number of intracellular parasites in BeWo cells [37]. The inhibition of caspase-8 decreases parasite-induced cellular differentiation and apoptotic cell death, but not cellular proliferation [11, 37].

2.4. The trophoblast and the innate immune cellular response against *T. cruzi*

The innate immune response against pathogens is initiated by pathogen pattern recognition receptors (PRRs), which include *Toll*-like receptors (TLRs) that recognize and bind highly conserved sequences known as pathogen-associated molecular patterns (PAMPs). The human trophoblast expresses all ten of the known functional TLRs [7], and *T. cruzi* is recognized by TLR-2, TLR-4, TLR-7, and TLR-9. Surface TLRs (TLR-2 and TLR-4) recognize glycosylphosphatidylinositol (GPI)-anchored mucin-like glycoproteins from *T. cruzi* surface [16, 38, 39]. We have shown that *T. cruzi* infection is related to TLR-2, but not to TLR-4 and TLR-9, expression, and activation [16]. The binding of TLR-2 to its ligands leads to activation of signaling pathways and upregulation of genes involved in the innate immune response including cytokines and chemokines [7, 16]. *T. cruzi* induces the secretion of IL-1β, IL-6, IL-8, IL-10, and TNF-α in HPCVE [16]. Interestingly, IL-1β, IL-6, and TNF-α secretions are also associated with cellular proliferation and differentiation in the trophoblast [40, 41], and inhibition of TLR-2 impairs trophoblast turnover (manuscript under review in "*Placenta*"). However, up to now, we do not know whether the activation of TLRs occurs mainly in the trophoblast or if other placental cells are also involved in this matter that should be addressed in the future. Importantly, as a consequence of our results, the TLR-2-initiated cytokine profile should also be considered as a local placental defense mechanism.

2.5. Other placental defense mechanisms against *T. cruzi*

The placenta, and particularly the trophoblast, expresses many noncoding RNAs including microRNAs (miRNAs) that regulate placental development function. Moreover, different miRNAs exhibit specialized functions during normal and pathological pregnancies. Placental miRNAs, packaged within exosomes and other vesicles or bound in protein complexes, are capable of communicating distinctive signals to maternal and fetal tissues [5]. Placenta-specific and trophoblast-derived miRNAs, encoded in the chromosome 19 miRNA cluster (C19MC), are released within exosomes and confer resistance to viral infection in other mammalian cells [42]. Preliminary results from our laboratory show that *T. cruzi* induces in HPCVE a specific C19MC-encoded miRNA profile. Some of those miRNAs are involved in the regulation of immune functions, particularly those of TLR-mediated pathways [43]. Studies on *T. cruzi*-induced miRNAs and exosomes are currently ongoing, being of particular interest since miRNA pathways are potential diagnostic tools and targets for therapeutic control of parasitic diseases [44] and other pathologies, including placenta-derived ones [5]. Targeting miRNAs constitute a promising possibility for the treatment of different diseases due to the facts that (i) miRNAs are regulators of gene expression, (ii) are relatively easy to manipulate, (iii) can be administrated in vivo, and (iv) present an apparent lack of adverse effects when administered intravenously. Moreover, *miRNAs are detectable in biological fluids, thus offering real potential as noninvasive biomarkers*, providing new diagnostic and therapeutic options during pregnancy and for several diseases as well [45, 46].

In summary, the studies about the placental defense mechanism that determines the probability of infection, together with parasite, maternal, and fetal/newborn factors, are of outstanding interest since they are potential diagnostic, prognostic, and therapeutic tools.

Author details

Castillo Christian, Ana Liempi, Lisvaneth Medina, Ileana Carrillo and Ulrike Kemmerling*

*Address all correspondence to: ukemmerling@uchile.cl

Instituto de Ciencias Biomédicas, Facultad de Medicina, Universidad de Chile, Santiago, Chile

References

[1] Altemani AM, Bittencourt AL, Lana AM. Immunohistochemical characterization of the inflammatory infiltrate in placental Chagas' disease: A qualitative and quantitative analysis. The American Journal of Tropical Medicine and Hygiene. 2000;**62**(2):319-324

[2] Shippey 3rd SH, Zahn CM, Cisar MM, Wu TJ, Satin AJ. Use of the placental perfusion model to evaluate transplacental passage of *Trypanosoma cruzi*. American Journal of Obstetrics and Gynecology. 2005;**192**(2):586-591

[3] Liempi A, Castillo C, Duaso J, Droguett D, Sandoval A, Barahona K, et al. *Trypanosoma cruzi* induces trophoblast differentiation: A potential local antiparasitic mechanism of the human placenta? Placenta. 2014 Dec;**35**(12):1035-1042

[4] Liempi A, Castillo C, Carrillo I, Munoz L, Droguett D, Galanti N, et al. A local innate immune response against *Trypanosoma cruzi* in the human placenta: The epithelial turnover of the trophoblast. Microb Pathog. 2016 Oct;**99**:123-129

[5] Arora N, Sadovsky Y, Dermody TS, Coyne CB. Microbial vertical transmission during human pregnancy. Cell Host & Microbe. 2017;**21**(5):561-567

[6] Mor G, Cardenas I. The immune system in pregnancy: A unique complexity. American Journal of Reproductive Immunology. 2010;**63**(6):425-433

[7] Koga K, Aldo PB, Mor G. Toll-like receptors and pregnancy: Trophoblast as modulators of the immune response. The Journal of Obstetrics and Gynaecology Research. 2009;**35**(2):191-202

[8] Kemmerling U, Bosco C, Infection GN. Invasion mechanisms of *Trypanosoma cruzi* in the congenital transmission of Chagas' disease: A proposal. Biological Research. 2010; **43**(3):307-316

[9] Carlier Y, Truyens C. Congenital Chagas disease as an ecological model of interactions between *Trypanosoma cruzi* parasites, pregnant women, placenta and fetuses. Acta Tropica. 2015;**151**:103-115

[10] Hermann E, Berthe A, Truyens C, Alonso-Vega C, Parrado R, Torrico F, et al. Killer cell immunoglobulin-like receptor expression induction on neonatal CD8(+) T cells in vitro and following congenital infection with *Trypanosoma cruzi*. Immunology. 2010;**129**(3): 418-426

[11] Liempi A, Castillo C, Carrillo I, Munoz L, Droguett D, Galanti N, et al. A local innate immune response against *Trypanosoma cruzi* in the human placenta: The epithelial turnover of the trophoblast. Microbial Pathogenesis. 2016;**99**:123-129

[12] Pérez-Molina JA, Molina I. Chagas disease. Lancet. 2018 Jan 6;**391**(10115):82-94

[13] Duaso J, Yanez E, Castillo C, Galanti N, Cabrera G, Corral G, et al. Reorganization of extracellular matrix in placentas from women with asymptomatic chagas disease: Mechanism of parasite invasion or local placental defense? J Trop Med. 2012;**2012**:758357

[14] Duaso J, Rojo G, Cabrera G, Galanti N, Bosco C, Maya J, et al. *Trypanosoma cruzi* induces tissue disorganization and destruction of chorionic villi in an *ex vivo* infection model of human placenta. Placenta. 2010;**31**(8):705-711

[15] Lujan CD, Triquell MF, Sembaj A, Guerrero CE, Fretes RE. *Trypanosoma cruzi*: Productive infection is not allowed by chorionic villous explant from normal human placenta *in vitro*. Experimental Parasitology. 2004;**108**(3-4):176-181

[16] Castillo C, Munoz L, Carrillo I, Liempi A, Gallardo C, Galanti N, et al. *Ex vivo* infection of human placental chorionic villi explants with *Trypanosoma cruzi* and *Toxoplasma*

gondii induces different Toll-like receptor expression and cytokine/chemokine profiles. American Journal of Reproductive Immunology. 2017 Jul;**78**(1-8)

[17] Furukawa S, Kuroda Y, Sugiyama A. A comparison of the histological structure of the placenta in experimental animals. Journal of Toxicologic Pathology. 2014;**27**(1):11-18

[18] Janeway Jr CA, Medzhitov R. Innate immune recognition. Annual Review of Immunology. 2002;**20**:197-216

[19] Hazlett L, Wu M. Defensins in innate immunity. Cell and Tissue Research. 2011;**343**(1): 175-188

[20] Diaz-Lujan C, Triquell MF, Castillo C, Hardisson D, Kemmerling U, Fretes RE. Role of placental barrier integrity in infection by *Trypanosoma cruzi*. Acta Tropica. 2016;**164**: 360-368

[21] Diaz-Lujan C, Triquell MF, Schijman A, Paglini P, Fretes RE. Differential susceptibility of isolated human trophoblasts to infection by *Trypanosoma cruzi*. Placenta. 2012;**33**(4):264-270

[22] Robbins JR, Zeldovich VB, Poukchanski A, Boothroyd JC, Bakardjiev AI. Tissue barriers of the human placenta to infection with *Toxoplasma gondii*. Infection and Immunity. 2012;**80**(1):418-428

[23] Huppertz B, Borges M. Placenta trophoblast fusion. Methods in Molecular Biology. 2008;**475**:135-147

[24] Mayhew TM. Turnover of human villous trophoblast in normal pregnancy: What do we know and what do we need to know? Placenta. 2014;**35**(4):229-240

[25] Huppertz B, Gauster M. Trophoblast fusion. Advances in Experimental Medicine and Biology. 2011;**713**:81-95

[26] Carlier Y, Sosa-Estani S, Luquetti AO, Buekens P. Congenital Chagas disease: An update. Memórias do Instituto Oswaldo Cruz. 2015;**110**(3):363-368

[27] Drewlo S, Baczyk D, Dunk C, Kingdom J. Fusion assays and models for the trophoblast. Methods in Molecular Biology. 2008;**475**:363-382

[28] Droguett D, Carrillo I, Castillo C, Gomez F, Negrete M, Liempi A, et al. *Trypanosoma cruzi* induces cellular proliferation in the trophoblastic cell line BeWo. Experimental Parasitology. 2017;**173**:9-17

[29] Wang SC. PCNA: A silent housekeeper or a potential therapeutic target? Trends in Pharmacological Sciences. 2014;**35**(4):178-186

[30] Duaso J, Rojo G, Jana F, Galanti N, Cabrera G, Bosco C, et al. *Trypanosoma cruzi* induces apoptosis in ex vivo infected human chorionic villi. Placenta. 2011;**32**(5):356-361

[31] Baergen KBPKR. Pathology of the Human Placenta. 5th ed. Springer Science-Business Media, Inc.; 2006. p. 1065

[32] Castillo C, Villarroel A, Duaso J, Galanti N, Cabrera G, Maya JD, et al. Phospholipase C gamma and ERK1/2 mitogen activated kinase pathways are differentially modulated by

Trypanosoma cruzi during tissue invasion in human placenta. Experimental Parasitology. 2013;**133**(1):12-17

[33] Forbes K, Westwood M. Maternal growth factor regulation of human placental development and fetal growth. The Journal of endocrinology. 2010;**207**(1):1-16

[34] Gauster M, Siwetz M, Huppertz B. Fusion of villous trophoblast can be visualized by localizing active caspase 8. Placenta. 2009;**30**(6):547-550

[35] Gauster M, Moser G, Orendi K, Huppertz B. Factors involved in regulating trophoblast fusion: Potential role in the development of preeclampsia. Placenta. 2009;**30**(Suppl A): S49-S54

[36] Pidoux G, Gerbaud P, Cocquebert M, Segond N, Badet J, Fournier T, et al. Review: Human trophoblast fusion and differentiation: Lessons from trisomy 21 placenta. Placenta. 2012;**33**(Suppl):S81-S86

[37] Carrillo I, Droguett D, Castillo C, Liempi A, Munoz L, Maya JD, et al. Caspase-8 activity is part of the BeWo trophoblast cell defense mechanisms against *Trypanosoma cruzi* infection. Experimental Parasitology. 2016;**168**:9-15

[38] Tarleton RL. Immune system recognition of *Trypanosoma cruzi*. Current Opinion in Immunology. 2007;**19**(4):430-434

[39] Gravina HD, Antonelli L, Gazzinelli RT, Ropert C. Differential use of TLR2 and TLR9 in the regulation of immune responses during the infection with *Trypanosoma cruzi*. PLoS One. 2013;**8**(5):e63100

[40] Haider S, Knofler M. Human tumour necrosis factor: Physiological and pathological roles in placenta and endometrium. Placenta. 2009;**30**(2):111-123

[41] Hamilton ST, Scott G, Naing Z, Iwasenko J, Hall B, Graf N, et al. Human cytomegalovirus-induces cytokine changes in the placenta with implications for adverse pregnancy outcomes. PLoS One. 2012;**7**(12):e52899

[42] Bayer A, Delorme-Axford E, Sleigher C, Frey TK, Trobaugh DW, Klimstra WB, et al. Human trophoblasts confer resistance to viruses implicated in perinatal infection. American Journal of Obstetrics and Gynecology. 2015;**212**(1):71e1-71e8

[43] Zhou A, Li S, Wu J, Khan FA, Zhang S. Interplay between microRNAs and host pathogen recognition receptors (PRRs) signaling pathways in response to viral infection. Virus Research. 2014;**184**:1-6

[44] Zheng Y, Cai X, Bradley JE. MicroRNAs in parasites and parasite infection. RNA Biology. 2013;**10**(3):371-379

[45] Donker RB, Mouillet JF, Chu T, Hubel CA, Stolz DB, Morelli AE, et al. The expression profile of C19MC microRNAs in primary human trophoblast cells and exosomes. Molecular Human Reproduction. 2012;**18**(8):417-424

[46] Sadovsky Y, Mouillet JF, Ouyang Y, Bayer A, Coyne CB. The function of TrophomiRs and other microRNAs in the human placenta. Cold Spring Harbor Perspectives in Medicine. 2015;**5**(8):a023036

10

New Approaches for Chagas Disease Chemotherapy

Guadalupe García Liñares

Abstract

The latest advances concerning drug design and chemotherapy development to combat the Chagas' disease are discussed. This chapter is based on the metabolic differences between the pathogenic parasite and mammal hosts that led to the progress in the search for novel metabolic pathways in parasites that may be essential for parasite's survival but with no counterpart in the host. There is a considerable amount of work in the search of more promising molecular targets for drug design. However, the chemotherapy for this disease remains unsolved. It is based on old and fairly not specific drugs associated with long-term treatments, severe side effects, drug resistance, and different strains' susceptibility. Herein, a thorough analysis of selected molecular targets is described in terms of their potential usefulness for drug design. Therefore, rational approaches to the chemotherapeutic control of American trypanosomiasis describing some useful metabolic pathways are covered. Enzymes involved in ergosterol biosynthesis (squalene synthase, HMG-CoA reductase, farnesyl diphosphate synthase (FPPS), sterol 24-methyltransferase, and sterol 14α-demethylase), trypanothione system (glutathionyl-spermidine synthetase, trypanothione synthetase, and trypanothione reductase), cysteine proteases, trans-sialidase, and so on are discussed. The design of specific inhibitors of these metabolic activities as possible means of controlling the parasites without damaging the hosts is presented.

Keywords: *Trypanosoma cruzi*, drug development, molecular targets

1. Introduction

Chagas' disease or American trypanosomiasis is among the most prevalent parasitic diseases worldwide [1–3]. It has been estimated that around 20 million people are infected and over 40 million individuals are facing the risk of infection by the hemoflagellates protozoan *Trypanosoma cruzi*, the responsible agent of Chagas' disease. This disease is endemic in Latin

American countries, but the migration of individuals and blood transfusions have made possible the occurrence of the Chagas' disease in developed countries. Currently, no vaccine is available, so the control of the disease is limited to its detection, vector control, screening of blood banks and organ donors, and case finding of infected pregnant women. Moreover, the development of a safer and more effective chemotherapeutic intervention is crucial for the treatment of Chagas disease.

This disease is characterized by three phases: (1) an early acute phase in which trypomastigotes circulate in blood and infect cells transforming into the asexually-multiplying amastigotes; (2) a subsequent intermediate phase where the cells are broken, parasites are released to the blood and infect other cells (in this phase there are unspecific symptoms like fever, allergic reactions, acute heart failure, or meningoencephalitis); (3) a late chronic phase, a prolonged, and asymptomatic indeterminate phase, where parasites establish in their target organs (during this stage patients may have nonspecific clinical manifestations or present major complications such as cardiomyopathy and/or megaesophagus and megacolon syndromes [4]. The absence of adequate treatment in the acute phase results in the development of the above-mentioned stages of the disease.

The existing chemotherapy remains deficient; it is based on two old drugs empirically discovered, (**1**) nifurtimox, actually discontinued, and (**2**) benznidazole (**Figure 1**). Although both of these compounds are able to cure at least 50% of recent infections, they present important drawbacks such as selective drug sensitivity on different *T. cruzi* strains, serious side effects including vomiting, anorexia, peripheral neuropathy, allergic dermopathy, and long-term treatment [2, 5, 6]. Moreover, these compounds are not effective in the chronic stage of the disease. Consequently, the development of novel, safe, and affordable compounds with potent antiparasitic activity is urgently needed [7, 8]. The existence of *T. cruzi* populations naturally resistant to benznidazole and nifurtimox led to the search for compounds with a different mechanism of action [2, 8]. The development of new drugs that are more effective and safer than those currently available is urgently necessary.

There is a considerable amount of work in the search of unique aspects of the biochemistry and physiology of *T. cruzi* intending to find specific molecular targets for drug design [9]. It can be thought that the selective inhibition of a biosynthetic pathway that leads to a crucial metabolite for parasite survival would not have any significant toxic effect on the host. Based on these facts, this chapter will discuss the search for new approaches based on metabolic differences between the pathogenic parasite and mammal hosts and the development of new potential antiparasitic drugs in the last years.

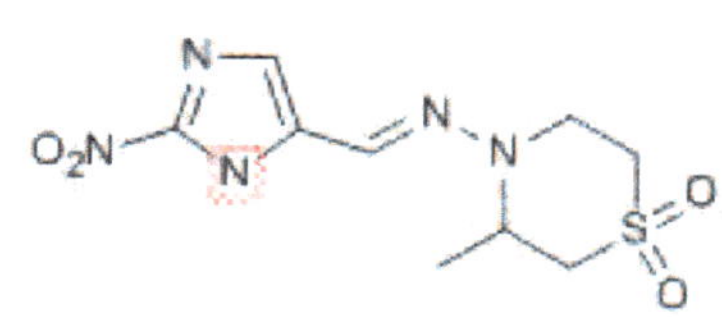

Nifurtimox, 1

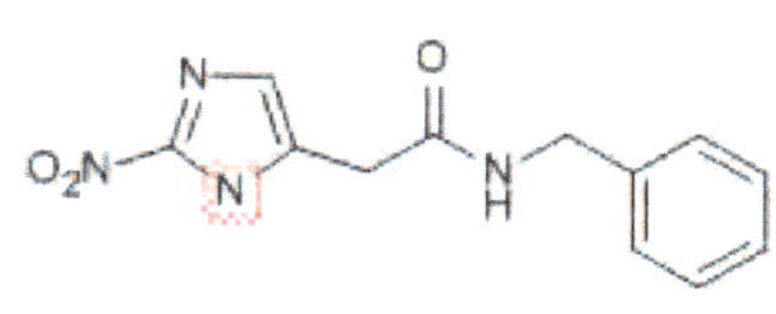

Benznidazole, 2

Figure 1. Drugs currently used for Chagas' disease treatment.

2. Molecular targets

There are many metabolic pathways and enzymes unique to *Trypanosoma cruzi* that constitute excellent molecular targets for drug development. However, despite the specificity of new compounds targeting parasite molecules, the effect of these drugs on mammalian metabolism must be carefully evaluated. A few of the most studied compounds targeting specific *T. cruzi* enzymes will be reviewed here.

2.1. Sterol biosynthesis

Isoprenoid biosynthetic pathway constitutes one of the most important metabolic pathways of all organisms because isoprenoids are essential for numerous biochemical functions. In trypanosomatides diverse enzymes of this biosynthetic pathway are involved in key process. Sterol biosynthesis in parasites differs from that in mammalian hosts since the final product is ergosterol instead cholesterol, the main sterol present in the mammals. As *T. cruzi* is entirely dependent on endogenously produced sterols for survival and proliferation, the sterol biosynthetic pathway constitutes an attractive target for drug development.

Reduction of endogenous sterols induces inhibition of the multiplication of *T. cruzi*. Then, the restriction of an enzyme of this biosynthetic pathway will inhibit the growth of the parasite [10, 11]. Sterol composition in *T. cruzi* is very similar to fungi with ergosterol and 24-ethylergosterol being the primary mature sterols in the epimastigote stage. Fungisterol and 24-ethylfurgisterol are the major sterols produced by the amastigote stage. In consequence, antifungal drugs are potentially capable of decreasing pathogen growth.

There are several interesting enzymes in the pathway as potential targets for anti-trypanosomal chemotherapy. For example, sterol 14α-demethylase, sterol 24-methyltransferase, farnesyl diphosphate synthase, squalene synthase, and HMG-CoA reductase.

2.1.1. Sterol 14α-demethylase (CYP51)

Sterol 14α-demethylase is a CYP monooxygenase that catalyzes the removal of the 14α-methyl group from eburicol. Unlike other hemoproteins, the hemo cofactor in CYP51 is coordinated to cysteine residue instead of histidine. Since it is an essential enzyme in sterol biosynthesis, the activity inhibition could be lethal in organisms requiring sterols for membrane function [12]. This enzyme constitutes an interesting target as it has the advantage of being inhibited by antifungal agents currently in clinical use. Azoles are the most efficient antifungal drugs and there have been reported numerous examples of its antiparasitic effects [13–15].

The first azoles such as ketoconazole (**3**), miconazole (**4**), or fluconazole (**5**) (**Figure 2**) were found to have potent *in vitro* activity but did not cure the *T. cruzi* infection. The mechanism of action involves binding to *T. cruzi* CYP51 and a disruption of sterol biosynthesis resulting in accumulation of 14-methylated sterols [16]. New azole drugs developed to combat fungal infections have been evaluated for the activity against *T. cruzi*. The experimental azole drug D0870 (**6**) was the first to cure the chronic infection in mice [17]. Unfortunately, D0870 was discontinued as an antifungal agent due to undesired side effects.

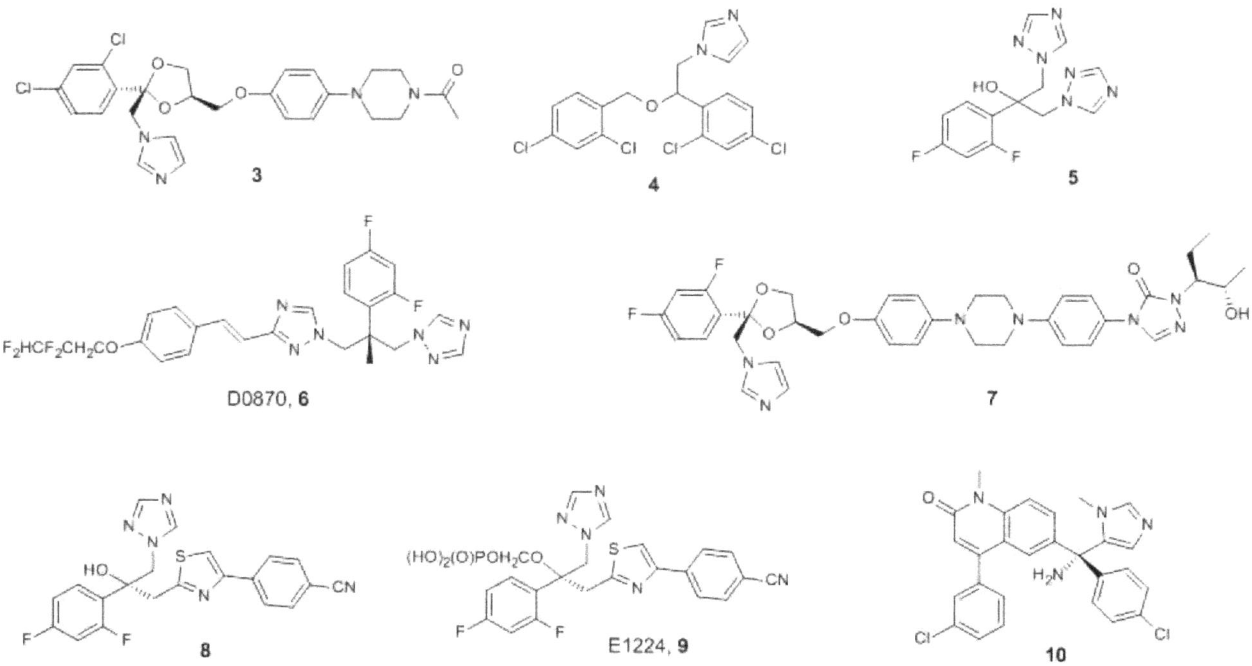

Figure 2. Structures of sterol 14α-demethylase (CYP51) inhibitors.

Among second-generation azoles, posaconazole (**7**) is the most potent drug against *T. cruzi*; because of its broad-spectrum antifungal activity, it could potentially be repurposed for use in Chagas' disease (**Figure 2**) [14]. It has been demonstrated that posaconazole is curative in the chronic murine model. In addition, it has potent activity against benznidazole and nifurtimox resistant *T. cruzi* strains [18]. Recently, a case was reported in Spain, describing the cure of chronic infection by treatment with posaconazole in an immunosuppressed patient. This compound is currently in phase II clinical trial for Chagas' disease. [19, 20] Unfortunately, posaconazole is a very expensive drug, so its application becomes impractical for patients with limited resources.

Ravuconazole (**8**) is another azole antifungal drug that has been evaluated as an antiparasitic agent and it appeared to be very efficient in restraining the parasitemia *in vitro* against *T. cruzi* in murine models [21]. However, since the half-life is much longer in humans than in mice, it is possible that this drug has curative effects. In fact, a prodrug of ravuconazole (E1224 **9**) is in a phase II trial [20]. In addition, ravuconazole has a simpler chemical structure than posaconazole, so the cost might be lower (**Figure 2**).

Tipifarnib (**10**) is an antitumor agent inhibiting human protein farnesyl transferase (**Figure 2**). It has considerable *in vitro* activity against *T. cruzi*. It was determined that the drug produces restriction of sterol biosynthesis by inhibition of CYP51 [22]. Analogs of tipifarnib have been designed and synthesized with improved CYP51 inhibitory activity and excellent pharmacokinetic properties [23].

2.1.2. Sterol 24-methyltransferase (24-SMT)

This enzyme catalyzes the methenylation of zymosterol, an important step for the biosynthesis of ergosterol and other related 24-alkylated sterols, which are the main sterols found in cell membranes of *T. cruzi* [24]. Azasterols are sterol compounds containing a nitrogen atom in the positions 23, 24, or 25 of the side chain. It was reported that these compounds inhibit the enzyme 24-SMT and demonstrated antiproliferative effects against trypanosomatids. 22, 26-azasterol (AZA, **11**), and 24, 25-epiminolanosterol (EIL, **12**) were the first azasterols reported to have trypanocidal activity [24, 25]. Different azasterols with modifications on their basic structure have been designed, synthesized, and biologically evaluated as antiparasitic agents [26, 27]. An important observation to take into account is that the 3β-OH group must be acylated. On the other hand, the nitrogen atom in the side chain can be located at the 23–25 position. The side chain can be attached via amine or amide bond and the presence of an ester moiety increased the activity [27]. General structures (**13**) of compounds, which have been developed as inhibitors of 24-SMT are shown in **Figure 3**.

2.1.3. 3-Hydroxy-3-methyl-glutaryl-coenzyme a reductase (HMG-CoA reductase)

The enzyme HMG-CoA reductase is involved in the first step in the pathway of isoprenoid biosynthesis and catalyzes the reduction of 3-hydroxy-3-methyl-glutaryl-coenzyme A to mevalonate. Therefore, HMG-CoA reductase is a key enzyme and constitutes a valid molecular target since its inhibition will also prevent the synthesis of compounds of the mevalonate pathway.

Current cardiovascular drugs have been tested for the treatment of Chagas' disease but new therapeutic drugs based on statins with a new anti-inflammatory approach have arisen as potential antiparasitic agents. Statins are thought to be associated with their ability to reduce cholesterol synthesis [28]. It was observed that lovastatin (**14**) and simvastatin (**15**) (**Figure 4**) have inhibited the growth of epimastigotes of *T. cruzi* and simvastatin could potentially inhibit HMG-CoA reductase both in epimastigotes and trypomastigotes [29]. Moreover, the combination of lovastatin with ketoconazole allowed the elimination of the presence of parasites into the blood flow and, in this way, prevented host death [30].

2.1.4. Farnesyl diphosphate synthase (FPPS)

The enzyme farnesyl pyrophosphate synthase, also known as farnesyl diphosphate synthase (FPPS) belongs to the E-family of the prenyltransferases and it has a key role in the isoprenoid biosynthetic pathway. Isopentenyl diphosphate (IPP) and its isomer dimethylallyl diphosphate (DMAPP) are synthesized via mevalonate pathway from acetyl-CoA [31]. DMAPP is the precursor for the biosynthesis of different and very important isoprenoids like sterols, ubiquinones, triterpenoids, and prenylated proteins.

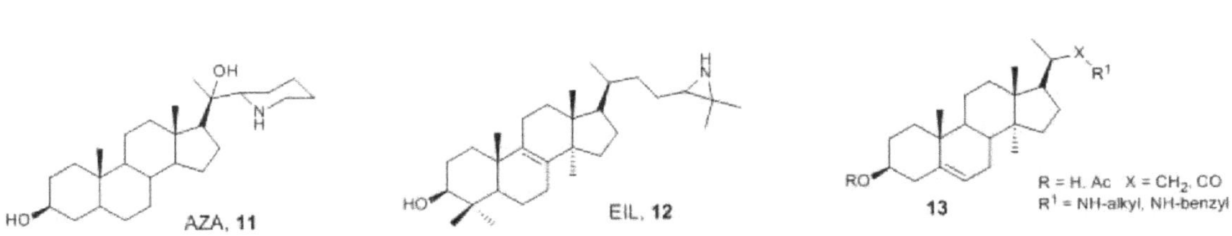

Figure 3. General structures of inhibitors of 24-SMT.

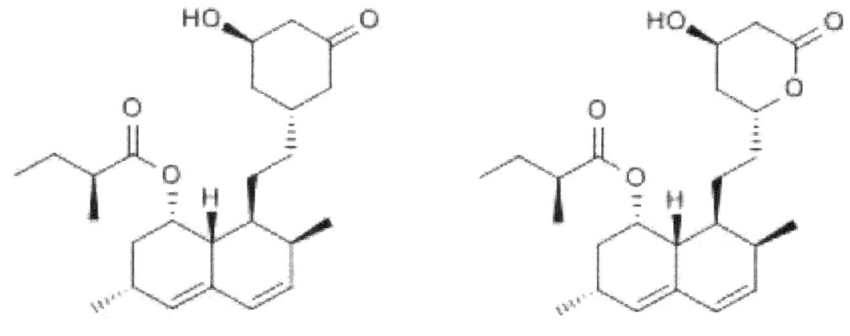

14 15

Figure 4. Chemical structures of inhibitors of the enzymatic activity of HMG-CoA reductase.

FPPS catalyzes two sequential steps: the addition of DMAPP to isopentenyl diphosphate (IPP) to form geranyl diphosphate (GPP) and the addition of DMAPP to geranyl diphosphate to produce farnesyl pyrophosphate (FPP). The inhibition or alteration of FPPS activity can regulate the isoprenoid metabolism. Therefore, FPPS has been selected as an excellent target for different disorders and anticancer, antibacterial, and antiparasitic drugs design among others [32–34].

Bisphosphonates act as inhibitors of bone resorption binding to the bone mineral. They are currently used for the treatment of several bone disorders like osteoporosis, Paget's disease, and hypercalcemia [35]. Bisphosphonates were the first FPPS inhibitors known and were reported as potent antiparasitic agents. Nitrogen-containing bisphosphonates like pamidronate (**16**), alendronate (**17**), risedronate (**18**), and ibandronate (**19**) were originally found to be effective against *T. cruzi* without toxicity to the host cells (**Figure 5**) [36]. Risedronate has shown a significantly increased survival of *T. cruzi*-infected mice *in vivo*. It was also found that diverse bisphosphonate derivatives were effective growth inhibitors of other pathogenic trypanosomatids and apicomplexan parasites [32, 37, 38].

Bisphosphonates have the disadvantage that they are highly polar and are rapidly removed from the circulatory system. Therefore, more lipophilic derivatives were developed (**20**) [38–40]. Bisphosphonates have a great potentiality as antiparasitic agents with characterized mechanisms of action involving the inhibition of FPPS, being very proper candidates to control and treat American trypanosomiasis. In addition, bisphosphonates have the advantage of being inexpensively synthesized and many compounds are FDA-approved drugs for the long-term treatment of several diseases.

2.1.5. Squalene synthase (SQS)

Squalene synthase (SQS) is also a key enzyme of ergosterol biosynthesis, which catalyzes the condensation of two farnesyl pyrophosphate molecules to form presqualene diphosphate and the subsequent loss of diphosphate, rearrangement, and reduction by NADPH to form squalene. Then, squalene epoxidase catalyzes the epoxidation of squalene affording oxidosqualene, which is cyclized by oxidosqualene cyclase to form lanosterol [41, 42]. Therefore,

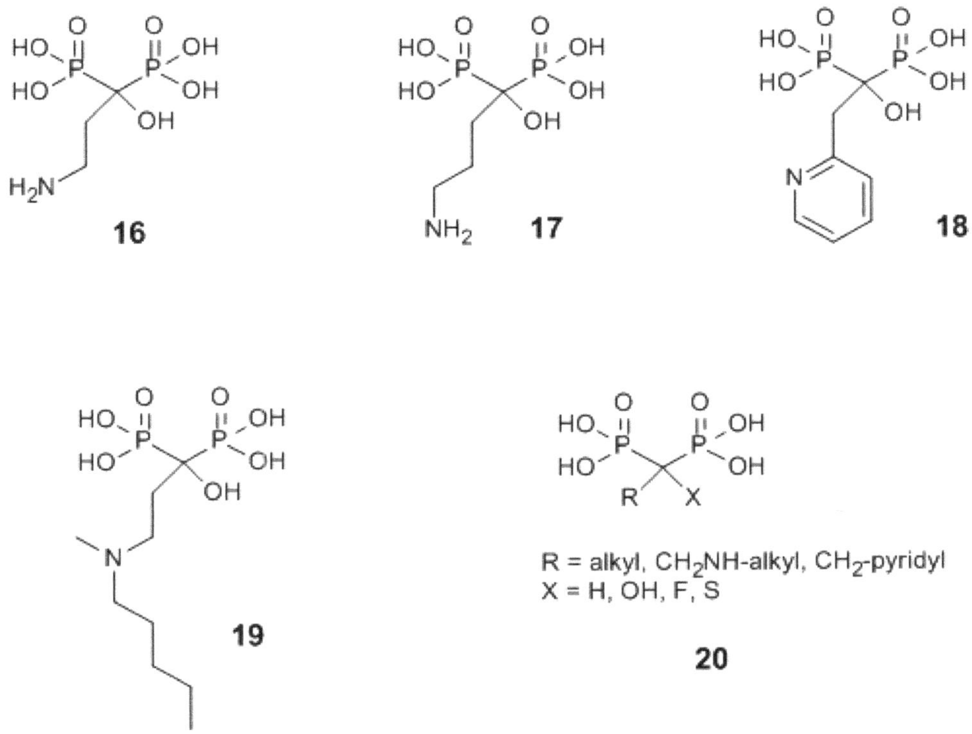

Figure 5. Chemical structures of representative bisphosphonates targeting FPPS.

any of these enzymes constitute an excellent molecular target for antitrypanosomal agent's development. SQS is also under intense study as a possible target for cholesterol-lowering drugs in humans [41].

Quinuclidines were developed as cholesterol-decreasing agents but actually, they also turned out to be potent SQS inhibitors. However, they showed poor SQS selectivity. It has also been reported that this class of compounds eliminated the parasite both *in vitro* and *in vivo* [43, 44].

SQ109 (**21**, **Figure 6**), an ethylenediamine currently in phase II clinical trials for the treatment of tuberculosis, is of great interest for the etiological treatment of Chagas' disease [45]. Studies have conveyed that SQ109 was an inhibitor of dehydrosqualene synthase from *Staphylococcus aureus*, a protein very similar to squalene synthase, suggesting that SQ109 might also inhibit *T. cruzi* SQS [46]. In fact, recently, it was determined that SQ109 is active against all life cycle stages of *T. cruzi*, detecting the most potent activity against the highly infective trypomastigote form. Furthermore SQ109 showed synergism with posaconazole [47].

Other very interesting SQS inhibitors that have been discovered include thiocyanates like WC-9 (**22**), which proved to be a potent inhibitor of this enzyme [48]. Fluorine-containing thiocyanate derivatives exhibited higher efficacy as inhibitors of *T. cruzi* proliferation (**23,24**) (**Figure 4**) [49]. Recently, the structures of human SQS and *T. cruzi* SQS bound to a substrate-like inhibitor were reported suggesting an interesting alternative for the development of selective drugs [50].

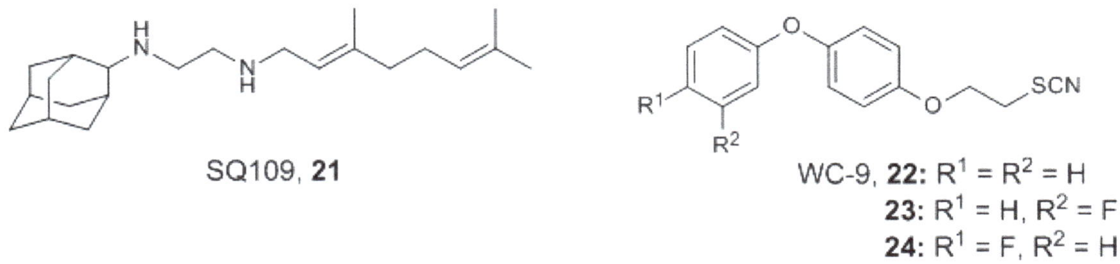

Figure 6. Chemical structures of inhibitors of the enzymatic activity of squalene synthase.

2.2. Cruzipain

Cruzipain is the main cysteine proteinase of *T. cruzi*, which is essential for the survival of the parasite. This enzyme is involved in different cellular functions such as nutrition, penetration into the host cell, defense, and differentiation processes [51]. It has been extensively studied as a valid target for new drug development [52, 53]. There are several three-dimensional structures of cruzipain with different inhibitors allowing the identification of structural regions of this enzyme that will enable the design of new agents [54, 55].

Numerous structurally varied compounds that inhibit proliferation of *T. cruzi* by inhibiting the enzymatic activity of cruzipain have been reported. Among the compounds tested, K777 (**25**), a vinyl sulfone derivative was active against a wide range of susceptible and resistant strains (**Figure 7**). Moreover, it was able to cure *T. cruzi* acute and non-acute infection in mice, showing also synergistic activity with benznidazole [56, 57].

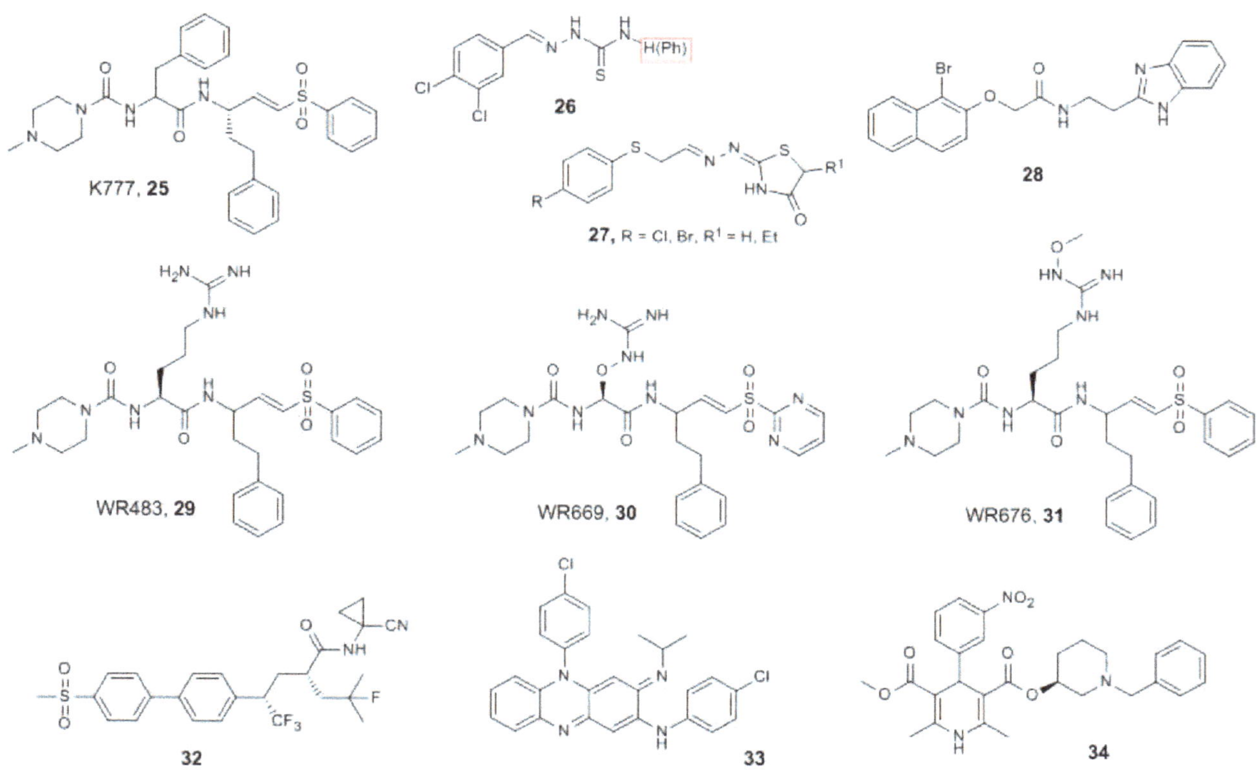

Figure 7. Structures of inhibitors of cruzipain activity.

Molecules containing thiosemicarbazones have been extensively explored [58–60]. Among these, 3, 4-dichlorophenyl thiosemicarbazone (**26**) is one of the most potent cruzipain inhibitor [61]. Recently, thiazolidinone derivatives (**27**) were identified as strong antiparasitic compounds (**Figure 7**) [62, 63].

Benzimidazoles have also been studied as cruzipain inhibitors and various derivatives have been synthesized and evaluated. *N*-(2-(1H-benzo[d]imidazol-2-yl) ethyl)-2-(1-bromonaphthalene-2-yloxy) acetamide (**28**) was the most potent enzyme inhibitor but it showed moderate trypanocidal activity [64, 65].

Other very potent cruzipain inhibitors have been developed such as oxyguanidine derivatives WRR-483, WRR-669, and WRR-676 (**29–31**). Some of these compounds showed suitable metabolic stability and a remarkable trypanocidal activity [66].

Very recently a series of peptidyl nitroalkenes was designed, synthesized, and evaluated as cruzipain inhibitors. Several compounds showed high activity against the enzyme observing the peptidic nature to be the determinant for their inhibitory activity [67].

Odanacatib (**32**), clofazimine (**33**), and benidipine (**34**) are examples of drug repurposing for the development of novel therapeutics for the Chagas' diseases (**Figure 5**). Odanacatib is a cathepsin K inhibitor used for the treatment of postmenopausal osteoporosis; it is a potent cysteine protease inhibitor, which is in Phase III clinical trials [68]. Clofazimine is an antibiotic applied to the treatment of leprosy [69] and benidipine is a calcium channel-blocking agent employed in the treatment of hypertension [70]. Clofazimine and benidipine were recently tested in a murine model of chronic Chagas' disease infection. Both compounds have reduced the parasitemia and the inflammatory effects have been well tolerated [71].

2.3. *Trans*-sialidase

The enzyme *trans*-sialidase (TS) belongs to the group of enzymes that are secreted by the parasite involved in the processes of cell invasion and immune evasion [72]. *T. cruzi* incorporates sialic acid (**35**) from exogenous sialoglycoconjugates by a trans-glycosylation reaction [73]. TS catalyze this transfer from host sialoglycoconjugates to glycoconjugates or mucins, which are attached to the cell membrane of *T. cruzi* via glycophosphatidylinositol anchors [74, 75]. Added to its important role, the absence of this enzyme in mammalian organisms makes it an excellent molecular target.

Within TS' inhibitors it can be mentioned fluorinated compounds like 9-benzoyl-3-fluoro-N-acetylneuraminic acid (**36**), and 3-fluorosialyl fluoride (**37**) selectively bind to the active site of the enzyme [76]. Sulfonamide-containing hydroxylated chalcones (**38**) and quinolones (**39**) are also specific inhibitors of *T. cruzi* TS, being dihydroxylated more potent than monohydroxylated derivatives (**Figure 8**) [77].

Some approved FDA drugs were evaluated on trypomastigotes deriving out of a computational screening protocol. The anti-inflammatory sulfasalazine (**40**) showed potent antiparasitic effects in *in vivo* assays, but with moderate TS inhibition. However, this drug and sulfonamide-containing compounds could be used as leading drugs in the development of new TS inhibitors [78].

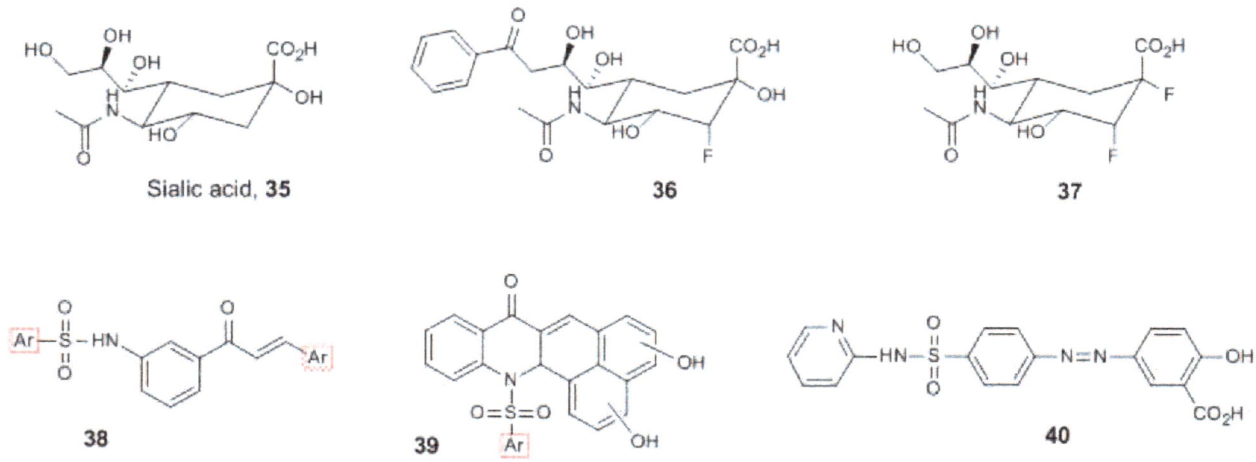

Figure 8. Representative inhibitors of *trans*-sialidase.

2.4. Trypanothione system

Trypanothione ($T[SH]_2$ or N^1, N^8-bis-(glutathionyl)spermidine, (**41**)) is a dithiol, which is responsible for the thiol metabolism in trypanosomatids by maintaining the intracellular redox balance [79]. Trypanothione is responsible for the protection against oxidative stress in *T. cruzi* trapping reactive oxygen species [80].

The protective reactions involve two key enzymes, which keep the trypanothione system operating: trypanothione reductase (TryR), homologous to mammal glutathione reductase and trypanothione synthetase (TryS) [81]. TryR catalyzes the reduction of trypanothione disulfide ($T[S]_2$, **42**) to $T[SH]_2$ (**Figure 9**); TryS catalyzes the synthesis of $T[SH]_2$ from glutathione and spermidine, keeping the amount of total trypanothione constant [82]. Taking into account the fact that trypanothione system is essential to the survival of parasites, these enzymes emerge as valid molecular targets for the search of new chemotherapeutics agents. In addition, TryS has no counterpart in mammals, making even more interesting to the design more specific and safer inhibitors [2].

Various reports have conveyed that different classes of compounds have selective enzyme inhibition activity such as tricyclic ring structures, bicyclic, and heterocyclic compounds or polyamines among others.

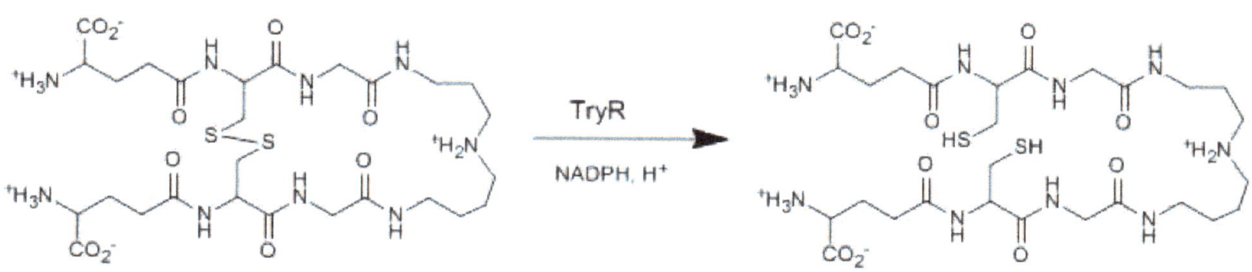

42 **41**

Figure 9. Structures of the oxidized and reduced forms of trypanothione.

Mepacrine (**43**) is a tricyclic antimalarial, which showed TryR inhibition without affecting human glutathione reductase and several mepacrine derivatives have been prepared. Although these derivatives presented greater potency, they turned out to be toxic to human cells [83].

Tricyclic phenothiazine-containing drugs are currently used as an antidepressant and have additionally exhibited antimicrobial activity [84]. Some phenothiazines demonstrated inhibitory activity against TryR [85]. Within them, thioridazine (**44**) is one of the most potent TryR inhibitors as investigations have suggested [86]. Clomipramine (**45**) [87] is another psychiatric drug with inhibiting action towards TryR. Both thioridazine and clomipramine seem to have *in vivo* effects against *T. cruzi* (**Figure 10**).

Library screening has allowed the identification of other classes of inhibitors that could be useful for the development of more potent TryR inhibitors. Some examples of these compounds are indatraline (**46**), a monoamine transporter inhibitor, 1-(2-(benzhydryloxy)ethyl)-4-(3-phenylpropyl)piperazine (GBR-12935, **47**) and a benzothiophene-piperidine derivative (BTCP **48**) [88]. Other or additional, studies allowed finding analogs of these compounds, which have increased the potency against TryR exhibiting higher selectivity [89]. The most interesting compounds were a piperazine-phenothiazine derivative of GBR-12935 (**49**) and a diaryl sulfide BTCP derivative [50, 88, 90].

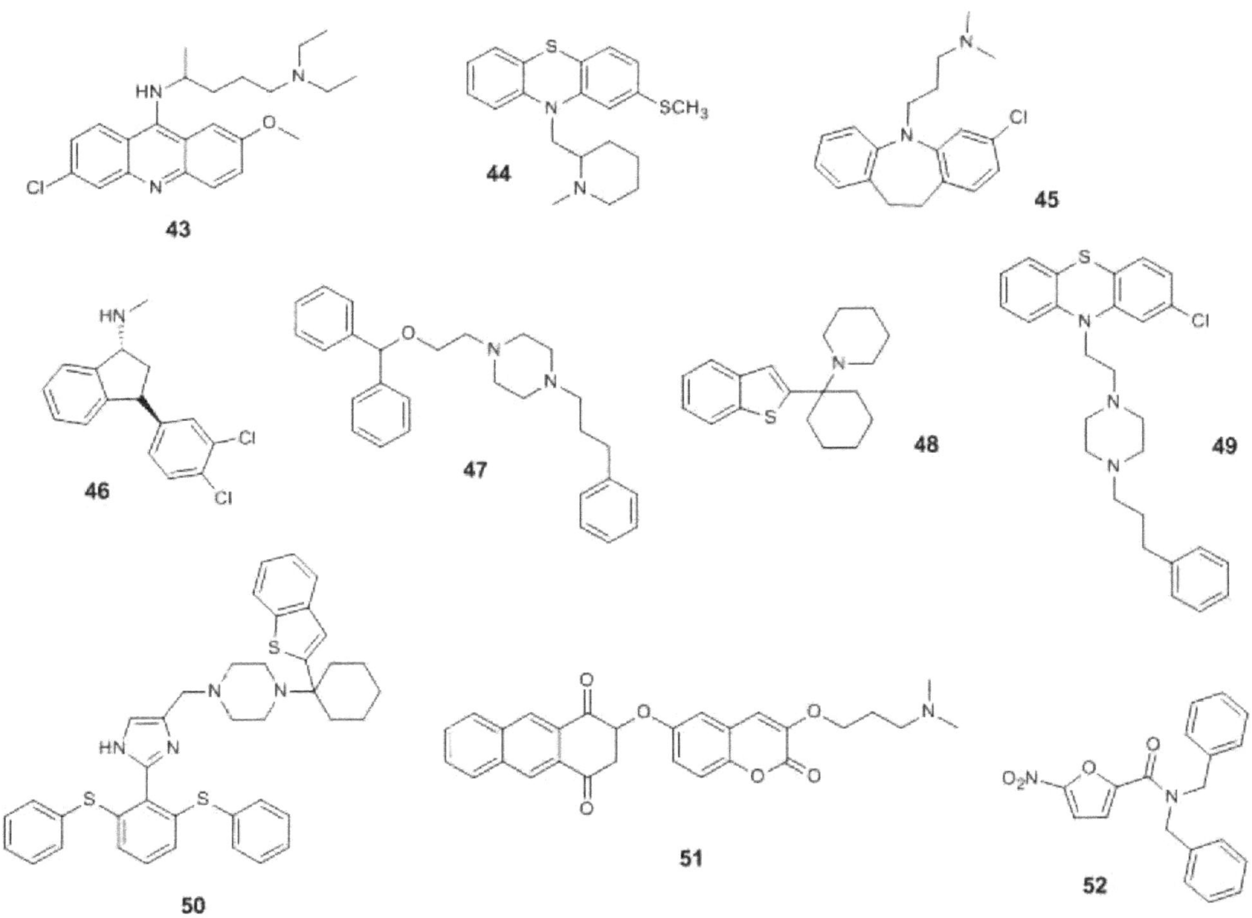

Figure 10. Chemical structures of relevant compounds targeting trypanothione reductase.

Different compounds can behave as TryR inhibitors when turning into reactive radical species through the reduction single-electron step [83, 91]. Within these structures, 1, 4 naphthoquinones and nitrofurans have been largely studied [92, 93]. The most potent derivative of 1,4 naphthoquinone was a quinone–coumarin hybrid [51] despite showing toxicity against rat skeletal myoblasts [94].

Between nitrofurans compounds, several 5-nitrofuroic acid derivatives have been synthesized and evaluated against *T. cruzi*. The best compound was 5-nitro-furan-2-carboxylic acid dibenzyl amide [52], which it significantly increased the trypanocidal nifurtimox activity being TryTR your molecular target [95].

3. Conclusions

Currently, the chemotherapy of American trypanosomiasis remains a serious problem in the field of neglected tropical diseases. There are no vaccines, and chemotherapy is limited to old drugs, which present important drawbacks. Taking into account that this disease is associated with poor populations and bad housing conditions, pharmaceutical companies have no economic motivations. Therefore, all efforts to the development of new drugs must be made by academic and/or governmental institutions and new chemotherapies are needed urgently. In order to search new, safer and efficient drugs for the Chagas' treatment, an overview of possible molecular targets based on specific features of the biochemistry of *Trypanosoma cruzi* was given. Although there are numerous potentially valid targets, only the more representative ones were discussed here. Furthermore, some of the new potential antiparasitic drugs as well as drugs applied to other human illness were described in this work. However, despite numerous efforts and progress in the searching of new or repositioned compounds for American trypanosomiasis chemotherapy, no ideal drugs are yet available for human treatment

Author details

Guadalupe García Liñares

Address all correspondence to: linares@qo.fcen.uba.ar

Departamento de Química Orgánica y UMYMFOR, Facultad de Ciencias Exactas y Naturales, Universidad de Buenos Aires, Buenos Aires, Argentina

References

[1] Second W. Report on Neglected Tropical Diseases. Sustaining the Drive to Overcome the Global Impact of Neglected Tropical Diseases; 2013

[2] Linares GE, Ravaschino EL, Rodriguez JB. Progresses in the field of drug design to combat tropical protozoan parasitic diseases. Current Medicinal Chemistry. 2006;**13**(3):335-360

[3] Pérez-Molina JA, Molina I. Chagas' disease. The Lancet. 2017;**391**(10115):82-94

[4] Coura JR, Borges-Pereira J. Chronic phase of Chagas' disease: Why should it be treated? A comprehensive review. Memórias do Instituto Oswaldo Cruz. 2011;**106**(6):641-645

[5] Bermudez J, Davies C, Simonazzi A, Real JP, Palma S. Current drug therapy and pharmaceutical challenges for Chagas' disease. Acta Tropica. 2016;**156**:1-16

[6] Morillo CA, Marin-Neto JA, Avezum A, Sosa-Estani S, Rassi A Jr, Rosas F, et al. Randomized trial of benznidazole for chronic Chagas' cardiomyopathy. The New England Journal of Medicine. 2015;**373**(14):1295-1306

[7] Moraes CB, Franco CH. Novel drug discovery for Chagas' disease. Expert Opinion on Drug Discovery. 2016;**11**(5):447-455

[8] Urbina JA, McKerrow JH. Drug susceptibility of genetically engineered *Trypanosoma cruzi* strains and sterile cure in animal models as a criterion for potential clinical efficacy of anti-*T. cruzi* drugs. Antimicrobial Agents and Chemotherapy. 2015;**59**(12):7923-7924

[9] Urbina J. New insights in Chagas' disease treatment. Drugs of the Future. 2010;**35**(5): 409-419

[10] Buckner FS, Urbina JA. Recent developments in sterol 14-demethylase inhibitors for Chagas' disease. International Journal for Parasitology: Drugs and Drug Resistance. 2012;**2**: 236-242

[11] Lepesheva GI, Villalta F, Waterman MR. Targeting *Trypanosoma cruzi* sterol 14α-demethylase (CYP51). Advances in Parasitology. 2011;**75**:65

[12] Lepesheva GI, Ott RD, Hargrove TY, Kleshchenko YY, Schuster I, Nes WD, et al. Sterol 14α-demethylase as a potential target for antitrypanosomal therapy: Enzyme inhibition and parasite cell growth. Chemistry & Biology. 2007;**14**(11):1283-1293

[13] Araújo M, Martins-Filho O, Pereira M, Brener Z. A combination of benznidazole and ketoconazole enhances efficacy of chemotherapy of experimental Chagas' disease. The Journal of Antimicrobial Chemotherapy. 2000;**45**(6):819-824

[14] Molina J, Martins-Filho O, Brener Z, Romanha AJ, Loebenberg D, Urbina JA. Activities of the triazole derivative SCH 56592 (posaconazole) against drug-resistant strains of the protozoan parasite *Trypanosoma* (Schizotrypanum) *cruzi* in immunocompetent and immunosuppressed murine hosts. Antimicrobial Agents and Chemotherapy. 2000;**44**(1): 150-155

[15] Urbina JA, Lira R, Visbal G, Bartrolí J. *In vitro* antiproliferative effects and mechanism of action of the new triazole derivative UR-9825 against the protozoan parasite *Trypanosoma* (Schizotrypanum) *cruzi*. Antimicrobial Agents and Chemotherapy. 2000;**44**(9):2498-2502

[16] Urbina JA, Payares G, Contreras LM, Liendo A, Sanoja C, Molina J, et al. Antiproliferative effects and mechanism of action of SCH 56592 against *Trypanosoma* (Schizotrypanum) *cruzi*: *in vitro* and *in vivo* studies. Antimicrobial Agents and Chemotherapy. 1998;**42**(7): 1771-1777

[17] Urbina JA, Payares G, Molina J, Sanoja C, Liendo A, Lazardi K, et al. Cure of short- and long-term experimental Chagas' disease using D0870. Science-New York then Washington. 1996;**273**:969-970

[18] Lepesheva GI, Hargrove TY, Anderson S, Kleshchenko Y, Furtak V, Wawrzak Z, et al. Structural insights into inhibition of sterol 14α-demethylase in the human pathogen *Trypanosoma cruzi*. The Journal of Biological Chemistry. 2010;**285**(33):25582-25590

[19] Pinazo M-J, Espinosa G, Gállego M, López-Chejade PL, Urbina JA, Gascón J. Successful treatment with posaconazole of a patient with chronic Chagas' disease and systemic lupus erythematosus. The American Journal of Tropical Medicine and Hygiene. 2010; **82**(4):583-587

[20] Clayton J. Chagas' disease: Pushing through the pipeline. Nature. 2010:S12

[21] de Figueiredo Diniz L, Caldas IS, da Matta Guedes PM, Crepalde G, de Lana M, Carneiro CM, et al. Effects of ravuconazole treatment on parasite load and immune response in dogs experimentally infected with *Trypanosoma cruzi*. Antimicrobial Agents and Chemotherapy. 2010;**54**(7):2979-2986

[22] Hucke O, Gelb MH, Verlinde CL, Buckner FS. The protein farnesyltransferase inhibitor Tipifarnib as a new lead for the development of drugs against Chagas' disease. Journal of Medicinal Chemistry. 2005;**48**(17):5415-5418

[23] Kraus JM, Tatipaka HB, McGuffin SA, Chennamaneni NK, Karimi M, Arif J, et al. Second generation analogues of the cancer drug clinical candidate tipifarnib for anti-Chagas' disease drug discovery. Journal of Medicinal Chemistry. 2010;**53**(10):3887-3898

[24] Urbina JA, Vivas J, Lazardi K, Molina J, Payares G, Pirns MM, et al. Antiproliferative effects of Δ24 (25) sterol methyl Transferase inhibitors on *Trypanosoma* (Schizotrypanum) *cruzi*: *In vitro* and *in vivo* studies. Chemotherapy. 1996;**42**(4):294-307

[25] Vivas J, Urbina JA, de Souza W. Ultrastructural alterations in *Trypanosoma* (Schizotrypanum) *cruzi* induced by Δ24 (25) sterol methyl transferase inhibitors and their combinations with ketoconazole. International Journal of Antimicrobial Agents. 1996;**7**(4): 235-240

[26] Gros L, Castillo-Acosta VM, Jiménez CJ, Sealey-Cardona M, Vargas S, Estévez AM, et al. New azasterols against *Trypanosoma brucei*: Role of 24-sterol methyltransferase in inhibitor action. Antimicrobial Agents and Chemotherapy. 2006;**50**(8):2595-2601

[27] Gigante F, Kaiser M, Brun R, Gilbert IH. Design and preparation of sterol mimetics as potential antiparasitics. Bioorganic & Medicinal Chemistry. 2010;**18**(20):7291-7301

[28] Quist-Paulsen P. Statins and inflammation: An update. Current Opinion in Cardiology. 2010;**25**(4):399-405

[29] Silva RR, Shrestha-Bajracharya D, Almeida-Leite CM, Leite R, Bahia MT, Talvani A. Short-term therapy with simvastatin reduces inflammatory mediators and heart inflammation during the acute phase of experimental Chagas' disease. Memórias do Instituto Oswaldo Cruz. 2012;**107**(4):513-521

[30] Urbina J, Lazardi K, Marchan E, Visbal G, Aguirre T, Piras M, et al. Mevinolin (lovastatin) potentiates the antiproliferative effects of ketoconazole and terbinafine against *Trypanosoma* (Schizotrypanum) *cruzi*: *in vitro* and *in vivo* studies. Antimicrobial Agents and Chemotherapy. 1993;**37**(3):580-591

[31] Lombard J, Moreira D. Origins and early evolution of the mevalonate pathway of isoprenoid biosynthesis in the three domains of life. Molecular Biology and Evolution. 2010;**28**(1):87-99

[32] Martin MB, Grimley JS, Lewis JC, Heath HT, Bailey BN, Kendrick H, et al. Bisphosphonates inhibit the growth of *Trypanosoma brucei*, *Trypanosoma cruzi*, Leishmania d onovani, *Toxoplasma gondii*, and *Plasmodium falciparum*: A potential route to chemotherapy. Journal of Medicinal Chemistry. 2001;**44**(6):909-916

[33] Reddy R, Dietrich E, Lafontaine Y, Houghton TJ, Belanger O, Dubois A, et al. Bisphosphonated benzoxazinorifamycin prodrugs for the prevention and treatment of osteomyelitis. ChemMedChem. 2008;**3**(12):1863-1868

[34] Miller K, Erez R, Segal E, Shabat D, Satchi-Fainaro R. Targeting bone metastases with a bispecific anticancer and antiangiogenic polymer–alendronate–taxane conjugate. Angewandte Chemie, International Edition. 2009;**48**(16):2949-2954

[35] Reszka AA, Rodan GA. Nitrogen-containing bisphosphonate mechanism of action. Mini Reviews in Medicinal Chemistry. 2004;**4**(7):711-719

[36] Urbina JA, Moreno B, Vierkotter S, Oldfield E, Payares G, Sanoja C, et al. *Trypanosoma cruzi* contains major pyrophosphate stores, and its growth *in vitro* and *in vivo* is blocked by pyrophosphate analogs. The Journal of Biological Chemistry. 1999;**274**(47):33609-33615

[37] Ghosh S, Chan JM, Lea CR, Meints GA, Lewis JC, Tovian ZS, et al. Effects of bisphosphonates on the growth of *Entamoeba histolytica* and *Plasmodium* species *in vitro* and *in vivo*. Journal of Medicinal Chemistry. 2004;**47**(1):175-187

[38] Szajnman SH, Garcıa GE, Li Z-H, Jiang C, Galizzi M, Bontempi EJ, et al. Synthesis and biological evaluation of 2-alkylaminoethyl-1, 1-bisphosphonic acids against *Trypanosoma cruzi* and *Toxoplasma gondii* targeting farnesyl diphosphate synthase. Bioorganic & Medicinal Chemistry. 2008;**16**(6):3283-3290

[39] Recher M, Barboza AP, Li Z-H, Galizzi M, Ferrer-Casal M, Szajnman SH, et al. Design, synthesis and biological evaluation of sulfur-containing 1, 1-bisphosphonic acids as antiparasitic agents. European Journal of Medicinal Chemistry. 2013;**60**:431-440

[40] Zhang Y, Cao R, Yin F, Hudock MP, Guo R-T, Krysiak K, et al. Lipophilic bisphosphonates as dual farnesyl/geranylgeranyl diphosphate synthase inhibitors: An X-ray and NMR investigation. Journal of the American Chemical Society. 2009;**131**(14):5153-5162

[41] Urbina JA, Concepcion JL, Rangel S, Visbal G, Lira R. Squalene synthase as a chemotherapeutic target in *Trypanosoma cruzi* and *Leishmania mexicana*. Molecular and Biochemical Parasitology. 2002;**125**(1):35-45

[42] Oldfield E. Targeting isoprenoid biosynthesis for drug discovery: Bench to bedside. Accounts of Chemical Research. 2010;**43**(9):1216-1226

[43] Urbina JA, Concepcion JL, Caldera A, Payares G, Sanoja C, Otomo T, et al. *In vitro* and *in vivo* activities of E5700 and ER-119884, two novel orally active squalene synthase inhibitors, against *Trypanosoma cruzi*. Antimicrobial Agents and Chemotherapy. 2004;**48**(7):2379-2387

[44] Sealey-Cardona M, Cammerer S, Jones S, Ruiz-Pérez LM, Brun R, Gilbert IH, et al. Kinetic characterization of squalene synthase from *Trypanosoma cruzi*: Selective inhibition by quinuclidine derivatives. Antimicrobial Agents and Chemotherapy. 2007;**51**(6):2123-2129

[45] Sacksteder KA, Protopopova M, Barry CE, Andries K, Nacy CA. Discovery and development of SQ109: A new antitubercular drug with a novel mechanism of action. Future Microbiology. 2012;**7**(7):823-837

[46] Lin F-Y, Liu Y-L, Li K, Cao R, Zhu W, Axelson J, et al. Head-to-head prenyl tranferases: Anti-infective drug targets. Journal of Medicinal Chemistry. 2012;**55**(9):4367-4372

[47] Veiga-Santos P, Li K, Lameira L, de Carvalho TMU, Huang G, Galizzi M, et al. SQ109, a new drug lead for Chagas' disease. Antimicrobial Agents and Chemotherapy. 2015; **59**(4):1950-1961

[48] Urbina JA, Concepcion JL, Montalvetti A, Rodriguez JB, Docampo R. Mechanism of action of 4-phenoxyphenoxyethyl thiocyanate (WC-9) against *Trypanosoma cruzi*, the causative agent of Chagas' disease. Antimicrobial Agents and Chemotherapy. 2003;**47**(6): 2047-2050

[49] Liñares GG, Gismondi S, Codesido NO, Moreno SN, Docampo R, Rodriguez JB. Fluorine-containing aryloxyethyl thiocyanate derivatives are potent inhibitors of *Trypanosoma cruzi* and *Toxoplasma gondii* proliferation. Bioorganic & Medicinal Chemistry Letters. 2007;**17**(18):5068-5071

[50] Shang N, Li Q, Ko T-P, Chan H-C, Li J, Zheng Y, et al. Squalene synthase as a target for Chagas' disease therapeutics. PLoS Pathogens. 2014;**10**(5):e1004114

[51] Sajid M, McKerrow JH. Cysteine proteases of parasitic organisms. Molecular and Biochemical Parasitology. 2002;**120**(1):1-21

[52] G Duschak V. A decade of targets and patented drugs for chemotherapy of Chagas' disease. Recent Patents on Anti-Infective Drug Discovery. 2011;**6**(3):216-259

[53] Martinez-Mayorga K, Byler KG, Ramirez-Hernandez AI, Terrazas-Alvares DE. Cruzain inhibitors: Efforts made, current leads and a structural outlook of new hits. Drug Discovery Today. 2015;**20**(7):890-898

[54] Brak K, Kerr ID, Barrett KT, Fuchi N, Debnath M, Ang K, et al. Nonpeptidic tetrafluorophenoxymethyl ketone cruzain inhibitors as promising new leads for Chagas' disease chemotherapy. Journal of Medicinal Chemistry. 2010;**53**(4):1763-1773

[55] Chen YT, Brinen LS, Kerr ID, Hansell E, Doyle PS, McKerrow JH, et al. *In vitro* and *in vivo* studies of the trypanocidal properties of WRR-483 against *Trypanosoma cruzi*. PLoS Neglected Tropical Diseases. 2010;**4**(9):e825

[56] McKerrow JH, Doyle P, Engel J, Podust L, Robertson S, Ferreira R, et al. Two approaches to discovering and developing new drugs for Chagas' disease. Memórias do Instituto Oswaldo Cruz. 2009;**104**:263-269

[57] Zingales B, Miles MA, Moraes CB, Luquetti A, Guhl F, Schijman AG, et al. Drug discovery for Chagas' disease should consider *Trypanosoma cruzi* strain diversity. Memórias do Instituto Oswaldo Cruz. 2014;**109**(6):828-833

[58] Espíndola JWP, de Oliveira Cardoso MV, de Oliveira Filho GB, e Silva DAO, Moreira DRM, Bastos TM, et al. Synthesis and structure–activity relationship study of a new series of antiparasitic aryloxyl thiosemicarbazones inhibiting *Trypanosoma cruzi* cruzain. European Journal of Medicinal Chemistry. 2015;**101**:818-835

[59] Fonseca NC, da Cruz LF, da Silva Villela F, do Nascimento Pereira GA, de Siqueira-Neto JL, Kellar D, et al. Synthesis of a sugar-based thiosemicarbazone series and structure-activity relationship versus the parasite cysteine proteases rhodesain, cruzain, and schistosoma mansoni cathepsin B1. Antimicrobial Agents and Chemotherapy. 2015; **59**(5):2666-2677

[60] Moreira DRM, Lima Leite AC, Cardoso MVO, Srivastava RM, Hernandes MZ, Rabello MM, et al. Structural design, synthesis and structure–activity relationships of Thiazolidinones with enhanced anti-*Trypanosoma cruzi* activity. ChemMedChem. 2014; **9**(1):177-188

[61] Carvalho L, Gomes M, Rocha B, de Oliveira R, Maria E, de Melo E. Anti-parasite effects of new thiosemicarbazones and their products thiazolidinone including cellular aspects of intracellular elimination of *Trypanosoma cruzi in vitro*. Journal of Developing Drugs 2014;**3**(126):10.4172

[62] Hernandes MZ, Rabello MM, Leite ACL, Cardoso MVO, Moreira DRM, Brondani DJ, et al. Studies toward the structural optimization of novel thiazolylhydrazone-based potent antitrypanosomal agents. Bioorganic & Medicinal Chemistry. 2010;**18**(22):7826-7835

[63] de Oliveira Filho GB, de Oliveira Cardoso MV, Espíndola JWP, Ferreira LFGR, de Simone CA, Ferreira RS, et al. Structural design, synthesis and pharmacological evaluation of 4-thiazolidinones against *Trypanosoma cruzi*. Bioorganic & Medicinal Chemistry. 2015;**23**(23):7478-7486

[64] Ferreira RS, Dessoy MA, Pauli I, Souza ML, Krogh R, Sales AI, et al. Synthesis, biological evaluation, and structure–activity relationships of potent noncovalent and Nonpeptidic Cruzain inhibitors as anti-*Trypanosoma cruzi* agents. Journal of Medicinal Chemistry. 2014;**57**(6):2380-2392

[65] Ferreira RS, Simeonov A, Jadhav A, Eidam O, Mott BT, Keiser MJ, et al. Complementarity between a docking and a high-throughput screen in discovering new cruzain inhibitors. Journal of Medicinal Chemistry. 2010;**53**(13):4891-4905

[66] Jones BD, Tochowicz A, Tang Y, Cameron MD, McCall L-I, Hirata K, et al. Synthesis and evaluation of oxyguanidine analogues of the cysteine protease inhibitor WRR-483 against Cruzain. ACS Medicinal Chemistry Letters. 2015;**7**(1):77-82

[67] Latorre A, Schirmeister T, Kesselring J, Jung S, Johé P, Hellmich UA, et al. Dipeptidyl nitroalkenes as potent reversible inhibitors of cysteine proteases Rhodesain and Cruzain. ACS Medicinal Chemistry Letters. 2016;**7**(12):1073-1076

[68] Ndao M, Beaulieu C, Black WC, Isabel E, Vasquez-Camargo F, Nath-Chowdhury M, et al. Reversible cysteine protease inhibitors show promise for a Chagas' disease cure. Antimicrobial Agents and Chemotherapy. 2014;**58**(2):1167-1178

[69] Cholo MC, Steel HC, Fourie PB, Germishuizen WA, Anderson R. Clofazimine: Current status and future prospects. The Journal of Antimicrobial Chemotherapy. 2011;**67**(2): 290-298

[70] Yao K, Nagashima K, Miki H. Pharmacological, pharmacokinetic, and clinical properties of benidipine hydrochloride, a novel, long-acting calcium channel blocker. Journal of Pharmacological Sciences. 2006;**100**(4):243-261

[71] Sbaraglini ML, Bellera CL, Fraccaroli L, Larocca L, Carrillo C, Talevi A, et al. Novel cruzipain inhibitors for the chemotherapy of chronic Chagas' disease. International Journal of Antimicrobial Agents. 2016;**48**(1):91-95

[72] Buschiazzo A, Amaya MF, Cremona ML, Frasch AC, Alzari PM. The crystal structure and mode of action of trans-sialidase, a key enzyme in *Trypanosoma cruzi* pathogenesis. Molecular Cell. 2002;**10**(4):757-768

[73] Previato J, Andrade A, Vermelho A, Firmino J, Mendonça-Previato L. Evidence for N-glycolylneuraminic acid incorporation by *Trypanosoma cruzi* from infected animal. Memórias do Instituto Oswaldo Cruz. 1990;**85**:38-39

[74] Cross GA, Takle GB. The surface trans-sialidase family of *Trypanosoma cruzi*. Annual Reviews in Microbiology. 1993;**47**(1):385-411

[75] Ferguson M, Brimacombe J, Cottaz S, Field R, Güther L, Homans S, et al. Glycosylphosphatidylinositol molecules of the parasite and the host. Parasitology. 1994;**108**(S1): S45-S54

[76] Buchini S, Buschiazzo A, Withers SG. A new generation of specific *Trypanosoma cruzi* trans-sialidase inhibitors. Angewandte Chemie, International Edition. 2008;**47**(14):2700-2703

[77] Kim JH, Ryu HW, Shim JH, Park KH, Withers SG. Development of new and selective *Trypanosoma cruzi* trans-Sialidase inhibitors from sulfonamide Chalcones and their derivatives. Chembiochem. 2009;**10**(15):2475-2479

[78] Lara-Ramirez EE, López-Cedillo JC, Nogueda-Torres B, Kashif M, Garcia-Perez C, Bocanegra-Garcia V, et al. An *in vitro* and *in vivo* evaluation of new potential trans-sialidase inhibitors of *Trypanosoma cruzi* predicted by a computational drug repositioning method. European Journal of Medicinal Chemistry. 2017;**132**:249-261

[79] Fairlamb AH, Cerami A. Identification of a novel, thiol-containing co-factor essential for glutathione reductase enzyme activity in trypanosomatids. Molecular and Biochemical Parasitology. 1985;**14**(2):187-198

[80] Brigelius-Flohé R, Flohé L. Basic principles and emerging concepts in the redox control of transcription factors. Antioxidants & Redox Signaling. 2011;**15**(8):2335-2381

[81] Flohé L. The trypanothione system and its implications in the therapy of trypanosomatid diseases. International Journal of Medical Microbiology. 2012;**302**(4):216-220

[82] Oza SL, Tetaud E, Ariyanayagam MR, Warnon SS, Fairlamb AH. A single enzyme catalyses formation of trypanothione from glutathione and spermidine in *Trypanosoma cruzi*. The Journal of Biological Chemistry. 2002;**277**(39):35853-35861

[83] Krauth-Siegel RL, Bauer H, Schirmer RH. Dithiol proteins as guardians of the intracellular redox milieu in parasites: Old and new drug targets in trypanosomes and malaria-causing plasmodia. Angewandte Chemie, International Edition. 2005;**44**(5):690-715

[84] Amaral L, Viveiros M, Kristiansen JE. "non-antibiotics": Alternative therapy for the management of MDRTB and MRSA in economically disadvantaged countries. Current Drug Targets. 2006;**7**(7):887-891

[85] Bernardes L, Zani C, Carvalho I. Trypanosomatidae diseases: From the current therapy to the efficacious role of trypanothione reductase in drug discovery. Current Medicinal Chemistry. 2013;**20**(21):2673-2696

[86] Presti MSL, Bazán PC, Strauss M, Báez AL, Rivarola HW, Paglini-Oliva PA. Trypanothione reductase inhibitors: Overview of the action of thioridazine in different stages of Chagas' disease. Acta Tropica. 2015;**145**:79-87

[87] Fauro R, Presti SL, Bazan C, Baez A, Strauss M, Triquell F, et al. Use of clomipramine as chemotherapy of the chronic phase of Chagas' disease. Parasitology. 2013;**140**(7):917-927

[88] Richardson JL, Nett IR, Jones DC, Abdille MH, Gilbert IH, Fairlamb AH. Improved tricyclic inhibitors of trypanothione reductase by screening and chemical synthesis. ChemMedChem. 2009;**4**(8):1333-1340

[89] Walton JG, Jones DC, Kiuru P, Durie AJ, Westwood NJ, Fairlamb AH. Synthesis and evaluation of Indatraline-based inhibitors for Trypanothione Reductase. ChemMedChem. 2011;**6**(2):321-328

[90] Eberle C, Lauber BS, Fankhauser D, Kaiser M, Brun R, Krauth-Siegel RL, et al. Improved inhibitors of trypanothione reductase by combination of motifs: Synthesis, inhibitory potency, binding mode, and antiprotozoal activities. ChemMedChem. 2011;**6**(2):292-301

[91] Gendron T, Lanfranchi DA, Davioud-Charvet E. Redox-active agents in reactions involving the Trypanothione/Trypanothione Reductase-based system to fight Kinetoplastidal parasites. Trypanosomatid Diseases: Molecular Routes to Drug Discovery. 2013:405-428

[92] Leroux AE, Krauth-Siegel RL. Thiol redox biology of trypanosomatids and potential targets for chemotherapy. Molecular and Biochemical Parasitology. 2016;**206**(1):67-74

[93] R Wilkinson S, Bot C, M Kelly J, S Hall B. Trypanocidal activity of nitroaromatic prodrugs: Current treatments and future perspectives. Current Topics in Medicinal Chemistry. 2011;**11**(16):2072-2084

[94] Belluti F, Uliassi E, Veronesi G, Bergamini C, Kaiser M, Brun R, et al. Toward the development of dual-targeted Glyceraldehyde-3-phosphate dehydrogenase/Trypanothione Reductase inhibitors against *Trypanosoma brucei* and *Trypanosoma cruzi*. ChemMedChem. 2014;**9**(2):371-382

[95] Arias D, Herrera F, Garay A, Rodrigues D, Forastieri P, Luna L, et al. Rational design of nitrofuran derivatives: Synthesis and valuation as inhibitors of *Trypanosoma cruzi* trypanothione reductase. European Journal of Medicinal Chemistry. 2017;**125**:1088-1097

11

Physiology and Pathology of Infectious Diseases: The Autoimmune Hypothesis of Chagas Disease

Armanda Moreira Mattoso-Barbosa,
Renato Sathler-Avelar,
Jordana Grazziela Alves Coelho-dos-Reis,
Olindo Assis Martins-Filho,
Andrea Teixeira-Carvalho and
Danielle Marchetti Vitelli-Avelar

Abstract

Infectious pathologies are a group of diseases that contribute with great impact on public health worldwide. Among the various diseases, some have a higher epidemiological importance, since their morbidity and mortality are very significant. In addition to the usual immune response, mounted against noxious agents, there is still the concept of infection-induced autoimmunity. Autoimmune diseases are defined as illnesses in which the evolution from benign to pathogenic autoimmunity takes place. However, proving a disease to be of autoimmune etiology is not a simple task. It is well known that both genetic influences and environmental factors trigger autoimmune disorders. However, some theories are still under great discussion. One of the most intriguing self-induced disorders is the hypothesis of autoimmunity during Chagas disease. Since the mid-1970s, the Chagas autoimmunity hypothesis has been considered an important contributor to the complex immune response developed by the host and triggered by *Trypanosoma cruzi*. New ideas and findings have strengthened this hypothesis, which has been reported in a series of publications from different groups around the world. The aim of this chapter is to discuss the mechanisms involving autoimmunity development during Chagas disease.

Keywords: Chagas disease, autoimmunity, *T. cruzi*, autoantibodies, immunology, cardiomyopathy

1. Introduction

Autoimmune diseases are chronic disabling disorders described as immune responses against self-antigens that comprise cells, tissues, and organs, resulting in devastating consequences for patients [1]. For over decades, the concept of autoimmune disease has been studied, and the relationship between infectious diseases and autoimmunity has been established. Among all illnesses, Chagas disease has caught the attention of many researchers worldwide. Along with all the possible pathogenic mechanisms involved in *Trypanosoma cruzi* infection, the autoreactive hypothesis has been discussed over the years and plays an important role in the cardiac damage presented by Chagas patients. This chapter intends to explore the *T. cruzi*-induced autoimmunity hypothesis by discussing its pathogenic mechanisms and its potential role in the tissue aggravation during Chagas disease.

2. Autoimmunity: an obscure immunological path

In order to understand autoimmunity, it is essential to go back into the first steps of T- and B-cell development, differentiation, and maturation. During the process of generation of new lymphocytic clones derived from a stem cell, a novel lymphocyte carrying a specific pattern of B-cell receptor (BCR) or T-cell receptor (TCR) is formed as revised recently [2, 3]. While B-lymphocytes may undergo full maturation in the bone marrow, T lymphocytes need thymic education, as can be observed in **Figure 1**.

After egressing the bone marrow, T lymphocytes undergo differentiation and maturation in the thymus in which they pass through a process called negative and positive selection [4, 5].

Positive selection occurs during classical thymic differentiation, in which thymocytes may generate naive conventional T lymphocytes. These cells migrate to peripheral tissues and further differentiate in response to encounter with nonself-antigens. The negative selection is based on the elimination or inhibition of "self-reactive" cells. Nevertheless, some of these self-reactive T cells could escape negative selection and might become activated during the inflammatory process. On the other hand, a second or agonist-driven thymic selection, was proposed in which specialized T-cell subsets are generated from thymocytes that bind with high avidity to self-antigens. In this case, these cells leave the thymus as antigen-experienced activated T cells, such as double-negative TCRαβ+ intestinal T cells, CD8αα+, invariant iNKT, Foxp3+ nTreg cells, TH17 cells [6] and possibly mucosal associated invariant T cells (MAIT) [7]. Two barriers for self-reactive cells exist, which are the central and peripheral tolerance [5]. Failure in these processes may allow the proliferation of self-reactive clones, thus establishing an autoimmune pathogenic disease. Genetic disorders as well as environmental conditions can trigger the failure on central or peripheral tolerance, [8–12]. In addition, other pathways can lead to autoimmunity such as molecular similarity or mimicry, specific epitope spreading, indirect or bystander activation, B- and T-cell polyclonal activation, infections, and self-inflammatory activation that trigger innate immunity [8, 13].

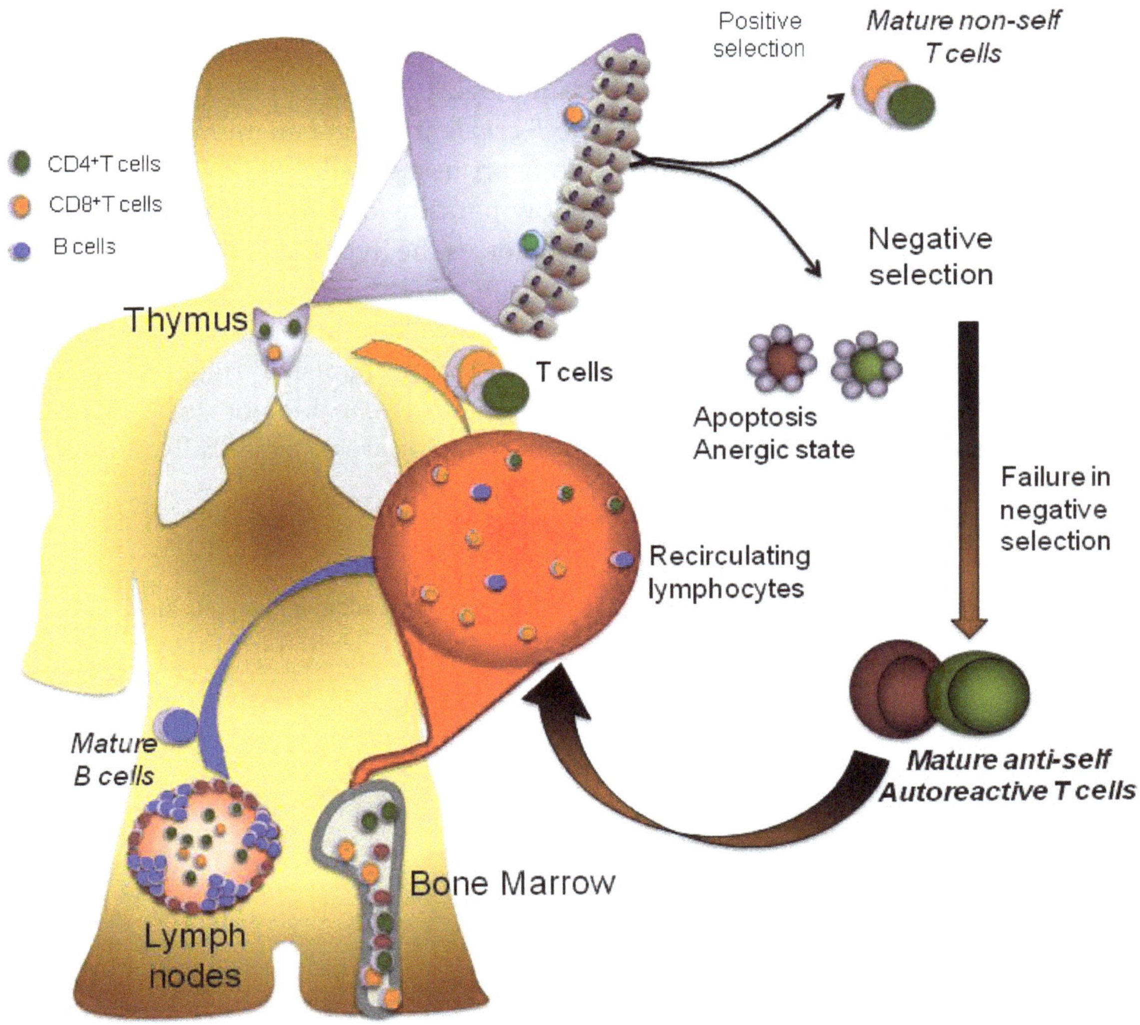

Figure 1. Dynamics of hematopoiesis, maturation and recirculation of newly generated lymphocytes as well as thymic selection of T-cell clones.

3. Chagas disease: an outburst of inflammatory events that may lead to autoimmunity

T. cruzi is a haemoflagellate parasite transmitted by several species of triatomine bugs. The best known mood of transmission is the vetorial via, which consists of vector insects ingesting contaminated blood meal containing bloodstream trypomastigotes. Later on, inside the insect's gut, the parasite differentiates into epimastigotes and replicates. The cycle is complete once the insect defecates, and releases metacyclic trypomastigotes forms which invade the host through the bite wound or mucosal membranes. Chagas disease progresses from a somewhat asymptomatic short acute phase to a chronic phase. Most individuals that progress to chronic phase remain asymptomatic, and the disease is detected by serological tests, but no clinical, radiologic, electrocardiographic, or echocardiographic evidenced. Overall, 20–40% of asymptomatic individuals develop clinically relevant Chagas heart disease, while approximately 10%

of the cases progress to digestive problems [14, 15]. In fact, the disease outcome toward differential clinical forms is related to many factors including the host-parasite interaction. Several studies have been proposed that the host immunological response plays a major role in the pathogenesis of Chagas disease [16]. Indeed, the *T. cruzi* can trigger an immune response, since parasite antigen has been consistently found in heart tissue infiltrated from cardiac patients [17, 18]. Nevertheless, the divergence between low parasite load in the tissue and severity of the lesions observed during the chronic phase reinforces the hypothesis that other factors than the immune response developed against the parasite might be involved in the development of Chagas pathology [19]. In this context, humoral and cellular autoimmune mechanisms are developed during Chagas disease [20–23]. Autoimmune mechanisms triggered during infection by *T. cruzi* may occur after bystander activation, parasite-cardiomyocyte harm, or molecular mimicry [24]. The mechanisms discussed in this chapter are schematically summarized in **Figure 2**.

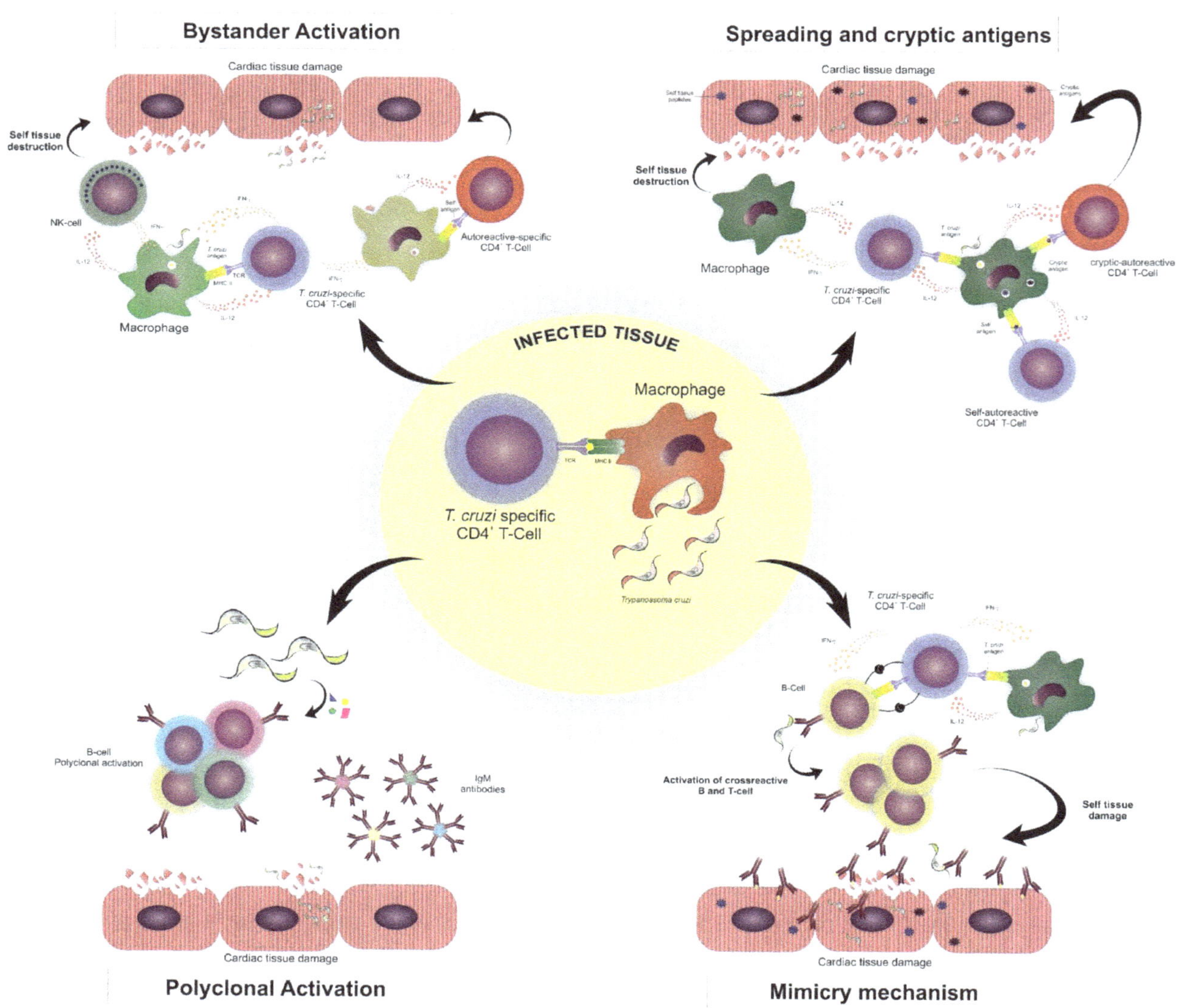

Figure 2. Scheme of the probable mechanisms involved in the autoimmune pathogenesis of Chagas disease.

Since *T. cruzi* presents a high variability of surface antigens, it is possible that the parasite causes polyclonal activation, which involves the T-independent stimulation of self-reactive B lymphocytes [25]. The lipopolysaccharide has been described as polyclonal activator, which induces the hypergammaglobulinemia phenomenon with higher secretion of autoantibodies, mainly IgM isotype [26]. Furthermore, *T. cruzi*-derived antigens can activate B1 lymphocytes before the development of T-cell-mediated immune response during the early stages of Chagas disease. [27, 28]. High percentage of B1 cells are found in the peripheral blood of chronic Chagas patients, as well as a significant decrease in the percentage of $CD3^+$ T cells [27, 28]. Additional studies have demonstrated that auto-anti-idiotypic antibodies (Ids) from chagasic cardiac disease patients preferentially stimulate B1 cells and $CD8^+$ T cells in magnified proportion as compared to indeterminate patients [29, 30]. The lower levels of T cells in the peripheral blood of chagasic cardiac patients suggest that T-cell-mediated immunity should be restricted to inflammatory foci, considering previous reports of the presence of T cells, mainly $CD8^+$ T lymphocytes, in the inflammatory infiltrate of cardiac tissue from individuals infected by *T. cruzi* [15]. A study using murine experimental model based on infection by *T. cruzi* demonstrated that the onset of cytokine production by T cells in the cardiac tissue is correlated with the local increase in the expression of cell adhesion molecules that is consistent with the T-lymphocyte migration to the inflammatory milieu [31]. In this study, the authors propose that chronic inflammation in the cardiac tissue from Chagas disease patients is highly active and is related to a permanent proinflammatory immune pattern that extends from the recent acute phase to the late stages of the chronic phase. Indeed, it is well accepted that the absence of pathology in individuals infected by *T. cruzi* is associated with the individual's ability to regulate the anti-*T. cruzi* response, which is responsible for the control of persistent parasitemia and tissue inflammatory damage, characteristic of Chagas disease [16, 32–34]. Certainly, the tissue inflammatory damage should be more severe in the absence of regulatory mechanisms involving both innate and adaptive immune responses. Indeed, our group has reported that in the indeterminate clinical form of Chagas disease, there is a higher frequency of $CD4^+CD25^{High}$ T cells and NKT lymphocytes than individuals with cardiac disease [35, 36]. As $CD4^+CD25^{High}$ T cells and NKT lymphocytes showed an important role in modulating the activation of $CD8^+$ T cells via apoptosis, as well as throughout the secretion of regulatory cytokines, it is possible that these cells during indeterminate clinical state further contribute to the control of the cytotoxic activity and deleterious events mediated by $CD8^+$ T cells [37, 38]. It is worth to mention that a fine equilibrium between inflammatory and regulatory cytokines represents a crucial element in the establishment of distinct clinical forms of chronic Chagas disease [33, 38]. It has been demonstrated that in the severe cardiac clinical status, leucocytes produce more IFN-gamma, while IL-10 is predominantly produced by PBMCs from indeterminate [38, 39].

In this regard, the functional role of peripheral blood leukocytes in patients infected by *T. cruzi*, after antigen stimulation has demonstrated that the main source of IFN-γ in cardiac patients is $CD4^+$ T lymphocytes, while monocytes are responsible for the production of high levels of IL-10 in patients with indeterminate status, favoring the regulation of the immune response and the control of disease morbidity [40]. It is possible that regulatory T cells are involved in this process, since they can inhibit the synthesis of IFN-γ, which could explain the low levels of this cytokine produced by T cells from indeterminate Chagas disease patients. In this context, it is important to reinforce that the inflammatory environment and cell destruction induced by *T. cruzi* infection could alter and induce antigen processing/presentation in such a way that novel self-epitopes are generated and recognized by the immune system, namely, cryptic epitope [41]. In steady state, the cryptic epitope displays low affinity for MHC molecules and is rarely presented by somatic cells, while dominant peptides show a high affinity for MHC molecules and are frequently presented by somatic cells. Furthermore, $CD8^+$ T cells specific for cryptic epitope could escape from the negative selection process in central tolerance [42]. Despite the fact that this process during *T. cruzi* infection is not yet clearly understood, this mechanism has been demonstrated to be involved in the pathogenesis of other autoimmune diseases [43]. Moreover, it has been shown that antigen processing and presentation were altered after the in vitro IFN-γ treatment, strengthening the hypothesis that the higher levels of IFN-γ in cardiac patients may favor the establishment of autoimmune mechanisms during Chagas disease. Indeed, the bystander activation mechanism caused by massive host antigens released in a proinflammatory environment may stimulate autoimmunity during *T. cruzi* infection.

4. The autoimmunity during Chagas disease: theories, concepts, and mechanisms triggered by *Trypanosoma cruzi*

Starting from the innate response, the human organism defends itself in a variety of ways. Physical barriers, phagocytic cells, (such as macrophages and dentritic cells), natural killer cells, neutrophils and the complement system are just a few examples of how precise and efficient our body reacts. Besides the innate response, the immune system is comprised of the adaptive response, a complex compartment of defense. Leucocytes (T and B lymphocytes), antibodies, and many other molecules are constantly working in order to keep the homeostasis. Furthermore, another important mechanism that is part of the immunological system is the autoimmunity concept. The autoimmunity concept started when researchers proposed that *T. cruzi* infection promoted rejection of allogeneic heart cell transplants and that T lymphocytes from *T. cruzi*-infected animals rapidly destroyed embryonic cardiomyocytes in culture [44]. However, reports that protective *T. cruzi*-specific T-cell-mediated immunity could be induced without eliciting pathogenic autoimmunity were soon published.

The debate about a role for autoimmunity in Chagas disease continued. Autoreactive T cells and antibodies were identified in individuals with chronic Chagas disease, and several specific antigens abundant in the myocardium were identified as targets of autoreactive responses [22, 45, 46]. Inflammatory factors present in the local environment, such as cytokines and nitric oxide, were also found to promote the activation of potentially autoreactive T cells encountering major histocompatibility complex-bound cognate antigen [21, 47, 48]. In this context, the autoimmune hypothesis plays a crucial role in the pathogenesis of many infectious diseases, including Chagas. The mechanisms proposed in this section for the generation of autoimmunity during Chagas disease are mimicry, indirect or bystander activation, and epitope spreading.

Mimicry is defined by the development of immune responses against foreign antigens that share sequence or structural similarities with self-antigens. This is due to the fact that immune responses can be directed against peptides with similar charge distribution and shape [8].

This mechanism suggests that *T. cruzi*-induced cardiac damage and/or molecular mimicry between parasite and host antigens leads to a breakdown in self-tolerance, resulting in eventual tissue damage [49]. Two cardiac molecules that have been related to the induction of Chagas autoimmune responses are myosin and troponin I [50, 51]. Troponin I have been recently described in *T. cruzi*-naturally infected macaques, which present high titers of troponin I autoantibodies in their circulatory system. In regards to myosin, it is the most abundant protein in the heart and may represent a significant cardiac antigen. Several studies have demonstrated the presence of autoantibodies against this protein circulating in the sera of Chagas disease experimental models [41, 52, 53]. Its potential to become an antigen mimicry candidate has been under discussion for over decades, especially considering several studies, which have linked it to the autoimmune hypothesis. Furthermore, a robust myosin-specific autoimmunity as well as immune tolerization to myosin suppresses parasite-specific immunity [41, 53]. However, it seems that myosin-specific autoimmunity itself is not essential to establish an inflammation [54].

In addition, other host antigens have been studied and proved to cross-react with *T. cruzi* proteins, such as B1 and B2 adrenoreceptors, lymphocyte, neuronal tissues, muscle antigens, m2 muscarinic acetylcholine receptors, small nuclear ribonucleoprotein, and Cha, a novel autoantigen [22, 55]. Moreover, some *T. cruzi* proteins have also been identified as potential antigen mimicry candidates, like epitopes of B13, 24-kDa, 36-kDa, 38-kDa, ribosomal P1 and P2 proteins, the shed acute-phase antigen (SAPA), and the *T. cruzi* cysteine protease cruzipain [22, 51, 55–59]. Worthy of mentioning was the identification of three regions of homologous linear sequence among cruzipain and myosin as well as the partial homology displayed in ribosomal P protein internal peptide sequence between *T. cruzi* and humans. These findings provide more evidence that the molecular mimicry mechanism may stimulate autoimmunity and strengths the hypothesis.

An additional concept of great discussion is the bystander activation. During microbial infection, toll-like receptors (TLRs) and pattern recognition receptors present on antigen-presenting cells (APCs) are stimulated leading to the synthesis and release of proinflammatory mediators. Together with self-antigens, coming from tissue destruction and creating a milieu of proinflammatory factors, all of these mediators may defeat self-tolerance by decreasing the threshold of activation enough to activate potentially autoreactive T cells and trigger autoimmunity. Furthermore, $CD8^+$ T cells may also initiate bystander activation by proliferating in response to self-antigen presented by APCs [21, 49, 60]. Hyland et al. [61] have shown that a reduction in parasitemia via treatment with Benznidazole, decreased or eliminated myosin-specific autoimmunity. They hypothesized that reduction of parasitemia consequently reduces release of host antigens and also dampens the inflammatory environment lessening bystander activation. Altogether, these data bring great perspectives to elucidate the autoimmune hypothesis of Chagas disease.

Subsequent to bystander activation, there is the development of autoimmune responses to endogenous epitopes secondary to the release of self-antigens, the so-called epitope spreading. It results from a change in protein structure, for example, changing of an amino acid from arginine to citrulline, which may succumb in an immune reaction against either the original protein or the citrullinated protein. Some of the mechanisms involved in epitope spreading are endocytic processing, antigen presentation, and somatic hypermutation, all culminating in broadening the immune response in autoimmune pathologies. Several authors have demonstrated the epitope spreading against many cardiac proteins, such as myosin, Cha protein, desmin, actin, myoglobin, tubulin, and B1 adrenergic receptor [49, 55, 62]. Still, more studies must be conducted in order to prove that this mechanism fully contributes to the propagation of autoimmunity in Chagas disease.

5. Final remarks

Chagas disease afflicts millions of people each year worldwide. Some individuals present mild to moderate symptoms during the chronic phase, while others develop severe and life-threatening cardiac and digestive conditions. There have been great advances in understanding the physiopathology of Chagas heart disease, which may contribute to the evolution in the field of drug development and therapy approaches. Apparently the auto-reactive cells are great responsible for destruction of the cardiac tissue leading to cardiac failure, the most severe consequence of the disease. Although the data describing the existence of *T. cruzi*-induced autoimmunity continues to grow, there is still lack of direct evidencere ported in the literature. Elucidating the autoimmune hypothesis of Chagas disease may help to solve potential complications for Chagas disease treatments involving autoimmunity, as well as to better understand many questions that remain unanswered about Chagas disease pathogenesis. Moreover, this hypothesis may serve as a model for studying infection-induced autoimmunity, which may be applicable to proposing and investigating new immune therapies for autoimmune diseases.

Acknowledgements

OAMF and ATC received fellowship from Conselho Nacional de Desenvolvimento Científico e Tecnológico (CNPq). JGCdR received fellowship from Programa Nacional de Pós-Doutorado funded by Coordenação de Aperfeiçoamento de Pessoal de Nível Superior (CAPES).

Author details

Armanda Moreira Mattoso-Barbosa[1], Renato Sathler-Avelar[1*],
Jordana Grazziela Alves Coelho-dos-Reis[1,2], Olindo Assis Martins-Filho[2],
Andrea Teixeira-Carvalho[2] and Danielle Marchetti Vitelli-Avelar[2]

*Address all correspondence to: renatosavelar@gmail.com

1 Faculdade de Minas – FAMINAS-BH, Belo Horizonte, Brazil

2 Grupo Integrado de Pesquisas em Biomarcadores, Centro de Pesquisas Rene Rachou, FIOCRUZ, Belo Horizonte, Brazil

References

[1] Kapsogeorgou EK, Tzioufas AG. Autoantibodies in autoimmune diseases: Clinical and critical evaluation. The Israel Medical Association Journal. 2016;**18**(9):519-524

[2] García-Muñoz R, Panizo C. Follicular lymphoma (FL): Immunological tolerance theory in FL. Human Immunology. 2017;**78**(2):138-145. DOI: 10.1016/j.humimm.2016.09.010

[3] Miller JF. The golden anniversary of the thymus. Nature Reviews Immunology. 2011;**11**(7):489-495. DOI: 10.1038/nri2993

[4] Oftedal BE, Ardesjö Lundgren B, Hamm D, Gan PY, Holdsworth SR, Hahn CN, et al. T cell receptor assessment in autoimmune disease requires access to the most adjacent immunologically active organ. Journal of Autoimmunity. 2017;**81**. DOI: 10.1016/j.jaut.2017.03.002. [Epub ahead of print]

[5] Bour-Jordan H, Esensten JH, Martinez-Llordella M, Penaranda C, Stumpf M, Bluestone JA. Intrinsic and extrinsic control of peripheral T-cell tolerance by costimulatory molecules of the CD28/B7 family. Immunology Reviews. 2011;**241**(1):180-205. DOI: 10.1111/j.1600-065X.2011.01011.x

[6] Cheroutre H, Mucida D, Lambolez F. The importance of being earnestly selfish. Nature Immunology. 2009;**10**:1047-1049. DOI: 10.1038/ni1009-1047

[7] Moreira ML, Tsuji M, Corbett AJ, Araújo MSS, Teixeira-Carvalho A, Martins-Filho OA, et al. MAIT-cells: A tailor-made mate in the ancient battle against infectious diseases? Immunol Lett. 2017;**187**:53-60

[8] Floreani A, Leung PSC, Gershwin ME. Environmental basis of autoimmunity. Clinical Reviews in Allergy and Immunology. 2016;**50**(3):287-300. DOI: 10.1007/s12016-015-8493-8

[9] Ermann J, Fathman CG. Autoimmune diseases: Genes, bugs and failed regulation. Nature Immunology. 2001;**2**(9):759-761

[10] Vojdani A, Pollard KM, Campbell AW. Environmental triggers and autoimmunity. Autoimmune Diseases. 2014;**2014**:798029

[11] Selmi C, Leung PS, Sherr DH, Diaz M, Nyland JF, Monestier M, et al. Mechanisms of environmental influence on human autoimmunity: A National Institute of Environmental Health Sciences expert panel workshop. Journal of Autoimmunity. 2012;**39**(4):272-284. DOI: 10.1016/j.jaut.2012.05.007

[12] Vojdani A. A potential link between environmental triggers and autoimmunity. Autoimmune Diseases. 2014;**2014**. DOI: 10.1155/2014/437231

[13] Root-Bernstein R, Fairweather D. Complexities in the relationship between infection and autoimmunity. Current Allergy and Asthma Reports. 2014;**14**(1):407. DOI: 10.1007/s11882-013-0407-3

[14] Tanowitz HB, Machado FS, Spray DC, Friedman JM, Weiss OS, Lora JN, Nagajyothi J, Moraes DN, Garg NJ, Nunes MC, Ribeiro AL. Developments in the management

of Chagas cardiomyopathy. Expert Rev Cardiovasc Ther. 2015;**13**(12):1393-1409. DOI: 10.1586/14779072.2015.1103648

[15] Menezes C, Costa GC, Gollob KJ, Dutra WO. Clinical aspects of Chagas disease and implications for novel therapies. Drug Development Research. 2011;**72**(6):471-479. DOI: 10.1002/ddr.20454

[16] Machado FS, Dutra WO, Esper L, Gollob KJ, Teixeira MM, Factor SM, Weiss LM, Nagajyothi F, Tanowitz HB, Garg NJ. Current understanding of immunity to *Trypanosoma cruzi* infection and pathogenesis of Chagas disease. Seminars Immunopathology. 2012;**34**(6):753-770. DOI: 10.1007/s00281-012-0351-7

[17] Nitz N, Gomes C, Rosa AC, D'Souza-Ault MR, Moreno F, Lauria-Pires L, et al. Heritable integration of kDNA minicircle sequences from *Trypanosoma cruzi* into the avian genome: Insights into human Chagas disease. Cell. 2004;**118**:175-186

[18] Williams JT, Mubiru JN, Schlabritz-Loutsevitch NE, Rubicz RC, VandeBerg JL, Dick EJ Jr, et al. Polymerase chain reaction detection of *Trypanosoma cruzi* in Macaca fascicularis using archived tissues. The Am J Trop Med Hyg. 2009;**81**(2):228-234

[19] Dutra WO, Rocha MO, Teixeira MM. The clinical immunology of human Chagas disease. Trends in Parasitology. 2005;**21**(12):581-587

[20] Pellegrini A, Carrera-Silva EA, Arocena A, Cano RC, Aoki MP, Gea S. *Trypanosoma cruzi* antigen immunization induces a higher B cell survival in BALB/c mice, a susceptible strain, compared to C57BL/6 B lymphocytes, a resistant strain to cardiac autoimmunity. Med Microbiol Immunology. 2011;**200**:209-218. DOI: 10.1007/s00430-011-0192-3

[21] Bonney KM, Taylor JM, Daniels MD, Epting CL, Engman DM. Heat-killed *Trypanosoma cruzi* induces acute cardiac damage and polyantigenic autoimmunity. PLoS One. 2011;**6**(1). DOI: 10.1371/journal.pone.0014571

[22] Bonney KM, Engman DM. Autoimmune pathogenesis of Chagas heart disease: Looking back, looking ahead. The American Journal of Pathology. 2015;**185**(6):1537-1547. DOI: 10.1016/j.ajpath.2014.12.023

[23] Iwaia LK, Julianoc MA, Julianoc L, Kalila J, Cunha-Neto E. T-cell molecular mimicry in Chagas disease: Identification and partial structural analysis of multiple cross-reactive epitopes between *Trypanosoma cruzi* B13 and cardiac myosin heavy chain. Journal of Autoimmunity. 2005;**24**:111-117. DOI: 10.1016/j.jaut.2005.01.006

[24] Bonney KM, Gifford KM, Taylor JM, Chen CI, Engman DM. Cardiac damage induced by immunization with heat-killed *Trypanosoma cruzi* is not antibody mediated. Parasite Immunology. 2013;**35**(1):1-10. DOI: 10.1111/pim.12008

[25] Bermejo DA, Amezcua Vesely MC, Khan M, Acosta Rodriguez EV, Montes CL, Merino MC, et al. *Trypanosoma cruzi* infection induces a massive extrafollicular and follicular splenic B-cell response which is a high source of non-parasite-specific antibodies. Immunology. 2011;**132**(1):123-133. DOI: 10.1111/j.1365-2567.2010.03347.x

[26] Cardoso MS, Reis-Cunha JL, Bartholomeu DC. Evasion of the immune response by *Trypanosoma cruzi* during acute infection. Frontiers in Immunology. 2016;**18**(6):659. DOI: 10.3389/fimmu.2015.00659

[27] Sathler-Avelar R, Lemos EM, Reis DD, Medrano-Mercado N, Araujo-Jorge TC, Antas PRZ, et al. Phenotypic features of peripheral blood leucocytes during early stages of human infection with *Trypanosoma cruzi*. Scandinavian Journal of Immunology. 2003;**58**:655-663

[28] Dutra WO, Olindo A, Martins-Filho AO, Cancado JR, Pinto-Dias JC, Brener Z, Freeman Jr GL, et al. Activated T and B lymphocytes in peripheral blood of patients with Chagas' disease. Int Immunol. 1994;**6**(4):499-506

[29] Dutra WO, Colley DG, Pinto-Dias JC, Gazzinelli G, Brener Z, Pereira MES, et al. Self and nonself stimulatory molecules induce preferential expansion of $CD5^+$ B cells or activated t cells of chagasic patients, respectively. Scandinavian Journal of Immunology. 2000;**51**(1):91-97

[30] Reis DD, Gazzinelli RT, Gazzinelli G, Colley DG. Antibodies to *Trypanosoma cruzi* express idiotypic patterns that can differentiate between patients with asymptomatic or severe Chagas' disease. The Journal of Immunology. 1993;**150**(4):1611-1618

[31] Fuenmayor C, Higuchi ML, Carrasco H, Parada H, Gutierrez P, Aiello V, Palomino S. Acute Chagas' disease: Immunohistochemical characteristics of T cell infiltrate and its relationship with *T. cruzi* parasitic antigens. Acta Cardiologica. 2005;**60**(1):33-37

[32] Sathler-Avelar R, Vitelli-Avelar DM, Mattoso-Barbosa AM, Perdigão-de-Oliveira M, Costa RP, Elói-Santos SM, et al. Phenotypic features of circulating leukocytes from non-human primates naturally infected with *Trypanosoma cruzi* resemble the major immunological findings observed in human Chagas disease. PLoS Negl Trop Dis. 2016;**10**(1). DOI: 10.1371/journal.pntd.0004302

[33] Vitelli-Avelar DM, Sathler-Avelar R, Mattoso-Barbosa AM, Gouin N, Perdigão-de-Oliveira M, Valerio-dos-Reis L, et al. *Cynomolgus macaques* naturally infected with *Trypanosoma cruzi*-I exhibit an overall mixed pro-inflammatory/modulated cytokine signature characteristic of human Chagas Disease. PLoS Negl Trop Dis. 2017;**11**(2). DOI: 10.1371/journal.pntd.0005233

[34] Vitelli-Avelar DM, Sathler-Avelar R, Dias JCP, Pascoal VPM, Teixeira-Carvalho A, Lage PS, et al. Chagasic patients with indeterminate clinical form of the disease have high frequencies of circulating $CD3^+$ $CD16^-$ $CD56^+$ Natural Killer T Cells and $CD4^+$ CD25High regulatory T lymphocytes. Scandinavian Journal of Immunology. 2005;**62**:297-308. DOI: 10.1111/j.1365-3083.2005.01668.x

[35] Vitelli-Avelar DM, Sathler-Avelar R, Massara RL, Borges JD, Lage PS, Lana M, et al. Are increased frequency of macrophage-like and natural killer (NK) cells, together with high levels of NKT and $CD4^+$ CD25high T cells balancing activated $CD8^+$ T cells, the key to control Chagas' disease morbidity? Clinical and Experimental Immunology. 2006;**145**:81-92. DOI: 10.1111/j.1365-2249.2006.03123.x

[36] Godfrey DI, Kronenberg M. Going both ways: Immune regulation via CD1d-dependent NKT cells. The Journal of Clinical Investigation. 2004;**114**(10):1379-1388

[37] Murray DA, Crispe IN. TNF-α controls intrahepatic T cell apoptosis and peripheral T cell numbers. The Journal of Immunology. 2004;**173**(4):2402-2409

[38] Vitelli-Avelar DM, Sathler-Avelar R, Teixeira-Carvalho A, Dias JCP, Gontijo ED, Faria AM, et al. Strategy to assess the overall cytokine profile of circulating leukocytes and its association with distinct clinical forms of human chagas disease. Scandinavian Journal of Immunology. 2008;**68**:516-525. DOI: 10.1111/j.1365-3083.2008.02167.x

[39] Bahia-Oliveira LM, Gomes JA, Rocha MO, Moreira MC, Lemos EM, Luz ZM, et al. IFN-gamma in human Chagas' disease: Protection or pathology? Brazilian Journal of Medical and Biological Research. 1998;**31**(1):127-131

[40] Gomes JAS, Bahia-Oliveira LMG, Rocha MOC, Martins-Filho AO, Gazzinelli G, Correa-Oliveira R. Evidence that development of severe cardiomyopathy in human Chagas' disease is due to a th1-specific immune response. Infection and Immunity. 2003;**71**(3):1185-1193

[41] Leon JS, Engman DM. The significance of autoimmunity in the pathogenesis of Chagas heart disease. Frontiers in Bioscience. 2003;**8**:315-322

[42] Horiuchi Y, Takagi A, Uchida T, Akatsuka T. Targeting cryptic epitope with modified antigen coupled to the surface of liposomes induces strong antitumor CD8 T-cell immune responses in vivo. Oncology Reports. 2015;**34**(6):2827-2836. DOI: 10.3892/or.2015.4299

[43] Warnock MG, Goodacre JA. Cryptic T-cell epitopes and their role in the pathogenesis of autoimmune diseases. British Journal of Rheumatology. 1997;**3**:1144-1150

[44] Santos-Buch CA, Teixeira AR. The immunology of experimental Chagas' disease. 3. Rejection of allogeneic heart cells in vitro. The Journal of Experimental Medicine. 1974;**140**(1):38-53

[45] Soares MBP, Pontes-De-Carvalho L, Ribeiro-Dos-Santos R. The pathogenesis of Chagas'disease: When autoimmune and parasite-specific immune responses meet. Anais da Academia Brasileira de Ciências. 2001;**73**(4):547-559

[46] Pontes-de-Carvalho L, Santana CC, Soares MB, Oliveira GG, Cunha Neto E, Ribeiro-dos-Santos R. Experimental chronic Chagas' disease myocarditis is an autoimmune disease preventable by induction of immunological tolerance to myocardial antigens. Journal of Autoimmunity. 2002;**18**:131-138

[47] Cunha-Neto E, Kalil J. Heart-infiltrating and peripheral T cells in the pathogenesis of human Chagas disease cardiomyopathy. Autoimmunity. 2001;**34**:187-192

[48] Engman DM, Leon JS. Pathogenesis of Chagas heart disease: Role of autoimmunity. Acta Tropica. 2002;**81**:123-132

[49] Bonney KM, Engman DM. Chagas heart disease pathogenesis: One mechanism or many? Curr Mol. 2008;**8**(6):510-518

[50] Pisharath H, Zao CL, Kreeger J, Portugal S, Kawabe T, Burton T, et al. Immunopathologic characterization of naturally acquired *Trypanosoma cruzi* infection and cardiac sequelae in *Cynomolgus macaques* (macaca fascicularis). Journal of the American Association for Laboratory Animal Science. 2013;**52**(5):545-552

[51] Kierszenbaum F. Views on the autoimmunity hypothesis for Chagas disease pathogenesis. FEMS Immunology and Medical Microbiology. 2003;**37**:1-11

[52] Leon JS, Godsel LM, Wang K, Engman DM. Cardiac myosin autoimmunity in acute Chagas'heart disease. Infection and Immunity. 2001;**69**(9):5643-5649

[53] Leon JS, Wang K, Engman DM. Myosin autoimmunity is not essential for cardiac inflammation in acute Chagas' disease. The Journal of Immunology. 2003;**171**:4271-4277

[54] Leon JS, Daniels MD, Toriello KM, Wang K, Engman DM. A cardiac myosin-specific autoimmune response is induced by immunization with *Trypanosoma cruzi* proteins. Infection and Immunity. 2004;**72**(6):3410-3417

[55] Gironès N, Rodríguez CI, Basso B, Bellon JM, Resino S, Muñoz-Fernández MA, Gea S, Moretti E, Fresno M. Antibodies to an epitope from the Cha human autoantigen are markers of Chagas' disease. Clin Diagn Lab Immunol. 2001;**8**(6):1039-1043

[56] Giordanengo L, Maldonado C, Rivarola HW, Iosa D, Girones N, Fresno M, et al. Induction of antibodies reactive to cardiac myosin and development of heart alterations in cruzipain-immunized mice and their offspring. European Journal of Immunology. 2000;**30**(11):3181-3189

[57] Cunha-Neto E, Coelho V, Guilerme L, Fiorelli A, Stolf N, Kalil J. Autoimmunity in Chagas' disease. Identification of cardiac myosin-B13 *Trypanosoma cruzi* protein cross-reactive T cell clones in heart lesions of a chronic Chagas' cardiomyopathy patient. The Journal of Clinical Investigation. 1996, 15;**98**(8):1709-1712

[58] Kaplan D, Ferrari I, Bergami PL, Mahler E, Levitus G, Chiale P, Hoebeke J, et al. Antibodies to ribosomal P proteins of *Trypanosoma cruzi* in Chagas disease possess functional autoreactivity with heart tissue and differ from anti-P autoantibodies in lupus. Proc Natl Acad Sci of the United States of America. 1997;**94**(19):10301-10306

[59] Gironès N, Rodríguez CI, Carrasco-Marín E, Hernáez RF, de Rego JL, Fresno M. Dominant T- and B-cell epitopes in an autoantigen linked to Chagas' disease. The Journal of Clinical Investigation. 2001;**107**(8):985-993

[60] Teixeira ARL, Hecht MM, Guimaro MC, Sousa AO, Nitz N. Pathogenesis of Chagas' disease: Parasite persistence and autoimmunity. Clinical Microbiology Reviews. 2011;**24**(3):592-630

[61] Hyland KV, Leon JS, Daniels MD, Giafis N, Woods LM, Bahk TJ, Wang K, Engman DM. Modulation of autoimmunity by treatment of an infectious disease. Infection and Immunity. 2007;**75**(7):3641-3650

[62] Smulski C, Labovsky V, Levy G, Hontebeyrie M, Hoebeke J, Levin MJ. Structural basis of the cross-reaction between an antibody to the *Trypanosoma cruzi* ribosomal P2beta protein and the human beta1 adrenergic receptor. The FASEB Journal. 2006;**20**(9):1396-1406

Permissions

All chapters in this book were first published in CDBIC, by InTech Open; hereby published with permission under the Creative Commons Attribution License or equivalent. Every chapter published in this book has been scrutinized by our experts. Their significance has been extensively debated. The topics covered herein carry significant findings which will fuel the growth of the discipline. They may even be implemented as practical applications or may be referred to as a beginning point for another development.

The contributors of this book come from diverse backgrounds, making this book a truly international effort. This book will bring forth new frontiers with its revolutionizing research information and detailed analysis of the nascent developments around the world.

We would like to thank all the contributing authors for lending their expertise to make the book truly unique. They have played a crucial role in the development of this book. Without their invaluable contributions this book wouldn't have been possible. They have made vital efforts to compile up to date information on the varied aspects of this subject to make this book a valuable addition to the collection of many professionals and students.

This book was conceptualized with the vision of imparting up-to-date information and advanced data in this field. To ensure the same, a matchless editorial board was set up. Every individual on the board went through rigorous rounds of assessment to prove their worth. After which they invested a large part of their time researching and compiling the most relevant data for our readers.

The editorial board has been involved in producing this book since its inception. They have spent rigorous hours researching and exploring the diverse topics which have resulted in the successful publishing of this book. They have passed on their knowledge of decades through this book. To expedite this challenging task, the publisher supported the team at every step. A small team of assistant editors was also appointed to further simplify the editing procedure and attain best results for the readers.

Apart from the editorial board, the designing team has also invested a significant amount of their time in understanding the subject and creating the most relevant covers. They scrutinized every image to scout for the most suitable representation of the subject and create an appropriate cover for the book.

The publishing team has been an ardent support to the editorial, designing and production team. Their endless efforts to recruit the best for this project, has resulted in the accomplishment of this book. They are a veteran in the field of academics and their pool of knowledge is as vast as their experience in printing. Their expertise and guidance has proved useful at every step. Their uncompromising quality standards have made this book an exceptional effort. Their encouragement from time to time has been an inspiration for everyone.

The publisher and the editorial board hope that this book will prove to be a valuable piece of knowledge for researchers, students, practitioners and scholars across the globe.

List of Contributors

Luís Gaspar
Instituto de Investigação e Inovação em Saúde, University of Porto, Portugal
Institute for Molecular and Cell Biology, University of Porto, Porto, Portugal

Nilmar Silvio Moretti and Sergio Schenkman
Departament of Microbiology, Imunology and Parasitology, Escola Paulista de Medicina, Federal University of São Paulo, São Paulo, Brazil,

Terry K. Smith
Biomedical Sciences Research Complex, The University, St. Andrews, Fife, Scotland, UK

Anabela Cordeiro-da-Silva
Instituto de Investigação e Inovação em Saúde, University of Porto, Portugal
Institute for Molecular and Cell Biology, University of Porto, Porto, Portugal
Departament of Biological Sciences, Faculty of Pharmacy of University of Porto, Porto, Portugal

Mauricio Canals Lambarri
Programa de Salud Ambiental, Escuela de Salud Pública, Facultad de Medicina, Universidad de Chile, Chile
Departamento de Medicina, Facultad de Medicina, Universidad de Chile, Chile

Andrea Canals Cifuentes
Programa de Bioestadística, Escuela de Salud Pública, Facultad de Medicina, Universidad de Chile, Chile
Dirección Académica, Clínica santa María, Chile

Salvador Ayala
Departamento de Asuntos Científicos, Instituto de Salud Pública, Chile

Valentina Tapia-Garay and Dante Cáceres Lillo
Programa de Salud Ambiental, Escuela de Salud Pública, Facultad de Medicina, Universidad de Chile, Chile

María Elena Villagran-Herrera, Hebert Luis Hernández-Montiel, Ricardo Francisco Mercado-Curiel and Nicolás Camacho-Calderón
Department of Biomedical Research, Faculty of Medicine, Autonomous University of Queretaro, Santiago de Querétaro, Queretaro, Mexico
José Alejandro Martínez-Ibarra
Area of Medical Entomology, University Center of the South, University of Guadalajara, Guadalajara, Jalisco, Mexico

Manuel Sánchez-Moreno
Laboratory of Molecular Biology of Parasites, Faculty of Science, University of Granada, Granada, Spain

José Antonio de Diego-Cabrerade
Department of Preventive Medicine, Public Health and Microbiology, Faculty of Medicine, Autonomous University of Madrid, Madrid, Spain

Rodolfo A Kölliker-Frers
Parasitology Unit, José María Ramos Mejía Hospital, Buenos Aires, Argentina
Laboratory of Cytoarchitecture and Neuronal Plascíticy, Institute of Cardiological Research, "Prof. Dr. Alberto Taquini", ININCA-UBA-CONICET, Buenos Aires, Argentina

Matilde Otero-Losada
Laboratory of HPLC, Institute of Cardiological Research, University of Buenos Aires, National Research Council, ININCA-UBA-CONICET, Buenos Aires, Argentina

Gabriela Razzite and Mariela Calvo
Parasitology Unit, José María Ramos Mejía Hospital, Buenos Aires, Argentina

Justo Carbajales
Cardiology Unit, José María Ramos Mejía Hospital, Buenos Aires, Argentina

Francisco Capani
Laboratory of Cytoarchitecture and Neuronal Plascíticy, Institute of Cardiological Research, "Prof. Dr. Alberto Taquini", ININCA-UBA-CONICET, Buenos Aires, Argentina

Wilton H. Kawaguchi, Leticia Bonancio Cerqueira, Mariana Millan Fachi, Michel L. Campos and Roberto Pontarolo
Department of Pharmacy, Federal University of Paraná, Curitiba, Paraná, Brazil

Iara J. Messias Reason
Clinical Hospital, Federal University of Paraná, Curitiba, Paraná, Brazil

Rosa Lidia Solís-Oviedo
Faculty of Chemical Sciences, Autonomous University of Chihuahua, Chihuahua, Mexico

Víctor Monteon and Ruth López
Centre for Biomedical Research, Autonomous University of Campeche, Campeche, Mexico

Ángel de la Cruz Pech-Canul
CONACyT – Faculty of Chemical Sciences, Autonomous University of Chihuahua, Chihuahua, Mexico

Javier Varela and Mercedes González
Grupo de Química Orgánica Medicinal, Facultad de Ciencias, Universidad de la República, Montevideo, Uruguay

Hugo Cereceto
Grupo de Química Orgánica Medicinal, Facultad de Ciencias, Universidad de la República, Montevideo, Uruguay
Área de Radiofarmacia, Centro de Investigaciones Nucleares, Universidad de la República, Montevideo, Uruguay

Edgar Alfonso Paredes González and Jesús Ortega-García
Universidad de Sonora, Unidad regional Norte Caborca México, Mexico

Gerardo Álvarez Hernandez
Universidad de Sonora, Departamento de Ciencias Químicas, Unidad Centro Hermosillo Sonora, Mexico

Castillo Christian, Ana Liempi, Lisvaneth Medina, Ileana Carrillo and Ulrike Kemmerling
Instituto de Ciencias Biomédicas, Facultad de Medicina, Universidad de Chile, Santiago, Chile

Guadalupe García Liñares
Departamento de Química Orgánica y UMYMFOR, Facultad de Ciencias Exactas y Naturales, Universidad de Buenos Aires, Buenos Aires, Argentina

Armanda Moreira Mattoso-Barbosa and Renato Sathler-Avelar
Faculdade de Minas – FAMINAS-BH, Belo Horizonte, Brazil

Jordana Grazziela Alves Coelho-dos-Reis
Faculdade de Minas – FAMINAS-BH, Belo Horizonte, Brazil
Grupo Integrado de Pesquisas em Biomarcadores, Centro de Pesquisas Rene Rachou, FIOCRUZ, Belo Horizonte, Brazil

Olindo Assis Martins-Filho, Andrea Teixeira-Carvalho and Danielle Marchetti Vitelli-Avelar
Grupo Integrado de Pesquisas em Biomarcadores, Centro de Pesquisas Rene Rachou, FIOCRUZ, Belo Horizonte, Brazil

Index

A

Actin-dependent, 137-138

Amastigote, 4-5, 14, 16, 60, 72, 90, 104, 132-133, 137, 139, 142, 145, 148, 183, 193

Animal Model Studies, 132

Apoptotic Cell Death, 182, 186

Autoantibodies, 81, 84-87, 97, 211, 215, 217, 219, 223

B

Benznidazole, 2, 4, 64, 101-103, 105-106, 117-118, 120-122, 127, 130-131, 146, 192, 194, 198, 203, 217

Bystander Activation, 212, 214, 216-217

C

C-reactive Protein, 92, 98-100

Cardiomyopathy, 59, 63, 77-79, 81, 86-88, 91, 93-95, 97-100, 105, 109, 120-121, 124-125, 192, 203, 211, 220, 222-223

Cardiovascular Risk, 77-78, 81, 89-90, 94-95, 97-98

Cell Differentiation, 185-186

Chagas Disease, 1, 3, 14, 16-21, 24, 36-42, 46-53, 55, 57-60, 62-64, 73-82, 85, 87, 92-93, 95-99, 101-103, 109, 111-113, 118-121, 123-131, 135, 139, 144-147, 149-150, 152, 154-157, 161-163, 165, 178-183, 188-189, 192, 211-218, 220-223

Chemotherapy, 1, 20-21, 24, 31, 34-35, 74, 119-120, 123, 126-131, 146, 155-156, 158, 191-193, 202-209

Chronic Chagas Cardiomyopathy, 109, 124

Clomipramine, 115-116, 130, 201, 209

Congestive Heart Failure, 78-79

Connexivum, 40-41

Cruzipain, 102, 113, 115-116, 128-129, 136, 141, 198-199, 208, 217, 223

Cuticular Hydrocarbons, 161, 163-166, 168, 170, 172, 174, 177, 180

Cysteine Proteases, 129, 191, 206-208

Cytokine Profile, 141, 182, 186, 222

Cytoplasm, 12-13, 16, 80, 133

D

Drug Development, 18, 191, 193, 198, 218, 220

Drug Discovery, 1, 3-4, 14, 20-21, 33, 36, 100, 115, 128, 131, 157, 203-204, 206-207, 209

Dysautonomia, 79, 81-82, 109

E

Ecology, 37, 39, 42, 55, 151, 180

Epidemiology, 37, 39, 51, 57-58, 73, 95, 97, 124, 155

Epithelial Turnover, 182, 185, 188

F

Fibronectin, 134, 136, 141

G

Glycoproteins, 82-83, 136, 186

H

Heart Disease, 10, 38, 63, 74, 81, 86, 95, 97, 100-101, 121, 124-125, 213, 218, 220, 222-223

Hemolagellate Parasite, 60, 64

Heparan Sulfate, 134, 136

Host Cells, 5, 12, 14, 18, 133, 135-140, 196

Human Dwellings, 40, 51, 162, 165

I

Immune System, 5, 59, 65, 77-78, 82-84, 87, 89, 132, 134, 138, 182-183, 185, 188, 190, 216

Interleukin-17a, 91

K

Keratinocytes, 134

Kinetoplast, 60, 133

Kissing Bug, 56, 101

L

Leukopenia, 106, 146

Life Cycle, 12, 14, 16, 39, 60-61, 132, 135-136, 162, 197

Lysosomal-dependent, 137

M

Mammalian Cell, 25, 133, 143

Mass Spectrometry, 13, 23, 150, 158, 173

Megaesophagus, 38, 59, 192

Meningoencephalitis, 59, 145, 192

Metabolism, 9-10, 21, 23, 25, 27-29, 42, 89, 96, 99, 104, 122, 130, 139, 193, 196, 200

Metabolomics, 120, 144, 150, 155, 159

Metacyclogenesis, 14, 135-136, 140

Molecular Targets, 6, 79, 88, 147, 191-193, 200, 202

Mucous Membranes, 61, 105, 134

Murine Experimental Model, 215

Murine Model, 59-60, 66, 69, 71-72, 127, 130, 141, 152, 194, 199

Myocarditis, 59, 63, 77, 79, 82, 84-86, 90-91, 97, 108-109, 125, 145, 222

Myosin, 79, 95, 97, 217-218, 220, 223

N

Nicotinamide, 6-8, 15, 27, 34

Nifurtimox, 2, 4, 21, 58, 64, 101-107, 117, 120, 122-123, 130, 146, 192, 194, 202

Non-phagocytic, 132-133, 137-138

P

Parasite Interactions, 77, 81, 89, 94, 132

Parasitemia, 59, 63, 65-66, 69-72, 78, 80, 82, 84-85, 90, 98, 102, 108, 114-115, 117, 120, 137, 141, 149, 183, 194, 199, 215, 217

Parasitic Protozoa, 11, 15, 33, 75, 95

Peripheral Neuropathy, 106, 146, 192

Phagocytic Cells, 122, 137-138, 216

Pharmaceutical Companies, 1, 3-4, 202

Placebo, 105, 112-113, 122, 125, 127

Placenta, 182-190

S

Serology, 65, 71, 78, 95, 105

Sialic Acid, 82, 136, 199

Sirtuins, 1, 5-8, 10-19, 22-24, 27, 33

Symptomatic Treatment, 101, 108, 111, 117

T

Thrombocytopenic Purpura, 106, 146

Thromboembolism, 78, 109-110

Triatoma Rubida, 161-163, 165, 167-177, 179

Triatomine Specie, 136

Triatomines, 3, 42-45, 56, 63, 70, 72, 75, 161-165, 174, 177, 179-180

Trypanosoma Cruzi, 1-2, 8, 14, 20-21, 24, 36-37, 39, 45, 53-54, 56-61, 65-68, 70-71, 73-78, 95-98, 101, 114, 118, 120-123, 127-133, 135, 140-145, 156-158, 161-162, 177-180, 182-183, 187-191, 193, 202-212, 216, 220-223

Trypomastigotes, 5, 16, 37-38, 59, 61, 63, 68, 72, 83-84, 132-138, 141-142, 145, 148, 192, 195, 199, 213

V

Ventricular Arrhythmias, 78, 88-89, 94, 97, 110, 124

W

Wild Foci, 43, 51

www.ingramcontent.com/pod-product-compliance
Lightning Source LLC
LaVergne TN
LVHW060552210926
848485LV00005B/1300
* 9 7 8 1 6 3 9 8 7 1 0 0 1 *